The History of Medicine
in Alabama

THE HISTORY
OF MEDICINE
IN ALABAMA

Howard L. Holley, B.S., M.D.

Anna Lois Waters Professor of
Medicine in Rheumatology

The University of Alabama School of Medicine
Birmingham, Alabama

Produced and distributed for
The University of Alabama School of Medicine
by The University of Alabama Press
P.O. Box 2877
University, Alabama 35486

Library of Congress Cataloging in Publication Data

Holley, Howard L.
  The history of medicine in Alabama.

  Bibliography: p.
  Includes index.
  1. Medicine—Alabama—History. I. Title.
  [DNLM: 1. History of medicine—Alabama. WZ 70
  AA4 H7h]
  R155.H64   362.1'09761   81-10419
  ISBN 0-8173-0085-6   AACR2

This book is dedicated with affection to the young men and women of Alabama who choose the study of health sciences as a way of life. They are pioneers of the future.

"In today already walks tomorrow."
—Samuel Taylor Coleridge

Contents

Acknowledgments

This book is a compilation of the work of many individuals. Thanks are especially due to those who have generously made their findings available for inclusion in this book. It is my fear that I may fail to acknowledge many people who have assisted in writing this book, not only here in Birmingham but also in Montgomery and Mobile. "I am so grateful to so many—there are too many to thank."

Acknowledgment should be made to the following for kindly supplying photographs and permitting them to be used: The Lister Hill Library of the Health Sciences at The University of Alabama in Birmingham; the Amelia Gayle Gorgas Library, University of Alabama in Tuscaloosa; the Alabama State Department of Archives and History, and the Alabama Department of Public Health, Montgomery, Alabama; and the Heustis Medical Museum, Mobile, Alabama.

My very special thanks go to the Division of Clinical Immunology and Rheumatology of the Department of Medicine for allowing me time away from my duties there, without which it would have been impossible to write this volume, and to the Department of Medicine of the Medical Center for providing both encouragement and financial aid.

Invaluable assistance has been rendered me by Mrs. Sarah Brown, former Director, Mrs. Hilda Harris, Reference Librarian, and Jim Thompson, Circulation Librarian of the Lister Hill Library of the Health Sciences, The University of Alabama School of Medicine, The University of Alabama in Birmingham; Mrs. William Henson of the Huntsville Public Library; Mr. Velimir Luketic, who acted as a research assistant during the preparation of a portion of this manuscript; and Miss Lee Frommeyer, who has been a zealous researcher and critic. Miss Frommeyer, along with Dr. Julius Linn, Jr., were co-indexers of the manuscript. A special word of thanks is due Mrs. Nancy G. Riser for her aid in formulating the biographies.

I am indebted to Mrs. Lois T. Montgomery and Mrs. Renee Graves for deciphering my handwriting and for the typing of the manuscript. Without their assistance and patience my job would have been much more difficult. To Mrs. Patricia Hester, who typed and retyped the manuscript for publication, goes praise for an onerous task well done. To Miss Brenda Joyce Gosnell and Mrs. Anne Phelps Galloway goes appreciation for their typing of the manuscript, and to Mrs. Elizabeth Washington goes thanks for her excellent services as an archivist. To the quite remarkable Mrs. Mary T. Brown, of Browns, Alabama, goes a heartfelt thanks for her crisp, pertinent judgment in the final edition of this manuscript.

To Drs. Julius Linn, Jr., Bill Weaver, Sam Eichold, Gene Ball, and Mrs. Lyn Johns goes a special note of thanks for their critical reading of the manuscript.

Writing a book as a spare-time activity requires considerable forbearance from those who have to live with the author, and special gratitude is due for this alone to my wife. She has cheerfully shouldered the duties of secretary, cartographer, and literary adviser. Her part in the production of this book does not fall far short of coauthorship.

Foreword

For Alabama physicians and, indeed, for all others who take joy in the lovely language inherited by us from our British forebears, this book is both a classic and a "must."

Unlike Caesar's Gaul, it is divided into more than three parts. The Introduction includes quotations from wise individuals, each with the gift of expressing incisive thoughts in convincing words.

Among the divisions are chapters dealing with "Early Medicine," in which the efforts in medicine were feeble at best, "Irregular Practitioners," "Mental Health," "Public Health," "Dentistry," "Pharmacy," etc. The frivolous reader will enjoy the literary style, the studious one not only that but also the splendid depth of thought.

The book is for the ingestion of all and for the digestion of some. It displays not only Howard Holley's love of labor but his labor of love.

TINSLEY RANDOLPH HARRISON, M.D.
Birmingham, Alabama
August 1977

Introduction

Near the turn of the century Dr. Jerome Cochran of Mobile, who is considered "The Father of Public Health in Alabama," was asked to write a history of the medical profession in the state. In a footnote, he summed up his ideas of what such a history should contain. I have chosen to use his note as an introduction to this book.

I have undertaken to write a sketch of the medical history of Alabama. The first problem that presents itself for solution is to determine what things fall properly under the designation of medical history. Does it mean an account of the diseases, endemic and epidemic, which have afflicted the good people of the state since its foundation? Or does it mean a history of the medical profession of the state and of the great doctors who have made that profession illustrious? Or does it mean a history of the medical organization and the medical institutions[?] In the sketch that I have written I have construed it to mean all of these things; and accordingly all of them, under appropriate sub-heads, have been treated of as thoroughly as the time and space at my disposal would warrant. It has not been an easy thing to write this sketch, because it was very difficult to obtain the facts for the periods antedating the war. My medical brethren have been perfectly willing to help me; but their memories fail to reach back so far; and of printed records there are very few extant. I have done the best I could under the circumstances; and have packed the pages assigned me as full of facts as possible. It would have been very much easier to have filled them with fine writing flatteries, compliments, panegyrics—after the fashion of complaisant reporters for the daily press; but I think it will be admitted generally, or by judicious critics at any rate, that I have pursued the wiser course. I have used a great deal of care in the verification of the facts and details that I have made use of, and I am satisfied that almost without exception their accuracy may be depended upon.

Perhaps the most interesting part of the history of any profession is to be found in the study of the lives of its eminent men. I have therefore added to the formal accounts referred to above, biographical sketches of some of the leading members of the medical profession of Alabama, confining myself entirely to those who are no longer living. Many richly worthy of commemoration I have had to pass without mention, because I could not obtain for them the necessary materials for even short notices.[1]

Nearly two centuries have passed since the turn of the nineteenth century, and we look backward down a corridor of time to the earliest medical care in Alabama. Many hardships and dedicated efforts of those who seized the challenge of a frontier have faded and been forgotten.

1. Jerome Cochran, "The Medical Profession," *Memorial Record of Alabama: Historical and Biographical* (Madison, Wisconsin: Brant and Fuller, 1893), 2: 107.

We have lost touch with the reality of our pioneer physicians. They were living, aspiring, and struggling individuals, directly concerned with obtaining medical care for their patients. If this book can breathe life into the memory of those whose efforts provided Alabama with the foundations of good medical care, and if it can inspire hope for future achievement, it will have served its purpose.

Part I
Medical Practice in the State of Alabama

Chapter 1

Early Medical Practice in Alabama

Hostile Indians, inhospitable climate, lack of supplies, and poor communications were only a few of the problems faced by colonists on their arrival in what later became the state of Alabama. The greatest problem, in terms of both human and economic factors, was disease—which seemed to arrive in its most severe form along with the first settlers. The story of its depredation and the struggles against it form one of the most important chapters in Alabama history.

Military Medicine in Colonial Alabama

Although colonial governments were supposed to care for the medical needs of their troops and officials, their available funds were always inadequate and medical care suffered accordingly. One major problem in dealing with illness was the lack of competent medical personnel and facilities. It is impossible to say how many physicians were in French Mobile. The fact that Fort Toulouse, an important fort in the interior, was not assigned a surgeon until 1719, five years after it had been built, would seem to indicate a serious shortage of medical personnel.[1] The French did have a military hospital in the port of Mobile, but its facilities were poor. When the British took over in 1763, the building was lacking a chimney, a floor, and window frames. An inventory reveals sixteen small beds, thirteen Spanish hair mattresses, two large cupboards, one sideboard, and twenty-one worn bed sheets and blankets.[2] During the "sickly" season, Major Robert Farmar, the British officer in charge of Mobile, which had become part of West Florida, had to requisition housing for the sick and was forced to purchase at an exorbitant price a house to serve as an auxiliary hospital. Most of the time only one surgeon's mate was in charge of the Mobile facilities, there being one surgeon and six mates in all West Florida.[3] Later, the Spanish (1780–1813) and Americans faced similar shortages.

Most physicians during the Spanish regime were of French and English origin. The esteem in which they were held, probably because there were so few, can be inferred from their salaries. A typical surgeon was paid $360 per year, and a "practicante," a man who had not yet qualified as a physician, $300. In comparison, an army post commander's annual salary was $100.[4] The Americans at Fort Stoddard originally did not have a physician on their staff, and, ironically, when one did arrive, he found no instruments or medicines for use in treating the ill soldiers.[5]

Lack of medical supplies was another problem to be faced. Medicines commonly used in the colonies are recorded in several inventories of physicians' and pharmacists' stocks. Typical were two lists of medicines and supplies maintained for the use of the British troops in Mobile in 1764. Some of the drugs named, with their original spelling preserved, were:

Camphora.	. . . Rhabarb.
Cera flava.	. . . Radex Gentian.
Cortex Cinnamon.	Sal carthartic. amar.
Elixir Paregoric.	. . . Glauber. miral.
Flor. Chamomel.	semen Lini.
. . . Sulphur.	spiritus Vini retificat.
Magnesia alba.	Tinctura Thebaic.
Manna.	Unguent. Basilic.
Olea Chym.	. . . dialth.
Pulvis Cortic. Peruvian	. . . Mercurial fort.
. . . Jallap.	. . . alb.
. . . Radic. Ipecacuan.	Virtum ceret antimon.[6]

According to both British and Spanish sources, Glauber's salts, tartar emetic, and quinine were the drugs most frequently used.[7]

Drugs were usually imported from Europe or the West Indies and were frequently damaged in transit or deteriorated in the hot, humid climate once they reached their destination. For this reason, Major Farmar was forced to go to Jamaica in 1763 to purchase £52 6s. worth of medicines.[8]

The increasing need for medical supplies indicated that the already deplorable health situation was now growing worse. In 1765, General Thomas Gage had to dispatch a medicine chest to Dr. John Lorimer (?–1795) in Mobile although only two months earlier he had received two chests, "[each containing] sufficient [quantities] of drugs to last a regiment of one thousand men for years."[9] Fortunately, at least some of the deficiencies could be remedied at the local level.

Particularly frequent were purchases of alcoholic beverages. General Frederick Haldimand, governor of West Florida, believed that his good health was due to the regular drinking of Madeira wine, and between 1767 and 1769, he ordered $237 worth of Madeira for the use of convalescents in the hospital.[10] Similarly, Captain Bartholomew Schaumburgh, commanding officer at Fort Stoddard, purchased brandy, wine, and chocolate for use of the patients confined in the fort's hospital.[11] In addition, indigenous medicinal plants were often substituted for many drugs.

The British colonial authorities employed Bernard Romans from 1771 to 1776 and, later, Dr. John Lorimer as royal botanists. One of Romans's reports, dated 1773, mentioned the presence of many "antiscorbutics," "Jallop," and "Ipecacuanha." He also stated: "Besides these above mentioned, there is the Pistacia, Therebinthus, the Styrax, Officinale, Convuloulas [sic], Scammonia, Smilax China, Smilax Sarsaparilla, Pennica Granetum, Memordica Elateria, and innumerable others used by the Savages, and to us almost utterly unknown."[12]

In fact, many people preferred treatment by the Indians to the medications of their own physicians. One version of a common tale has been passed on to us by a French chronicler. Two men, suffering from the same disease, were being unsuccessfully treated by a French physician. One ran away, found an Indian doctor and was cured. The other died.[13] Another example is given by the botanist and traveler William Bartram, who reported that during his visit to Alabama, he suffered a bout with fever while visiting Major Farmar's plantation on the Taensa (Tensaw River). He searched "[for and found] a certain plant of extraordinary medicinal virtues, and [held] in high estimation with the [local] inhabitants."[14]

Health care for the civilian population must have been even worse than that for the military. It is known that under both the British and Spanish administrations, civilians were forbidden the use of military hospitals.[15] Although the French apparently allowed those without sufficient funds to be treated at the expense of the colonial government, there was never enough money available for this work. For example, in 1734, the colonial government complained, in a letter to Paris, that the 5,000 *livres* intended for care of the sick could not possibly meet the needs of all hospitals in the colony.[16]

One of these hospitals existed in Fort Louis de la Mobile and was operated by two nuns (lay nursing sisters) who had arrived on the *Pélican* in 1704.[17] No particulars concerning the size or equipment of the institution are known, nor is it known whether it ever had a regular physician.[18]

The situation was aggravated by quackery, which flourished in the area. To combat this, the French in the 1720s, and the Spanish in the 1780s, required that all physicians be licensed by colonial authorities.[19]

On the other hand, the authorities were not above taking advantage of the situation themselves, especially where medical supplies were concerned. Governor de Vandreuil of the Louisiana colony maintained a drugstore in his own house. His wife, who at times attended to the trade, acquired the reputation of a shrewd businesswoman by selling medicines at a large profit.[20]

Medical Practice in Alabama—1819–1860

Once Alabama had become a state (1819), there occurred a dramatic increase in population. In 1800, the Mississippi Territory, which included Alabama, had a population of 10,000, excluding slaves and Indians; twenty years later, Alabama alone had a population of 127,901.[21] Along with the increase in population, there was an increase in incidence of disease. Dr. Paul Hamilton Lewis (1814–1849) of Mobile, who was an early medical historian in Alabama, wrote that around 1820, when large areas of land were cleared and people settled on the land, the types and severity of disease were found to have increased rapidly.[22] These included such diseases as yellow fever and malarial fever. Particularly affected were the boom towns such as St. Stephens and Cahaba, two early capitals of the state. Situated along rivers, they were ravaged yearly by fevers until both were finally abandoned.

Under such circumstances, physicians were sorely needed and, indeed, many did settle in Alabama. Dr. John Young Bassett (1805–1851) of Huntsville estimated that in Madison County during the 1840s there were thirty physicians and six irregular or nondescript practitioners serving a population of 26,706.[23] However, only a few of them were well trained. During the 1820s and 1830s, Alabama was a frontier state where income was low. Only such cities as Mobile, Cahaba, Tuscaloosa, Huntsville, and the Black Belt counties (where many plantation owners paid well to insure the health of their slaves) could support even a small number of well-trained, full-time physicians. According to Dr. Bassett, the average income for physicians in 1849 was $1,000 per year.[24] As late as 1854, Dr. W. Taylor of Talladega registered the following complaint:

> The profession of Medicine, then, is a field of labor—it is one of action. It is a proud and noble calling; but it is devoid, in a great measure, of those secular advantages which men of other occupations enjoy—the accumulation of wealth. It is not a profession which will 'fill thy purse with gold.' No class of men in the world, considering the amount of capital expended in their education, and the amount of labour in their profession, are so poorly paid as the physician; and did a man make wealth solely his object, he would be more likely to succeed with a wood-saw and an axe, than with an education which cost him a dozen years' hard study, and all the money

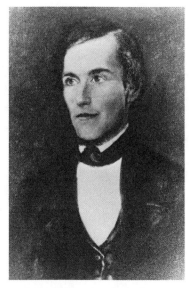

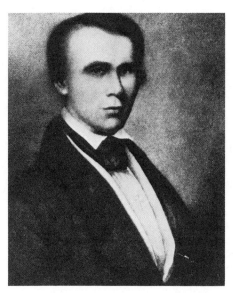

Paul Hamilton Lewis, M.D.,
1814–1849
(Courtesy of Mrs. Frank Moody)

John Young Bassett, M.D., 1805–1851

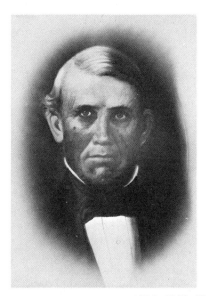

Thomas Fearn, M.D., 1789–1863 (Courtesy
of the Alabama State Department of
Archives and History)

he could procure. Lawyers sometimes get large fees, and are often called to honorable and lucrative stations. Divines, according to Freedley, if they do not get large salaries, have one secular advantage at least—they sometimes marry advantageously. Women have an idea that they make good husbands, and hence, with address, they may obtain serviceable fathers-in-law. But the profession of Medicine should be chosen from other and higher considerations than to obtain wealth.[25]

Many physicians worked their fields during the day and attended patients at night. One of these was Philip Madison Shepard (1812–1861), who came to Tallapoosa County a few years after the first settlers.[26] Others, such as Thomas Fearn (1789–1863), one of the most successful physicians in Huntsville, abandoned their profession entirely to engage in business.[27]

Thus, during this early period (1700–1840), few well-trained and established physicians were willing to leave older states to tackle the long hours and small income of rural practice in Alabama. Yet medical care was needed, and the high disease rate, together with the rapid increase in population, created a growing demand for physicians. Such conditions afforded an opening for hydropathy, homeopathy, and Thomsonianism, as well as other forms of quackery. (See Chapter 10, "Irregular Practice of Medicine.") Most of the settlers were Jacksonian populists and frontiersmen, who did not appreciate the value of professional training and, consequently, were not inclined to distinguish between regular and irregular practitioners. In 1859, an editorial in the *Dallas Gazette* stated the case succinctly:

> Here, the practice of Physic—like everything else—is a "free think"—the only qualifications required is to get patients, and these will allow no one but themselves to judge the competence of their doctor. It is one of the inalienable rights of free American citizens to be quacked to death by whomsoever he employs to do it.[28]

The situation that developed from these conditions was graphically described by Joseph G. Baldwin in his book *The Flush Times in Alabama and Mississippi* of 1853:

> Men dropped down into their places as from the clouds. Nobody knew who or what they were, except as they claimed, or as a surface view of their characters indicated. Instead of taking to the highway and magnanimously calling upon the wayfarer to stand and deliver, or to the fashionable larceny of credit without prospect or design of paying, some unscrupulous horse-doctor would set up his sign as "Physician and Surgeon," and draw his lancet on you, or fire at random a box of his pills into your bowels, with a vague chance of hitting some disease unknown to him, but with a better prospect of killing the patient, whom or whose administrator he charged some ten dollars a trial for his marksmanship.[29]

The irregular practice of medicine flourished everywhere. Some estimates show that in the early days of the state the number of irregular practitioners far exceeded the number of qualified physicians.[30] Among the thirty-six practitioners in Madison County mentioned by Dr. Bassett, there were a German root-doctor, a homeopathist, a steam doctor, and several black faith doctors.[31] As late as 1852, a professional census of the heavily populated Mobile County revealed that there were forty regular practitioners, two homeopathists, two hydropathists, three root-doctors, three Thomsonians, three quacks and one "idio-eclectopathist."[32] During the 1850s, the homeopathists and Thomsonians were so numerous that in 1854 and 1856 the Alabama General Assembly chartered separate licensing boards for the botanic doctors.[33] In 1854, the General Assembly chartered a Hydropathic Institute, planned for Rockford, Coosa County, although there is no evidence that it ever functioned.[34]

Many regular practitioners were little better than the irregulars whom they disliked. Dr. Bassett even had contempt for the majority of the regulars who had been active in Madison County as late as the twenties and thirties of the nineteenth century:

> These were principally young Virginians of good families, who had never offered for graduation, or who had been rejected by the Philadelphia and Baltimore Schools (for there was a time when our Medical Schools did reject some), and whose out-fit in life generally consisted of a pretty fair education, a genteel suit of clothes, a good horse and a mulatto servant; and whose object in life, to judge from their habitudes, was like that of our young preachers: to marry, and quit a profession they never loved, because they never knew.[35]

This judgment would seem excessively harsh if other writers did not agree. For example, until 1837, none of the Bibb County practitioners had ever heard a lecture in medicine, and it was not until 1849 that a graduate of a medical school began to practice in that county.[36] It certainly was not true, however, that either lectures and/or a degree guaranteed a competent physician.

There were outstanding schools in Baltimore, Philadelphia, and New York, but they were exceptions rather than the rule. Most medical schools were of the so-called proprietary type and were under the complete control of their faculties, who shared in the profits derived from matriculants' fees. There was no agency to regulate the standards, and abuses were frequent. (See Chapter 3, "Efforts in Medical Education.")

As a result of the inadequacy of medical care, many people treated themselves. In this respect, a daybook kept by Martin Marshall, who lived near Fort Claiborne from 1815 until 1865, is most illuminating.[37] Marshall was a weaver, blacksmith, and planter, and his book is a collection of useful household information covering everything from taking care of furniture and clothing to preserving food and getting rid of insects. Almost one-third of it is devoted to methods for dealing with various diseases. In these recipes, Marshall utilized indigenous plants that were thought to have medicinal qualities, patent medicines, and even dust from his own anvil. Thus, he used bearberry, Bear's whortle-berry, or wild cranberry leaves for

> the irritation of the stone gravel, and old cases of gonorrhea, menstrual discharges, also catarrhs and consumption; Samson's snake root for dyspepsia, indigestion, diarrhea and dysentery; a paste made of walnut and sassafras bark and red root for rheumatism, cachexy, dropsy, ague, cancerous ulcers, fever and worms; cows' urine, boiled down to a jelly, for "sore leg;" tincture of rhubarb, made of rhubarb, cardamon seeds or ginger, and brandy or rum, for a laxative; and honey and "the purest charcoal" for making the teeth white.[38]

It is not difficult to trace most of these "cures" to their origins. Many had been copied from newspapers, journals, and magazines; some had been developed by Marshall or his neighbors and friends, and others were derived from traditional Indian and slave formulas. Several prescriptions also had been recommended by a local physician, Dr. Caleb Lindsey. For example, he prescribed the following for indigestion: "Take 1 quart of clean Hickory ashes, and half a pint of clean [chimney] soot, put it into a Jug, with One Gallon of water, and shake it often—After three or four days a wine glass full to be taken three times a day."[39]

Poorly trained medical practitioners were a major obstacle in the fight against disease in early Alabama. But frequently not even the most educated physicians—men who had received the best training the United States and Europe had to offer and who continued to study the problems they encountered in their daily practices—could alleviate the sufferings brought on by most infectious diseases prevalent at that time. One of the main difficulties involved the then accepted theories concerning the nature and treatment of disease.

The most common view concerning the etiology of disease held in the eighteenth and early nineteenth centuries was succinctly stated by Bernard Romans in 1775: "It must be allowed, that all fevers however dissimilar in appearance, proceed from the same origin; nature only works with more or less violence to rid herself of what is detrimental to her."[40]

Dr. Jabez Wiggins Heustis (1784–1841), who practiced in Mobile during the twenties and thirties of the nineteenth century, was a prominent and prolific writer on all medical subjects.[41] He adhered to the same theory as Romans, who writing some fifty years later, stated:

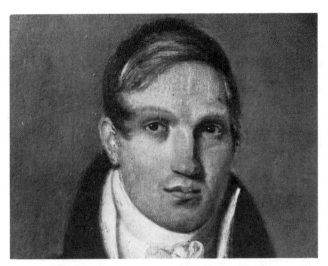

Jabez Wiggins Heustis, M.D., 1784–1841 (Portrait by Sully; Courtesy of Mrs. Francis Lowe, Mobile, Alabama)

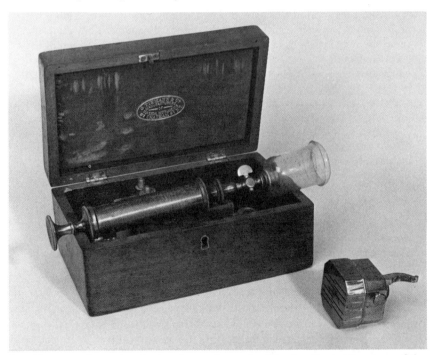

Scarificator and cupping device, formerly used to bleed patients (Courtesy of the Alabama Museum of the Health Sciences, Lister Hill Library, Medical Center, The University of Alabama in Birmingham)

> One of the most striking effects of a high temperature is the decomposition or destruction which it occasions in dead animal and vegetable substances. The immediate consequence of this decomposition is the escape of the elastic gases, and the corruption or [vitiation] of the surrounding atmosphere. The effect of this contamination . . . is the production of endemic and epidemic diseases.[42]

These ideas were in perfect accord with Dr. Heustis's theory of treatment. For if only one cause had to be blamed for all diseases, only one basic treatment need be devised to deal with it. Like so many of his contemporaries, Dr. Heustis, a follower of Dr. Benjamin Rush of Philadelphia, believed that he had found such a treatment in the use of venesection and purgation. His treatment of malarial fever and influenza was a typical "heroic" therapeutic regimen employed by early Alabama physicians and physicians throughout the country:

> I have sometimes taken away a quart of blood at a single operation, and with the best results. . . . In cases where blood-letting was not required, I commenced . . . by the exhibition of an emetic . . . in ordinary cases . . . tartarized antimony . . . till it produced five or six operations by vomiting. After the operation of the emetic, a cathartic was exhibited. Finding ten grains of jalap insufficient to carry calomel . . . through the bowels in the rapid manner I wished, I added fifteen grains of the former to ten of the latter; but even this dose was slow and uncertain in its operation. I then issued three doses . . . one to be given every six hours until they produced four or five large evacuations. The effects of this powder not only answered, but far exceeded my expectation. It perfectly cured four out of the first five patients. . . . I gave a purge every day while the fever continued. . . . I have sometimes been obliged to direct the administration of as many as thirty pills of calomel and jalap . . . directing two or three to be taken every ten or fifteen minutes.[43]

And influenza, he said,

> generally yielded to the fourth or fifth bleeding, to the extent of about a quart of blood at each venesection. After bleeding, a large blister plaster was applied to the affected region, and an active carthartic, as calomel and castor oil and jalap . . . with an infusion of Virginia snakeroot was exhibited.[44]

The adverse effect of such a regimen was incalculable. Dr. Bassett, in his medical reports, was characteristically short in his opinion of the practitioners who employed it: "Those who lived after it reflected great credit on the doctor, and gained him the reputation of being a 'bold practitioner.' "[45]

Dr. P. H. Lewis echoed these words:

> Armed with a box of those pills [drastic purgatives], the uninstructed practitioner went forth to conquer or to kill, and if perchance victory . . .

was the fortunate result . . ., great was the laudation and many the converts; but if, as was not [infrequently] the case, a much more aggravated form of disease than the original supervened, it was purely viewed as the will of fate.[46]

During the 1840s when these two men wrote, many thoughtful physicians began to question the value of such drastic treatment. Dr. Lewis further stated that "the diseases of Alabama presented new features from those they were accustomed to witness in the older States, and want of success in practice compelled them to abandon original theories, and to direct their thoughts in a new channel of speculation."[47]

Tragic experience was beginning to reveal that the treatment regimens according to "original theories" were a mistake. Thus, Dr. Lewis estimated that half of the typhoid fever cases treated with emetics had proven fatal.[48] Dr. William B. Ames of Montgomery reported in 1854 that no complication had developed in pneumonia patients who had not been bled while in many of those treated with mercury, emetic tartar, and bloodletting, "complications were produced by the deleterious agency of the remedies."[49]

Dr. William McFarland Boling (1811–1859) of Montgomery wrote that "among diseases treated principally with tartar emetic half as many deaths [had] occurred in consequence of gastro-enteritis—induced seemingly by the remedy—as from the primary disease itself."[50] A very good example of this revolutionary movement in medicine is evident in the developments in the use of quinine. After its general acceptance as an indispensable medication in the treatment of malarial fever around 1830, quinine came to be considered as a cure for all "fevers," especially when given in large doses (100 grains or more).[51] Although many medical men, including Dr. Bassett, had recognized that large doses could prove fatal even in the treatment of malaria, it was only much later, when quinine's lack of effectiveness in dealing with yellow and typhoid fevers was recognized, that physicians finally limited its use to the treatment of malaria.[52]

This lack of success among regular practitioners was in direct contrast to that of their greatest irregular competitors, the Thomsonians, who practiced a system of treatment based on the use of various herbs, primarily mild emetics. Around 1830, Thomsonianism became popular in Alabama. The Thomsonians made free use of stimulants externally and internally.[53] These stimulants were usually steam and red pepper, thus their nicknames, "steam doctors" and "red pepper gentlemen." Most of the regular physicians had only contempt for them and rarely talked about them without enumerating their failures.[54] Dr. Lewis gave an impression that this was due, at least in part, to professional jealousy. He stated that although their theory was false, the practice was much more appropriate to the kinds of disease found in this area and achieved signal success over the equally false theories and often fatal practices of those in the regular profession. In time, many physicians, while not adopting the complete regimen, did modify their treatment along the Thomsonian lines. For example, the first few issues of the *Transactions of the Medical Association of the State of Alabama*, the organ of the most prominent physicians in the state, were full of reports on the "indigenous botany" of Alabama. Dr. Philip Madison Shepard promised the students in his medical school that "Allopathy, Hydropathy, Homeopathy, and Botany would be taught scientifically."[55]

One irregular system of practice at this time recommended the administration of very small doses of drugs, which presumably produced the same symptoms as the disease. This was known as homeopathy. One doctor, who formerly gave calomel by the shovelful and castor oil by the quart, considered "Homeopathy a handsome satire . . . on our fraternity. 'Homeopaths,' according to an ironical yet instructive description, 'gave little, beautiful, and transcendental doses, potencies, triburations, shakes, globules, dilutions, and attenuations.' "[56] Homeopathy was practiced in the state until well after the turn of the century, but it appears to have had little impact on medicine in the state.

The pressure from the Thomsonians and other irregular systems of practice strengthened the movement away from the "heroic" treatment. Physicians, taught by experience, became much more conservative and began to use as few drugs as possible. Only a few continued to use the lancet, which came to be called the "sickle of death" instead of the instrument for successful treatment.[57] As early as 1844, Dr. William M. Boling said:

> a system of treatment much more judicious and successful [was] rapidly being adopted by the physicians of the South, and a number of those who [took] pride in boasting of their hundred grain dose of calomel or the number of drastic pills given in a [single] dose, [was] small, indeed.[58]

Two years later, Dr. P. H. Lewis claimed that the physicians of Mobile were "convinced beyond [doubt], that by the use of brandy alone, given at the proper time, hundreds, even [while] on the verge of the grave, [had] been rallied, sustained, and restored to life."[59]

By 1854, Dr. William Ames reported that "[of the] physicians of experience in this section of the country, . . . not one, . . . could be found who ever entertains a thought of following out the *Coup sur coup* plan."[60]

Indeed, Dr. Bassett was perfectly justified in stating in 1850:

> during the second lustrum of [Alabama's] political existence, the intellectual and professional character of [its] practicing physicians gradually

improved, [and that] there were men of proper education and undoubted genius occasionally among them.[61]

Alabama had become more populated, wealth had increased, and a much higher caliber physician had been attracted to the state. During the 1850s, few states in the Union could boast of such men as Osler's "Alabama Student," J. Y. Bassett; two future presidents of the American Medical Association, the world-renowned James Marion Sims (1813–1883) of Montgomery and William Owen Baldwin (1818–1886) of Montgomery; and the surgeon and natural historian Josiah Clark Nott (1804–1873) of Mobile. Under their leadership and with a conservative trend, medical practice in Alabama improved; and the public mistrust, which had burdened physicians in the earlier days, was gradually dispelled.

These improvements also influenced new theories of the etiology of disease and new approaches to its treatment. The appearance of typhoid fever and the frequent, increasingly virulent epidemics of yellow fever presented problems with which "heroic" treatment could not cope.

Dr. J. C. Nott exerted considerable influence on the changes in medical practice of the pioneer Alabama physicians. He used as few drugs as possible, thereby causing no harm by excessive and rash medication. He also appreciated the influence of the nervous system on body function and disease. Psychology played a large part in his therapeutics: his personality was the largest item in his drug kit. Probably more than today's physicians, he prescribed placebos. Nonetheless, he observed his patients closely and took a concerned interest in the various phases of their illnesses. These observations were the primary source of his extraordinary data on diseases.[62]

Infectious Diseases

Yellow Fever

In 1704, the *Pélican*, a ship from France, arrived at Fort Louis de la Mobile. The fort had been founded two years earlier as the capital of French Louisiana, and the eagerly awaited ship was bringing much needed supplies, colonists, soldiers, and two lay nursing sisters in charge of twenty-three girls, who were to be married to colonists already established there. Unfortunately, an uninvited passenger was also on board—yellow fever. The ship had stopped in Havana, and some of the crew and passengers had contracted the disease. Within a short time after arrival, half the ship's crew, thirty soldiers, some of the colonists, as well as the great explorer Enrico di Tonti, were dead.[63] This was the first and probably proportionately the most fatal epidemic of a disease that was to plague the settlers of Alabama for the next 200 years. The disease came to be known as "The Terrible Black Vomit," "The Great Plague of the Western Hemisphere," "The Terror of Terrors," "The Scourge of the South," and "Yellow Jack."

Inasmuch as there has not been sufficient research on the colonial medical history of the Gulf Coast states, it is almost impossible to document the occurrence and extent of yellow fever in the area that later became the state of Alabama. Only one other large-scale epidemic of this disease has been fully reported. The epidemic occurred in the early years of the colony and was brought to Mobile in 1765 by British soldiers from Jamaica. Throughout these years, yellow fever was also a frequent visitor in cities along the Atlantic Coast.[64] It appears to have originated in the West Indies from which it was brought by shipping to the Gulf ports. This was true of Mobile, which received most of its supplies by way of Santo Domingo and Cuba. Indeed, a description of yellow fever formed a large part of Bernard Romans's account of diseases in *A Concise Natural History of East and West Florida* published in 1775. The British, who occupied the area from 1763 until 1781, considered Mobile one of the most unhealthy places in the world. British Governor George Johnston wrote in 1765 "that [the] persisting in quartering of troops there [in Mobile and Pensacola] is a kind of war against Heaven, by piling up of dead bodies."[65]

A group of French Protestants settled upon a large land grant on the Escambia River in 1767. Among the colony of 278 inhabitants were several prominent families, all of whom seemed industrious and thrifty. Within a few months, the settlement was wiped out by yellow fever, and the few survivors migrated to Mobile and Pensacola.[66]

By the time Alabama had become a state, yellow fever appeared almost annually in Mobile. Fortunately, in most instances, there were only a few cases. Some years, however, it also occurred in epidemic form, attacking thousands of individuals and causing hundreds of deaths. In 1819, the number of fatalities was estimated at 274; in 1829 at 130; in 1837 at 350; in 1839 at 450; in 1843 at 750 (other accounts give the death total as 764); in 1853 at 1,191; in 1867 at 148; and in 1870 at 289.[67] When the number of deaths was compared to the total population exposed to yellow fever, the results were even more frightful. For example, in 1819, the fatalities were calculated to be between 25 and 40 percent of the population; in 1839, between 13 and 20 percent; and in 1853, when approximately one-third of the population fled from the city, nearly 17 percent of those who remained died from yellow fever.[68]

Mobile was not the only city in Alabama to suffer. As the population of the state increased, yellow fever began to spread inland to settlements along the navigable rivers. In 1819, it reached Fort St. Stephens and Fort Claiborne; in 1853, after ravaging Mobile, it spread to Selma, Montgomery, Cahaba, Demopolis, Fulton, and St. Stephens Road; and in 1878, during a severe epidemic, it occurred throughout the entire state. In the towns of Florence, Decatur, and Huntsville, yellow fever had been introduced by infected refugees from the Memphis epidemic.[69]

Improved means of transportation were partially responsible for the spread of the disease. The frightened populace fled the infected areas at the least sign of danger. Obviously, some of these individuals had already been infected, although they had few or no symptoms, and carried the disease with them. Dr. Jerome Cochran (1831–1896) of Mobile wrote in 1877: "A common danger did not inspire in all a common spirit of helpfulness, but rather a desperate selfishness, and a personal determination to escape from the plague, the motto of many being *sauve qui peut* [escape who can]."[70] Many difficulties experienced by the refugees were recorded. Friendless and treated as pariahs, these wretched people suffered untold hardships on their flight from the stricken city.[71]

The French inhabitants of Mobile moved to their plantations at the first sign of fever in the town.[72] Everyone who could afford to, fled the city. For example, in Mobile in 1819, 300 out of a population of 1,200 fled, and in 1853, 13,000 out of 25,000 fled.[73] Under the circumstances, it is not surprising that nearby communities often took extreme measures to protect themselves from the deadly malady. Usually, this was done by means of a proclamation issued by local authorities prohibiting the entrance of goods, people, trains, and ships from infected areas. Since such quarantines were frequently enforced with shotguns, many cities were almost completely isolated for the duration of the epidemic.[74]

Aside from the great loss of human life, there was much damage to the economy. The funds devoted to fighting this disease were calculated in millions of dollars.

It is difficult to imagine the terror that can possess an entire population threatened by this dread disease. The usual flow of human sympathy and philanthropy that ill fortune sometimes brings ceased to exist. The history of these epidemics is filled with instances of dreadful suffering due to the ravages of yellow fever. Whole families succumbed or, in some instances, all adult members were stricken and died, leaving little children who, having no one to care for them, frequently died from neglect.

Yellow fever came to be one of the diseases most discussed among Alabama physicians and was the source of frequent articles in such publications as *The New Orleans Medical and Surgical Journal* and *Southern Medical Reports*.

Some diseases presented specific differences in various sections of the state.[75] These differences provided physicians with the possibility that each disease had its own etiology, especially that there might be different types of "fevers." Dr. P. H. Lewis tried to explain this, attributing it "to some peculiarity attaching to the organic nature of each locality and region."[76] But others went beyond this. The most important of these was Dr. Josiah C. Nott. After studying medicine in South Carolina, Philadelphia, and Paris, Dr. Nott had settled in Mobile in 1836. He observed at first hand the measures taken to fight the yellow fever epidemics of 1837, 1839, and 1843. In 1847, he startled his colleagues by suggesting that the spread of both yellow fever and malaria could best be explained by the insect theory. (See Chapter 12, "The Development of Public Health in Alabama.")

The peculiar habits of insects, he believed, were the only possible means by which the erratic spread of yellow fever could be explained:

> It would certainly be quite as philosophical . . . to suppose that some insect or animalcule, hatched in the lowlands, like the mosquito, after passing through its metamorphoses, takes flight, and either from preference for a different atmosphere or impelled by one of those extraordinary instincts which many are known to possess, wings its way to the hill top to fulfil its appointed destiny.[77]

Dr. Nott thought this could also explain the belief that yellow fever struck more often at night: "Many of the Infusoria, as well as insects proper, are rendered inactive by too much light, heat, or dryness. They remain quiet during the day, and do their work at night."[78] Moreover, he speculated that the insect is only a carrier of the germ, and advanced a revolutionary theory of contagion, which explained why some people, although exposed to yellow fever, never contracted the disease:

> It is probable that [yellow] fever is caused by an insect or animalcule bred on the ground, and in what manner it makes its impression on the system, is by surmise—unless the animalcule is, like that of Psora, bred in the system, we could no more expect it to be contagious, than the bite of a serpent. We may therefore easily understand, that it can at the same time be transportable in the form of a germ, and yet not [be] contagious.[79]

If this theory had been accepted and acted upon, it would have revolutionized prevention and treatment of yellow fever fifty years before the work of Carlos Finlay, Walter Reed, and William Crawford Gorgas.[80]

Dr. Nott's contemporaries ridiculed his beliefs. Few could accept his ideas concerning contagion and the multiplicity of "morbific agents," or his theory that insects were responsible for the spread of malaria and yellow fever. Fortunately, these theories were accepted by Dr. Jerome Cochran, "The Father of Public Health in Alabama." He had started practice in Mobile after the Civil War and was closely associated with Dr. Nott in the work of the local medical association. Later, as Alabama's first State Public Health Officer, Dr. Cochran was responsible for putting many of Dr. Nott's ideas into practice.

CAN'T-GET-AWAY CLUB

It was during the 1839 epidemic that the "Can't-Get-Away Club" was organized in Mobile for the care of the sick in time of yellow fever epidemics.*[81] This local relief society, modeled after the Red Cross of Geneva, Switzerland, was in reality the "Won't-Get-Away Club" in that its heroic members declined to flee their city and were ever ready with physicians, medicine, food, and nursing care for those stricken and suffering with yellow fever. Many local physicians as well as civic-minded laymen lost their lives after becoming ill while attending those afflicted.

In 1838, the year prior to the formation of the Can't-Get-Away Club, the Samaritan Society had been organized to provide for care of the poor and unemployed during the crisis. Public works usually afforded employment for the able bodied. This society, along with the Can't-Get-Away Club worked together to alleviate suffering in the city during yellow fever epidemics.

In August, 1839, yellow fever occurred in Mobile and spread rapidly. Only three or four physicians were available, and the few nurses obtainable were charging ten dollars a day; therefore, the poor received little attention save what they could manage for themselves. A dozen citizens, meeting as was their daily custom in the Alhambra Hotel for luncheon, talked over the situation and began to raise a relief fund. Some of them suggested that an organization be formed, and this proved agreeable. It was decided that this should be purely a yellow fever relief association, leaving to other charitable organizations the general relief causes. John Hurtel was elected president of the club. It was incorporated later by an act of the General Assembly and approved by Governor John A. Winston (governor of Alabama, 1853–1857) on February 1, 1854.

Work for the sick and dying began at once, and never was there greater need. The disease had caused havoc in the little city as several thousand people were ill and many died. The worst was over, however, by mid-November, and the affliction was brought to an end by a frost.

Almost yearly a few instances of yellow fever would appear, but an epidemic did not occur again until 1843 when the organization served as before. In that year, Mobile suffered the most severe assault it had yet sustained. The deaths exceeded those of 1839 by 78, the total being 764. The next epidemic years were 1853, 1867, 1870, and 1878.

---

*In New Orleans, a similar society was organized and named the Howard Association, which did yeoman duty in time of epidemics. This society undoubtedly aided in the Mobile epidemics. John Duffy, ed., *The Rudolph Matas History of Medicine in Louisiana* (Baton Rouge: Louisiana State University Press, 1962), 2: 13–14, 131.

John Hurtel still directed the club's operation in the great epidemic of 1853 when "there were 20, 30 and then 50 deaths a day, until not enough well persons remained to care for the sick. The dead were carried to the cemetery in wagons and carts, and were buried without coffins."

The Can't-Get-Away Club was reorganized in the summer of 1865 for the first time after the Civil War. No epidemic of the fever occurred that year, but in 1867 and 1870, the disease returned with serious consequences.

In 1878, the club gave aid to other afflicted cities, principally Memphis; New Orleans; Vicksburg, Holly Springs, and Granada, Mississippi. The club sent physicians, nurses, and money. This assistance was given before yellow fever struck Mobile that year; nonetheless, the club gave aid not only to these cities but to its own until the epidemic was over.

The last yellow fever epidemic in Mobile occurred in 1897. In 1905, however, yellow fever recurred on the Gulf Coast, and there was a severe outbreak in New Orleans. Alabama reported three deaths, none of which were in Mobile or in Mobile County. Also, in 1905, a determined anti-mosquito campaign was undertaken in New Orleans, and for the first time, the fever was stamped out before the appearance of frost. Similar methods for prevention of yellow fever and its spread were adopted elsewhere, rendering the region at last free from this menace. The services of the Can't-Get-Away Club were no longer needed, and the organization was disbanded.

Malaria

Malarial fever was another of the illnesses with which inhabitants of Alabama had to contend, for the conditions that aided the spread of yellow fever were just as favorable for malaria. Alabama—with its long and humid summers, its many rivers, marshes, and stagnant pools—was an ideal breeding ground for the *Anopheles* mosquito. It was not surprising that malaria reached epidemic proportions in some parts of the state almost yearly and that as late as 1913, eighty-six fatalities were attributed to this disease in the Black Belt counties.[82]

The sheer number of names used to describe the summer and autumn fevers reveals how extensive malarial fever really was. Dr. John Lorimer, writing about health conditions in Mobile in 1769, employed the terms "bilious, remitting and intermittent fevers." A few years later, Bernard Romans discussed "continual, inflammatory, and ague fevers." In 1846, Dr. P. H. Lewis wrote an article entitled "Medical History of Alabama," in which he described malarial fever as "slow, swamp, continued and congestive fevers."[83] In addition, terms such as *miasmatic, marsh, river, lake, malignant,* and *chill* fevers were also used to describe malarial fever.[84]

Although malaria was not as fatal as yellow fever, it was much more disruptive in the long run. It incapacitated large segments of the population from June until the coming of cold weather and the disappearance of the mosquito in October. Dr. Lorimer stated in 1769 that there were few who were sick with fevers until the month of June. "The bilious, remitting and intermittent fevers then set in, and continued [with] repeated relapses throughout the months of July, August, and September."[85] These relapses were the most incapacitating aspects of malaria, because once the disease had been acquired there was a constant threat of renewed attack. Both Romans and Lewis, in writing about the treatment of malaria, warned physicians to be constantly aware of the possibility of a relapse during the protracted convalescent period.[86] Even earlier, Dr. Lorimer had observed that the primary problem in the treatment of fevers among soldiers stationed at Mobile was the practice of returning them to duty before they had completely recovered, a practice resulting in numerous relapses.[87] The British, in fact, frequently did not have enough healthy men to defend the fort during the summer months, a situation that had occurred previously at the French Fort Toulouse, and later at the American Fort Stoddard.[88]

The problem was compounded by the fact that the new immigrants to this area seemed to be particularly susceptible to malaria. For example, in 1763, the newly arrived British soldiers suffered vicious attacks of this disease, probably due in part to the debilitating effect of their long sea voyage, together with a poor ship's diet.[89] To prevent this type of occurrence, a group of British surgeons suggested that troops from England be brought to West Florida only during the winter and spring months in order that they might be "seasoned" to the climate before the advent of the deadly summer.[90] Similarly, Dr. Lewis noticed that between 1829 and 1843 the majority of yellow fever and malaria cases occurred among people who were recent settlers in the city of Mobile.[91]

In the 1820s, Dr. Jabez W. Heustis and others used Peruvian bark to treat malarial fever. Dr. Heustis "spoke of it with faint praise." After 1830, Alabama physicians used quinine; its "talismatic influence" received early recognition from some physicians, among whom were Drs. Lewis, Baldwin, Boling, and Fearn. Widespread acceptance of quinine as a therapeutic agent was truly a revolutionary development. Unfortunately, quinine was used to treat all fevers and also used in every size dose. In the 1840s, patients were given doses of 30, 50, and even 100 grains. It was typhoid fever and yellow fever that belatedly convinced the medical profession that quinine could not cure every fever.[92]

Typhus and Typhoid Fever

Although little is mentioned concerning typhus fever, there are some references to its occurrences in the *Transactions of the Medical Association of the State of Alabama.*[93] Evidently, it did not pose a serious problem in the antebellum era.

Typhoid fever was another disease altogether. This was the "continued fever" that is mentioned so often in the writings of the early physicians in Alabama, who apparently recognized its epidemic character. It appeared almost annually in many sections in Alabama. Typhoid was not confined to the river towns nor did it occur exclusively during the summer and fall months. It most likely had its origin in the mass movement westward of the country's population between 1820 and 1869. These early pioneers probably carried the disease with them.

There were a number of reports of typhoid fever occurring as an epidemic among plantation slaves, and the disease was often confined to one plantation.[94] It was also recognized that blacks were more susceptible and often more severely affected by this disease than were whites. On the other hand in "intermittent fever," that is, malarial fever, the blacks exhibited at least a partial immunity.

Treatment remained empirical. A number of physicians felt that a large dose of quinine used early would abort the attack.[95] Very little follow-up observation was possible to confirm this theory. On the whole, most physicians had developed a sane and conservative treatment regimen. Bleeding and purgation were unusual, and symptomatic therapy for the fever and discomfort was recommended. The restriction of food intake during the acute phase, as well as the recovery phase, was deemed worthwhile. Observations of hemorrhaging as well as perforation of the bowel were noted in typhoid fever. During recovery, the starving patient might intemperately ingest a large amount of food to his detriment, for perforation of the intestine might occur and usually resulted in peritonitis and death. Autopsies, which were occasionally performed, revealed mesenteric lymphadenopathy, splenomegaly, and ulcerations in the small intestines. In some cases, perforations and peritonitis were present.

Even though its occurrence was often confined to a single plantation, there was no indication that fecal contamination of water and milk was suspected. The recognition of typhoid fever was unquestionably obscured by the high incidence of malaria and other febrile illnesses in the same area. However, in 1852, Dr. L. H. Anderson of Sumter County presented a paper to the State Medical Association in which he detailed a differential diagnosis of typhoid and malarial fever that was amazingly accurate.[96]

Dengue

Dengue, another febrile disease, was reported as occurring in Mobile and the river towns in Alabama between 1850 and 1855.[97] It was usually characterized by a chill and mild fever associated with musculoskeletal pain and headache. Reference was made to the malignant type, which was considered to be a cross between yellow fever and dengue. No fatalities were reported. There is no evidence that the physicians were aware of its epidemiology. It did occur, however, in epidemic form on the Gulf Coast.[98]

Smallpox

Smallpox occurred sporadically in early Alabama settlements. Vaccination against this disease was introduced in the United States in 1800 by Benjamin Waterhouse, Harvard Professor of Medicine. The vaccine was responsible in large part for reducing the incidence of smallpox in this country. Unfortunately for the southern states and western territories, lack of communication often hindered and delayed the use of this preventive measure. Also, ignorance and superstition prevented widespread vaccination; therefore, smallpox still made periodic appearances, frequently with devastating results. Alabama had a law requiring quarantine of all persons suffering with smallpox, and this, plus the widely separated settlements and availability of vaccination, were probably responsible for its infrequent occurrence in epidemic form during this early period.[99]

With the increase in population, the situation changed. Smallpox occurred sporadically in Mobile, the Gulf Coast area, and the towns along the rivers during the antebellum era. Accounts of its occurrence were reported in the *Transactions* prior to 1855. Unquestionably, smallpox was introduced with foreign commerce, together with the influx of nonimmune immigrants and slaves.

The people in general had a healthy respect for smallpox and were usually zealous in obtaining vaccination, which was available at little or no cost. Treatment of the smallpox victim was symptomatic, and quarantine of all cases was strictly enforced.

Digestive Diseases

Dr. John Lorimer wrote that "at the approach of cold weather, the fevers abated, and [the people] then fell [victims of] fluxes, dropsies, and cachexias."[100] Digestive tract diseases, primarily diarrhea and dysentery, were considered by Alabama physicians to be the greatest cause of death. Bernard Romans, who himself had suffered from "hemorrhoidal flux" for eight years, wrote that this disease, if it became chronic, was "almost always a slow though sure harbinger of death, . . . draining to the very last drop of moisture from the sufferer, who, being left a [mere] skeleton, is as [if he] were carried off in the manner of an expiring candle-snuff."[101]

A similar situation was noted in 1847 by Dr. J. C. Nott, who, while surveying health conditions in the southern ports for insurance purposes, came to the conclusion that only 77 of every 100 children born in Alabama lived to be five years old. Death was most commonly caused by digestive diseases, mostly *cholera infantum.*[102] Many other physicians agreed, although they considered these figures conservative.[103] The number of children's graves in the early cemeteries of this area bears mute witness to the high mortality in infants and young children.

In addition, people of all ages, though particularly children, suffered greatly from "worm fever."[104] During most of the nineteenth century, physicians had little to say about this disease, although as late as 1896 some "two million people of sound English ancestry" living in the South suffered from its ravages. "Generations of these southern whites have craved dirt, have grown feeble, have had spasms, have bought carloads of patent medicines and have gone through the world 'shiftless' and 'lazy' without knowing what was the matter with them."[105] It was not until 1910 that, with the help of generous grants from the Rockefeller Foundation, a successful antihookworm campaign was launched. (See Chapter 12, "The Development of Public Health in Alabama.")

Respiratory Diseases

The occurrence of cold weather brought respiratory diseases to many people already debilitated from fevers and diarrhea. Bronchitis, influenza, pleurisy, and pneumonia appeared so rapidly that Dr. Lewis felt justified in naming one particular variety "congestive intermittent fever."[106]

These diseases seem to have been especially prevalent among and dangerous to blacks in the state. In 1848, Dr. John Y. Bassett observed that "the number of cases and the relative proportion of deaths among [blacks] from pneumonia [was] many times greater than among whites." This conclusion was made after making allowances for the fact that slaves were constantly exposed to inclement weather.[107] Also, tuberculosis, then known as "consumption," was especially hazardous to the black population.

Bernard Romans referred to the occurrence of tuberculosis and mentions that one of the cures was periodic short sea voyages.[108] During most of the nineteenth century, "consumption," which affected entire families, was considered a hereditary disease, and physicians who could offer little in the way of treatment had even less to say about it in published reports.

Diphtheria

The serious nature of diphtheria has always been fully appreciated. It was reported as having occurred in Wilcox County in 1849.[109] However, it is difficult to determine whether the physicians recognized its infectious nature. It did occur in several members of the same families, but apparently it was not considered an epidemiological problem. Often it was referred to as "membranous croupe." The treatment was symptomatic, and the death rate was surprisingly small.

Other Diseases

Insofar as other infectious diseases were concerned, measles, scarlet fever, and whooping cough were present every year. This can be concluded from reports of these diseases occurring in various parts of the state and published in the *New Orleans Medical and Surgical Journal*,

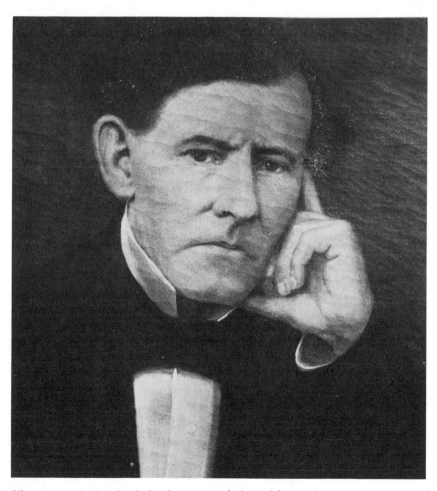

Silas Ames, M.D., ?–1859 (Courtesy of the Alabama State Department of Archives and History)

Southern Medical Reports, and the *Transactions of the Medical Association of the State of Alabama*.

Dr. George Augustus Ketchum (1825–1906) of Mobile reported in 1855 an epidemic of lead poisoning caused by the drinking water in Mobile being contaminated by lead pipes. His description of the disease is classic for lead colic.[110]

An epidemic of cerebrospinal meningitis was reported by Dr. Silas Ames (?–1859) in Montgomery in 1849. Postmortem examination showed that the pathologic lesions were those of meningitis. The meninges were inflamed, and there were no intestinal lesions.[111] Dr. W. P. Reese (1818–1878) described cerebromeningitis in both Selma and nearby Marion, Alabama.[112]

The Early Specialties

Obstetrics

Excessive modesty pertaining to the female genitalia and childbirth made obstetrical examination difficult and almost always uninformative. It took unusual skill for a physician to examine and treat a patient without being able to observe what he was doing. Fortunately, the advances in science brought an end to this false modesty. The introduction of the vaginal speculum was one of the factors that helped to do away with the secrecy attached to the female genital organs.

By the 1840s, there were a large number of midwives whose training was either strictly empirical or virtually nonexistent. As the population increased by leaps and bounds, the demand for midwives brought hundreds of ignorant and incapable white and black women into the field. The licensing laws for these parapractitioners were lax or nonexistent. The public health officials in Alabama, as well as other states, had observed that the high rate of infant and maternal deaths during childbirth was directly related to the use of untrained midwives. Their training and regulation, however, would require a long and determined struggle by physicians and public health officials.

A number of published reports gives evidence of the concern of the physicians of the state as to the inadequacies of the midwives' care. In the nineteenth century, there can be little doubt that some of the high mortality of parturient mothers could be attributed to treatment by incompetent midwives. *Trismus nascentium* or infant lockjaw was a form of tetanus frequently caused by infected navels.[113] One of the midwives' practices, after severing the umbilical cord, was that of spreading cow dung over the exposed navel area. This was thought to promote healing. One does not have to guess the origin of the tetanus. *Procidentia* or prolapse of the uterus was not unusual and was probably secondary to the use of excessive force during delivery by inexperienced midwives.[114]

Puerperal fever was an enigma with respect to etiology and treatment.[115] The idea of its being infectious and contagious was apparently not even considered. Venesection and purgation together with measures for counter irritation were used in its treatment and probably increased the possibility of a fatal termination. The long difficult labor often associated with the birth of the first child provided ample impetus for interference by ignorant physicians and midwives. Such examination increased the possibility of infection. The use of clean instruments or the simple washing of hands was a rare practice in the antebellum era. Oliver Wendell Holmes (1809–1894) and Ignaz Semmelweis (1818–1865) in the 1840s had suggested that these measures be used in an attempt to prevent puerperal sepsis. Unfortunately, it would require long and tragic experience before aseptic childbirth was practiced in Alabama. Indeed, puerperal sepsis remained a problem in the early part of the twentieth century and was a threat until the introduction of chemotherapy and antibiotic agents.

Physicians occasionally specialized in obstetrics, but for the most part they were only called in difficult cases. Forceps delivery was widely practiced. Instances of craniotomy, evisceration, and dismemberment of the fetus in pelvic deformity were reported. Pelvic deformities, not an uncommon finding, were attributed to widespread dietary deficiencies.

A case of *placenta previa* was reported.[116] Diagnosis and management appear to have been adequate, but blood loss resulted in death for both mother and child.

The use of venesection in prolonged difficult labor was a fairly widespread practice in Alabama, particularly in the rural areas prior to 1850.[117] It was believed that the bleeding relaxed the uterus and birth canal and thus made delivery easier. Cesarean sections were performed but usually proved fatal to the mother and child from loss of blood and shock. However, on a closer scrutiny of these reports, it would be fair to say that when the operation was finally performed, the patients had been in labor for a long period of time and were in extremis. In one instance, the uterus had ruptured, and the fetus and placenta were in the abdominal cavity.[118]

However, successful cesareans were performed in Alabama prior to the Civil War. In 1852, Dr. Zackery E. Nettles of Wilcox County performed a cesarean section on a black female with a narrow pelvis and an impacted head of the fetus. The patient and baby lived, but the child died at four months of age with a childhood disease.[119]

In 1857, Dr. James W. Stewart of Florence reported successfully performing a cesarean section.[120] In this instance, with a transverse position of the fetus, the mother lived but the baby died. In 1866, Dr.

Richard Fowler of Burnt Corn, Monroe County, Alabama, performed a cesarean section on a black female with a fetal shoulder presentation. The mother lived but the child died.[121]

Antebellum Surgery

The practice of medicine in rural Alabama was similar to that found elsewhere in a predominately rural South. The physicians for the most part were too isolated to keep abreast of new developments and had little time or incentive to do so. However, the quality of medicine and surgery practiced in the cities of Mobile, Montgomery, Tuscaloosa, Huntsville, and Selma was comparable to that in other large cities of the South. Interested and energetic physicians cooperated to improve their medical knowledge by organizing medical societies.

Dr. J. Marion Sims's contributions to medicine and surgery are well known. His outstanding achievements occurred in the relatively pioneer city of Montgomery from 1840 to 1850 and are even more remarkable when we consider that they came prior to the use of aseptic surgical techniques and anesthesia. Dr. Sims came to Alabama to practice in the village of Mount Meigs. His practice flourished until a severe attack of malaria forced him to move to the healthier climate in Montgomery. He was one of the first individuals in the state who was treated with quinine for malaria.

Dr. Sims was well trained, having finished the Medical College of South Carolina and the Jefferson Medical College in Philadelphia. He then enrolled in a course of regional and surgical anatomy. Dr. Sims later wrote that these experiences were instrumental in influencing his surgical career. He successfully treated with surgery a wide variety of difficult conditions, including clubfoot, strabismus, harelip, and removal of a malignant growth on the face and neck. Dr. Sims was a pioneer in gallbladder surgery and gave us the term cholecystotomy.[122]

The unique surgical operation that he developed was for the repair of vesicovaginal fistula.[123] This condition was usually secondary to difficult childbirth. Due to the resultant urinary and fecal incontinence, these individuals were considered pariahs in their families and social circles. Dr. Sims attempted to close vesicovaginal fistulas in three slave women and devoted all of his time, effort, and income to these individuals. He even paid their expenses during these procedures. Finally, after four years of trial and failure, he operated for the thirtieth time on one of the patients and successfully closed the fistula. He afterwards operated on the two other women and quickly restored them to health, confirming the success of his new technique.

To undertake this type of surgery, Dr. Sims devised the knee-elbow position (Sims's position), a special curved speculum (Sims's speculum), a new self-retaining catheter to keep the bladder empty while the fistula was healing, and finally silver sutures to keep infection to a minimum. This operation was performed without anesthesia and must have caused considerable pain.

At that time, Dr. Sims, along with many other surgeons, made a practice of giving large quantities of narcotics in some form in order to keep the intestines inactive so that the operation's success would not be endangered by bowel activity. According to his report, this "locking up" of the bowels went on for weeks—not less than ten to fifteen days and maybe as long as three to four weeks. Fortunately, he had no fatalities from this procedure.[124]

Dr. Sims's major breakthrough in gynecology did not bring him immediate fame. He was suffering from chronic diarrhea, and his impaired health prompted him to move from Montgomery to New York City in May, 1852. In New York, he successfully interested several influential women in founding the Woman's Hospital, which opened May 1, 1855.[125] This was a thirty-bed charity hospital.

In 1861, Dr. Sims went to Europe where he lived for the duration of the Civil War. As his surgical fame had preceded him to Europe, he was able to perform his vesicovaginal fistula operation and to use other techniques he had developed and introduced in Montgomery. The French government honored him by creating him a Knight of the Legion of Honor for his signal contributions to surgery.

Dr. Sims returned to New York in time to be the principal speaker at the first anniversary celebration of the Woman's Hospital in 1869. He was elected president of the American Medical Association in 1875 and served in 1876.

There is a memorial on the state capitol grounds in Montgomery to this extraordinary physician whose achievements in surgery were world famous.[126]

Dr. Sims was also instrumental in founding the New York Cancer Hospital. An anonymous donor had offered $150,000 to erect a pavilion for the exclusive care of cancer patients on the grounds of the Woman's Hospital.[127] Sims wanted desperately to devise a method of alleviating the suffering of cancer victims who, at that time, were doomed to die after months or a few years at most of agonizing pain. He believed the early operation (1883), "extirpation of the cancerous uterus" (hysterectomy), was the only method of curing uterine malignancy.[128] He was distressed that the Woman's Hospital, which had a policy of not admitting patients with cancer, was depriving these sufferers of their only hope to live.[129]

After much discussion, the anonymous financial offer was declined, but a new hospital specifically designed for the treatment of cancer was planned. The cornerstone of the New York Cancer Hospital was laid

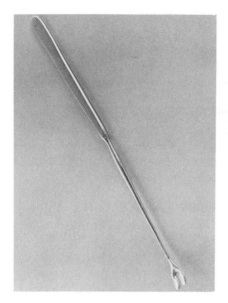 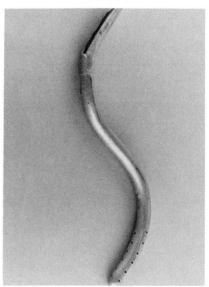

Instruments designed and used by Dr. J. Marion Sims: (*above*) shield for suturing in gynecological surgery (*left*), self-retaining catheter; (*below*) curved speculum (*left*), silver wire sutures with lead shot for anchoring the sutures (Courtesy of the Alabama Museum of the Health Sciences, Lister Hill Library, Medical Center, The University of Alabama in Birmingham)

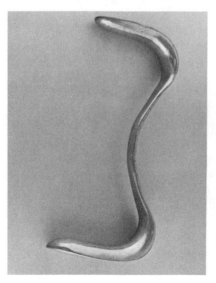 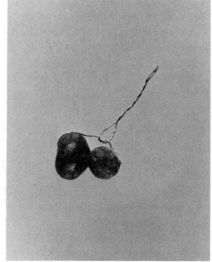

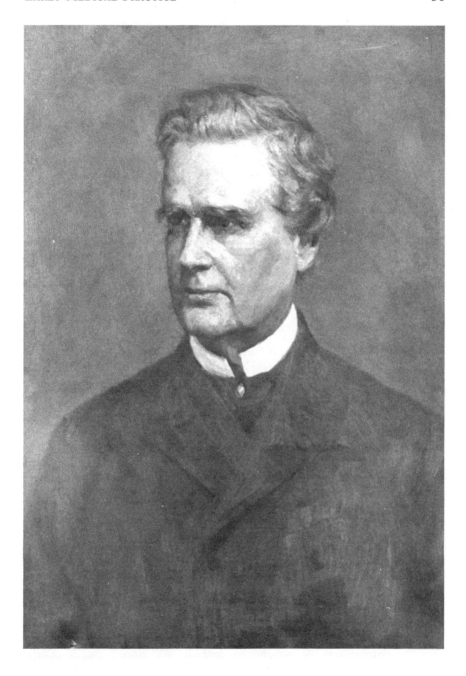

James Marion Sims, M.D., 1813–1883 (Courtesy of the Alabama State Department of Archives and History)

March 17, 1884. The anonymous donor was John Jacob Astor. Although Mr. Astor was instrumental in founding this hospital, it was originally Sims's idea.[130]

Dr. Nathan Bozeman (1825–1905), a native of Alabama, was educated in Louisville, Kentucky, and spent an apprenticeship in surgery as an assistant to the distinguished Dr. Samuel David Gross (1805–1884), a Louisville surgeon.[131] Dr. Bozeman became a well-trained surgeon, and on the recommendation of Dr. Gross, he was employed by Dr. Sims as an assistant. Dr. Sims had hoped that Dr. Bozeman would relieve him of some of the burden of his practice and free him for new investigations, but a misunderstanding arose over credit for some of the innovations from Dr. Sims's surgical techniques and caused an animosity that was to last a lifetime.[132] Dr. Bozeman devised a self-retaining vaginal speculum and an improved chair for use during surgery using the knee-chest position. In 1859, he performed a kolpokleisis as a means of surgical closure of vesicovaginal fistulas.[133]

From 1856 to 1858, Dr. Bozeman was associated with Dr. John Brown Gaston, II (1834–1913) of Montgomery. In 1861, he offered his services to the Confederate Army and served the Confederacy until the Civil War ended. After the war, Dr. Bozeman moved to New York City where he practiced gynecology; he became a surgeon at the Woman's Hospital where he was recognized as a skilled and learned gynecologist. In 1878, he was elected a Fellow in the American Gynecological Society, and in 1891, the University of Alabama conferred an honorary LL.D. degree upon him.[134]

Dr. William O. Baldwin, an eminent physician and surgeon of Montgomery, first described quinine-induced amblyopia, which he had observed during his investigation of the use of "heroic" doses of quinine in treatment of malarial fever. Although little public enmity had existed between the physicians of the North and South during the Civil War, there were somewhat strained relationships afterward. Dr. Samuel D. Gross of Philadelphia felt that the election of a Southerner to the presidency of the American Medical Association (AMA) would do much to heal the breach. Dr. Baldwin was elected in the fall of 1868 and served as president of the AMA in 1869.[135]

Possibly one of the most outstanding of these Southerners was Dr. Josiah Clark Nott. A surgeon by training and widely known for his contributions in surgery, he is best remembered for his work in epidemiology. He was a life-long friend and colleague of Dr. Sims. In 1844, in the *New Orleans Medical and Surgical Journal*, Nott described the condition of coccygodynia. As early as 1832, Dr. Nott first performed a coccygectomy for "severe and intractable neuralgia." In 1859, he

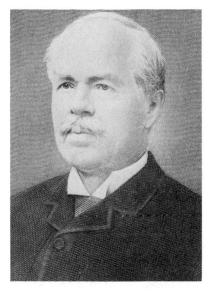

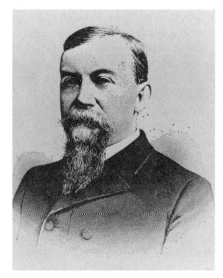

Nathan Bozeman, M.D., 1825–1905

John Brown Gaston II, M.D., 1834–1913
(Courtesy of the Alabama State Department of Archives and History)

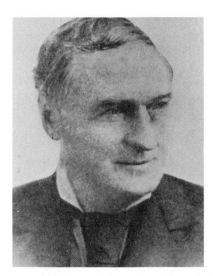

William Owen Baldwin, M.D., 1818–1886

founded the Medical College of Alabama in Mobile and became Professor of Surgery there.[136]

Dr. Henry S. Levert (1804–1864) of Mobile demonstrated the innocuous character of lead, gold, silver, and platinum wire for ligating arteries in his experiments on dogs. Dr. Levert's nephew, Dr. C. H. Mastin (1826–1898) of Mobile, successfully tied the external iliac artery with silver wire in 1866.[137]

Dr. Seneca Powell (1847–?), a native of Wilcox County, Alabama, became a New York surgeon. It was he who demonstrated the fact that pure alcohol instantly neutralizes the caustic effect of carbolic acid and who introduced the carbolic acid treatment of chronic leg ulcers.[138]

Among the surgical procedures carried out in Alabama and reported in the *Transactions* before 1860 were the repair of strangulated inguinal hernia, varicose veins, lithotomy, trephine with evacuation of subdural hematoma, removal of bilateral congenital cataracts, arterial ligation for the treatment of aneurysm of the subclavian artery, and the excision of anal fistula. A number of amputations were also reported.

Although both ether and chloroform were widely used after 1850—with ether used most frequently—some of these procedures were performed without anesthesia.[139]

The Advent of Anesthesia

The improvements in surgical techniques during the first half of the nineteenth century did little to alleviate the fears and apprehensions of prospective surgical patients. In the days before anesthesia, operations were always painful and frequently fatal. One can understand why it was not unusual for patients to permit tumors to reach enormous size before finally resorting to surgery.

Elective surgery was very rare and done only as a last resort. Five years before the introduction of anesthesia, elective operations at the Massachusetts General Hospital in Boston averaged about three operations a month.[140]

The surgeon of this era was depicted as bold, strong, dexterous, and quick in his actions—all essential qualities for the surgeon of his day. Indeed, physical strength and audacity were among the prime requisites for a successful surgeon. The good surgeon was of necessity the quick one, as in any very lengthy operation it was thought that the patient could die from shock due to the agonizing pain. Sometimes limbs were amputated in less than a minute, but the operation was not complete. The blood vessels still had to be tied and the wound closed. Patients appeared to suffer as intensely at this stage as they did during the amputation so that the ligation and suturing had to be done equally as fast.

Prior to the use of anesthesia, surgical patients often were not mechanically restrained. Instead they were held by strong attendants. Even these were not always able to cope with some patients in the agony caused by the cautery and scalpel.

Dr. J. Marion Sims tells the story of a patient who had previously seen a Montgomery physician who had recognized and attempted to remove a tumor.[141] After the initial incision, however, the patient leapt from the chair and positively refused to undergo further surgery. When Dr. Sims was consulted, he advised removing the tumor. "In the presence of ten students and fifteen doctors (not to mention a portrait painter charged with the task of making sketches of various stages of the operation) he persuaded [the unfortunate man] to sit in a barber's chair; then, taking the [patient] momentarily unaware, he and his five assistants hastened to fasten him down by means of an elaborately constructed device involving a five-foot plank and surcingle webbing, with leather straps over his thighs, knees, ankles, abdomen, thorax, shoulders, elbows, wrists, and head."

By now the patient was much alarmed. Dr. Sims tried to ease the patient's apprehension by giving him 60 drops of laudanum. When the laudanum failed to work, he was given brandy and water during the operation. For forty minutes the patient sweated and suffered quite helplessly. Sims opened the cheek, dissected away the diseased mass, and then experimented with three different instruments before he found a chain saw that he thought could do the proper job of cutting away the diseased bone. Yet, in the end, the patient had reason to be grateful for his ordeal. After a long convalescence, he returned home cured, but with a hideous scar on his cheek.

Dr. Sims, a perfectionist who was always trying to improve his surgical techniques, pondered on how such a scar might have been avoided. By the time he had to perform another operation on an osteosarcoma of the lower jaw, he had a plan. The patient was an elderly black man with an exceptionally large mouth. Dr. Sims was able to perform the entire operation, which included removal of most of the jawbone, by using a series of complicated maneuvers which caused no external mutilation and minimal scarring.[142]

Dr. Sims also described the case of an eighteen-year-old male slave who, without flinching, underwent surgery for the removal of a malignant tumor in the sinus back of his eye. However, in less than two months the tumor had reappeared and was twice its original size. At the patient's urgent request, Dr. Sims operated a second time, "probing for the diseased tissue in the deep dark recesses at the base of the brain, guided only by the sense of touch in his left forefinger." To help the patient through this agonizingly painful surgery, he was given brandy and water and "evidenced wonderful fortitude, but at the close his strength was almost exhausted, and often he would cry out in the bitterest agony: 'Oh! How long? How long will it last?' "[143] The operation lasted an hour and a half, but he suffered for naught. The tumor returned almost immediately, and the courageous man died in a few months.[144]

The pain of repairing dislocated joints and setting bone fractures was almost equal to that of the cutting operations. Physicians had found that the ingestion of alcohol or bleeding the patient to the point of extreme weakness was a fairly effective means of relaxing the muscles. When these procedures did not suffice, the affected limb was strapped and traction was applied with a mechanical block and tackle. The suffering this procedure entailed was often beyond endurance.[145]

Many attempts to prevent pain in surgical procedures were tried, but most were unsuccessful. Mesmerism was one of these early attempts, but it was not very effective. The best painkiller was found to be opium, and a large dose of laudanum was given before an operation in the 1840s. However, even this was insufficient to deaden the piercing pain of the cautery and scalpel. Another expedient method was to render the patient "dead drunk" with alcohol. This measure was also, for the most part, unsuccessful. Occasionally, cold compresses were applied to numb the nerves in order to prevent pain, but these too were inadequate. Chloroform, sulfuric ether, and nitrous oxide gas were beginning to revolutionize surgery in the 1850s, but were new and untried; therefore the surgeon was reluctant to use them. A credible theory is that fear of killing the patient with such little-known chemical agents was the principal restraining factor. Rendering a patient insensible with gas could be a hazardous procedure, particularly when the correct dosage, limits of toleration, and harmful side effects were unknown. The use of anesthesia was delayed altogether too long, but its use did come in time to help lessen the immense suffering that was brought about during the Civil War.[146]

Chloroform very early superseded ether as the standard anesthetic agent in Alabama. By 1849, it was used for obstetrical as well as surgical cases. Although deaths associated with chloroform anesthesia had been observed, this agent was at first much more widely used than ether. Probably one reason was the hazard of explosion associated with the latter. The facilities to prevent this calamity were not then available.

Unfortunately, the advent of anesthesia was not accompanied by surgical asepsis. After operating with unscrubbed hands and unsterilized instruments, surgeons saw, without knowing why, that many of their patients died of "blood poisoning," infections, abscesses, erysipelas, and gangrene.

The Beginning of Science–Based Medicine

By the middle of the nineteenth century, the era of rash methods of treatment was finally giving way to a period of comparatively conservative medicine. Though it is true that the profession often went to extremes in new treatment regimens, there is ample evidence that the physicians of the state were beginning to appreciate scientifically based medicine.

One cogent observer opined that accurate histories of patients were often unobtainable and physicians were frequently unable to observe either the effects of prescribed remedies or if indeed their instructions had been obeyed. Further, he lamented that too often the disease, because of neglect and delay, had become complicated and hopeless; and, finally, physicians were generally denied postmortem inspections.[147] Autopsies were performed, however, but were usually regional in nature, and only the gross appearance of organs was observed and described.

Better diagnosis and treatment were a result of the increasingly conservative attitudes toward disease. Improved communication through scientific publications and organization of medical societies resulted in more effective medical practice.

However, the advent of the Civil War with its bitter regional strife brought an end to this early trend toward scientifically based medicine. All scientific effort ceased, and the medical facilities were closed in the state. After the hostilities ceased, recovery was not an easy task. A long painful struggle was necessary before Alabama could regain its former position in the field of medicine.

Physicians' Charges

The physicians in Alabama published their fee schedules soon after the establishment of the local licensure boards. The fee schedules for Mobile, Montgomery, and Cahaba are extant. Listed below are those made public by the physicians of Cahaba on January 1, 1837 (original spelling preserved).[148] Those for Mobile and Montgomery are comparable. It is interesting to note that physicians were often called upon to extract teeth because dentists were not always available in these early towns.

Milage in daylight, fair weather, per mile,	$1.00
Milage in night or inclement,	2.00
Milage in night rain or snow,	3.00
Personal attendance in daylight, per hour,	2.00
Personal attendance in night, per hour,	3.00
Consultation fee,	10.00

Consultation fee, to attending Physician,	5.00
Rising at night, from 10 P.M. 'till daylight,	5.00
Visit in Town, and medicine, first visit,	3.00
Visit in Town, subsequent visits, each,	2.00
Clinical prescriptions,	2.00
Bleeding,	1.00
Extracting Teeth,	1.00
Cupping,	2.00
Arteriotomy,	2.00
Enemoe, each,	2.00
Blisters, from 50 cents to	1.00
Obstetrical cases, (natural labor,)	20.00
Artificial and instrumental, from 30 to	100.00
[Obstetrical delivery]	
Delivery of retained Placenta, (manual)	20.00
(Visits and attendance charged as above.)	
Amputations, from $10 to	50.00
Reducing Luxations, from $5 to	50.00
Setting simple fractures, from $10 to	20.00
Introducing Bougie or Catheter, (1st time,)	5.00
Introducing Bougie or Catheter, (subsequent)	3.00
Prescriptions in chronic cases, with written advice, from $5 to	10.00
Prescription in shop, from $1 to	5.00
For examination of slaves in relation to general health,	10.00
Prescriptions for slaves on plantations, from 50 cents to	1.00
Cure of Syphyllis, from $20 to	40.00
Cure of Acute Urithritis,	10.00
Cure of Chronic Urithritis,	20.00

Notes

1. Fort Toulouse was founded in 1714 by the French at the confluence of the Coosa and Tallapoosa rivers. The site of the old fort is near that of a later fort, Fort Jackson, not far from Wetumpka.

2. L. D. S. Harrell, "Colonial Medical Practice in British West Florida, 1763–1781," *Bull. Hist. Med.* 41 (1967): 540.

3. Robert R. Rea, " 'Graveyard for Britons,' West Florida, 1763–1781," *Fla. Hist. Quart.* 47 (1969): 346.

4. J. D. L. Holmes, "Medical Practice in the Lower Mississippi Valley During the Spanish Period, 1769–1803," *Ala. J. Med. Sci.* 1 (1964): 335 (hereafter cited as Holmes, "Medical Practice").

5. J. D. L. Holmes, ed., "Fort Stoddard in 1799: Seven Letters of Captain Bartholomew Schaumburgh," *Ala. Hist. Quart.* 26 (Fall & Winter 1964): 235 (hereafter cited as Holmes, "Fort Stoddard"). Fort Stoddard (also Stoddert) was built by the settlers in July, 1799, and was located at Ward's Bluff on the bank of the Mobile River. It was at this point that Americans could stop the Spaniards going up the river and collect customs duty.

6. Harrell, p. 541.

7. Ibid.; and Holmes, "Medical Practice," p. 334.

8. Harrell, p. 541.

9. Rea, p. 349. General Gage was commander of the British forces in America from 1763 until 1772. Dr. John Lorimer studied medicine at St. Andrews in Scotland and received his degree in 1764. A year later, he became the surgeon at Pensacola in the newly acquired British West Florida.

10. Rea, p. 352.

11. Holmes, "Fort Stoddard," p. 234.

12. Harrell, p. 549. Captain Bernard Romans was born in Holland about 1720 and educated in England. He was sent to America in 1755 as a civil engineer. Originally, he served in Georgia and East Florida. In 1769–1770, he was appointed chief deputy surveyor for the Southern District. Governor Peter Chester of West Florida obtained permission to appoint him the King's botanist in the province. Romans' *A Concise Natural History of East and West Florida*, 1775, is an important account of life in this area: Bernard Romans, *A Concise Natural History of East and West Florida* (New York: n.p., 1775; reprint ed., New Orleans: Pelican Publishing Co., 1961), Introduction.

13. Milo B. Howard, Jr., "Health Problems in Colonial Alabama," *J.M.A. Ala.* 39 (1970): 1055.

14. William Bartram, *Travels Through North & South Carolina, Georgia, East & West Florida* (Philadelphia: James & Johnson, 1791), p. 411.

15. Harrell, p. 544; and Holmes, "Medical Practice," p. 337.

16. D. Rowland and A. G. Sanders, eds., *Mississippi Provincial Archives 1704–1743, French Dominion* (Jackson, Miss.: Press of the Mississippi Department of Archives and History, 1932), 3: 642.

17. Francois Ludger Diard, *The Tablet* 2 (Mobile, Ala.: n.p., April 1961): 1. Copy in the author's possession. Fort Louis de la Mobile, located at Twenty-Seven Mile Bluff, was about ten miles upstream from the present site of the city of Mobile. It was founded in 1702 and was abandoned in 1711.

18. Diard, p. 1.

19. Howard, p. 1052; and Holmes, "Medical Practice," p. 335.

20. Howard, pp. 1051–52.

21. Carey V. Stabler, "The History of the Alabama Public Health System" (Ph.D. diss., Duke University, 1944), p. 1 (hereafter cited as Stabler, "Dissertation").

22. P. H. Lewis, "Medical History of Alabama, Part 1," *New Orleans Med. & Surg. J.* (May 1847), p. 692.

23. John Y. Bassett, "Report on the Topography, Climate and Diseases of Madison County, Ala.," *South. Med. Reports* (1850), pp. 256–81. Reprinted in *The Medical Reports of John Y. Bassett, M.D.*, D. C. Elkin, ed., (Memaska, Wisconsin: Charles C. Thomas Pub., 1941), p. 5 (hereafter cited as Bassett, "Topography"). Bassett was memorialized by Sir William Osler in an essay, "An Alabama Student," in his book *An Alabama Student and Other Biographical Essays* (London: Oxford University Press, 1908).

24. Bassett, "Topography," pp. 29–30.

25. W. Taylor, "Valedictory Address," *Trans.* (1854), p. 154.

26. Roy H. Turner, "Graefenberg, The Shepard Family's Medical School," *Ann. Med. Hist.*, NS 5 (1933): 551. Philip Madison Shepard founded a "family" medical school in Dadeville in 1852.

27. Bassett, "Topography," p. 30.

28. *Dallas Gazette*, published in Cahaba, Dallas County, Alabama, 9 August 1859, p. 1.

29. Joseph G. Baldwin, *The Flush Times of Alabama and Mississippi* (New York: D. Appleton & Co., 1853), p. 89.

30. William H. Brantley, Jr., "Alabama Doctor," *Ala. Lawyer* 6 (1945): 248–49.

31. Bassett, "Topography," p. 5.

32. J. P. Barnes, "Report on the Number, Character, etc. of Practitioners of Medicine," *Trans.* (1852), p. 164.

33. Brantley, pp. 255–56. Until 1901, the State Senate and House of Representatives was known as the "General Assembly"; however, when the state constitution of 1901 was adopted, the combined bodies were designated, "The State Legislature."

34. Jerome Cochran, "The Medical Profession," *Memorial Record of Alabama: Historical and Biographical* (Madison, Wisconsin: Brant and Fuller, 1893), 2: 134 (hereafter cited as Cochran, "Medical Profession").

35. Bassett, "Topography," p. 8.

36. J. W. Crawford, "A Report on the Number and Character of Physicians of Bibb County," *Trans.* (1854), p. 148.

37. W. T. Jordan, *Ante-Bellum Alabama Town and Country* (Tallahassee: Florida State University, 1957), pp. 62–64. Fort Claiborne, founded (circa 1813) by General F. L. Claiborne during the Creek Indian War, was located in Monroe County at Weatherford Bluff on the Alabama River. County court was held at Fort Claiborne until 1832.

38. Jordan, pp. 78–81.

39. Ibid., p. 81.

40. Bernard Romans, *A Concise Natural History of East and West Florida* (New York: n.p., 1775; reprint ed., New Orleans: Pelican Publishing Co., 1961), p. 155.

41. Jabez Wiggins Heustis received his M.D. degree from the College of Physicians and Surgeons of New York City. He entered the United States Navy in 1808 and later joined the United States Army. He saw service under General Andrew Jackson in the campaign of the South. After the Civil War, he began private practice in Cahaba, Alabama. In 1835, he moved to Mobile where he became noted as a physician and surgeon. He was author of *Physical Observations and Medical Tracts and Researches, on the Topography and Diseases of Louisiana* and various other books and pamphlets on medical and kindred topics. Dr. Heustis is noted in particular for his vivid account of the ravages of scurvy among the American troops in Louisiana in 1809 and the disastrous results ensuing from the use of mercury to treat the scurvy patients. Thomas McAdory Owen, *History of Alabama and Dictionary of Alabama Biography* (Chicago: S. J. Clarke Pub. Co., 1921), 3: 804; and John Duffy, ed., *The Rudolph Matas History of Medicine in Louisiana* (Baton Rouge: Louisiana State University Press, 1958), 1: 310–11.

42. Stabler, "Dissertation," p. 12.

43. Carey V. Stabler, "Medicine—Forward March: Physicians and Preventive Medicine," TS, 1945, p. 2. Alabama Collection, Lister Hill Library, The University of Alabama in Birmingham, Birmingham, Ala. (hereafter cited as Stabler, "Medicine").

44. Ibid., p. 3.

45. Bassett, "Topography," p. 9.

46. P. H. Lewis, "Medical History of Alabama, Part 3," *New Orleans Med. & Surg. J.* (Sept. 1847), p. 169.

47. Ibid., p. 168.

48. Ibid., p. 171.

49. Stabler, "Medicine," p. 4.

50. Ibid.

51. Ibid., p. 5.

52. Bassett, "Topography," pp. 16–17; and Stabler, "Medicine," p. 5.

53. Lewis, Part 3, p. 171.

54. Bassett, "Topography," p. 17; and W. Boling, "Review of P. H. Lewis, 'Medical History of Alabama,' " *New Orleans Med. & Surg. J.* (1847), p. 485.

55. *Montgomery Advertiser and State Gazette*, 21 June 1859.

56. Stabler, "Dissertation," pp. 39–40.

57. Ibid., p. 41.

58. Stabler, "Medicine," p. 5.

59. Lewis, Part 3, p. 174.

60. Stabler, "Medicine," p. 4.

61. Bassett, "Topography," p. 9.

62. Stabler, "Dissertation," p. 40.

63. Peter J. Hamilton, *Colonial Mobile, A Historical Study* (New York: Houghton, Mifflin & Co.; Cambridge: Riverside Press, 1897), pp. 52, 55.

64. Jerome Cochran, "Yellow Fever in Relation to Its Cause," *Trans.* (1877), pp. 148–49.

65. Howard, p. 1056.

66. Albert Burton Moore, *History of Alabama* (Tuscaloosa: Alabama Book Store, 1951), pp. 48–49.

67. *Report on the Quarantine on the Southern and Gulf Coasts of the United States* (New York: n.p., 1873), p. 44 (hereafter cited as *Quarantine*); Cochran, "Medical Profession," p. 112; George Augustin, *History of Yellow Fever* (New Orleans: Searcy & Pfaff, Ltd., 1909), pp. 783–87; and Erwin Craighead, *Mobile: Fact and Tradition* (Mobile, Ala.: Powers Printing Co., 1930), p. 256.

68. Marie Bankhead Owen, *The Story of Alabama: A History of the State* (New York: Lewis Historical Pub. Co., Inc., 1949), 2: 560–61; *Quarantine*, p. 43; and William H. Anderson, "Report on the Diseases of Mobile," *Trans.* (1854), p. 42.

69. M. B. Owen, 2: 560–62; Augustin, pp. 781–90; Robert Partin, "Alabama's Yellow Fever Epidemic of 1878," *Ala. Rev.* 10 (1957): 31–51; and Benjamin Hogan Riggs, "The History of the Yellow Fever Epidemic in Selma in 1853," *Trans.* (1882), p. 422.

70. Caldwell Delaney, *Craighead's Mobile* (Mobile, Ala.: Haunted Bookshop, 1968), p. 94.

71. Ibid., pp. 94–100.

72. Romans, p. 7.

73. Augustin, p. 783; and William H. Anderson, *Trans.* (1854), p. 42. Other sources state that one-third of the population fled the city.

74. Partin, pp. 41–42.

75. Lewis, Part 1, p. 702.

76. Ibid.

77. J. C. Nott, "Yellow Fever Contrasted with Bilious Fever—Reasons for believing it a Disease *Sui Generis*—Its Mode of Propagation—Remote Cause—Probably Insect or Animalcular Origin, etc.," *New Orleans Med. & Surg. J.* (March 1848), p. 580.

78. Ibid., p. 581.

79. Ibid., p. 590.

80. Walter Reed served part of his military career at the Mount Vernon Military Barracks, Mount Vernon, Alabama, now the site of Searcy Hospital for the Insane. Dr. Nott was the attending physician at the birth of William Crawford Gorgas.

81. Craighead, pp. 253–59.

82. Stabler, "Dissertation," p. 3; and Glenn N. Sisk, "Diseases in the Alabama Black Belt, 1875–1917," *Ala. Hist. Quart.* 24 (Spring 1962): 58.

83. Hamilton, p. 206; Romans, pp. 154–61; and P. H. Lewis, "Medical History of Alabama," *New Orleans Med. & Surg. J.* Part 1 (May 1847), pp. 691–706; Part 2 (July 1847), pp. 1–34; Part 3 (Sept. 1847), pp. 151–77.

84. M. C. Mitchell, "Health and the Medical Profession in the Lower South, 1845–1860," *J. South. Hist.* 10 (1944): 433.

85. Hamilton, p. 206.

86. Romans, p. 160; and Lewis, Part 2, p. 11.

87. Hamilton, p. 208.

88. D. H. Thomas, "Fort Toulouse," *Ala. Hist. Quart.* 22 (1960): 169; and Holmes, "Fort Stoddard," p. 238.

89. Howard, p. 1056.

90. Rea, pp. 353–54.

91. P. H. Lewis, "Sketch of Yellow Fever of Mobile with a Brief Analysis of the Epidemic of 1843," *New Orleans Med. & Surg. J.* (1845), pp. 281–301, 413–34.

92. Stabler, "Dissertation," p. 41.

93. W. P. Reese, "Notes on Maramus, Pertussis and Typhoid Fever," *Trans.* (1850), pp. 112–17; and J. C. Harris, "Influence of Temperature in the Production of Various Forms of Fever," *Trans.* (1851), pp. 28–32. *The Transactions of the Medical Association of the State of Alabama* were printed from 1850 to 1855. Printing was discontinued in 1855 and resumed in 1869. The 1868 transactions were included in the 1869 transactions.

94. J. W. Crawford, "Report on the Diseases of Centreville and Vicinity," *Trans.* (1855), p. 54.

95. L. H. Anderson, "On the Summer and Autumnal Fevers of South Alabama: To which are appended some remarks on the Diagnosis and Treatment of Typhoid Fever," *Trans.* (1852), p. 132.

96. Ibid., pp. 97–157.

97. William H. Anderson, "Report on the Diseases of Mobile," *Trans.* (1850), pp. 71–73; and G. A. Ketchum, "Report on the Diseases of Mobile for 1854," *Trans.* (1855), p. 103.

98. William H. Anderson, *Trans.* (1850), p. 73.

99. Stabler, "Dissertation," p. 4.

100. Hamilton, p. 206.

101. Romans, p. 168.

102. J. C. Nott, "An Examination into Health and Longevity of the Southern Ports of the United States with Reference to the Subject of Life Insurance," *South. J. Med. & Pharm.* (1847–1848), p. 5. Cited in Stabler, "Dissertation," p. 4.

103. Stabler, "Dissertation," p. 4.

104. Romans, p. 170.

105. Sisk, pp. 58–59.

106. Lewis, Part 2, p. 9.

107. William Osler, *An Alabama Student* (London: Oxford University Press, 1908).

108. Romans, pp. 167–68.

109. E. D. McDaniel, "Report on the Topography, Climatology and Diseases, of Wilcox County," *Trans.* (1869), p. 101.

110. Ketchum, pp. 102–03.

111. Silas Ames, "Report on the Diseases of Montgomery County in 1849," *Trans.* (1851), pp. 39–41.

112. W. P. Reese, "Report of the Diseases of Selma for 1854," *Trans.* (1855), pp. 91–93.

113. John Duffy, ed., *The Rudolph Matas History of Medicine in Louisiana* (Baton Rouge: Louisiana State University Press, 1962), 2: 65.

114. Ibid., pp. 65–66.

115. Ibid., pp. 68–71.

116. H. V. Wooten, "Disease, etc. of Lowndesboro,' (Ala.) and Its Vicinity— Reported 1850," *Trans.* (1850), pp. 93–94.

117. Duffy, pp. 67, 69–70.

118. W. Taylor, "Report on Surgery—Talladega County," *Trans.* (1855), p. 90 (hereafter cited as Taylor, "Report on Surgery").

119. Robert P. Harris, "The Operation of Gastro-Hysterotomy (True Cesarean Section), Viewed in the Light of American Experience and Success; With the History and Results of Sewing Up the Uterine Wound; and a Full Tabular Record of the Cesarean Operations Performed in the United States, Many of them not Hitherto Reported," *Amer. J. Med. Sci.* 75 (April 1878): 336.

120. Ibid., p. 338.

121. Ibid.

122. Seale Harris, *Woman's Surgeon, The Life Story of J. Marion Sims* (New York: The Macmillan Company, 1950), pp. 344–47.

123. Ibid., pp. 99–102.

124. Ibid., p. 100.

125. T. M. Owen, 4: 1564.

126. Seale Harris, p. 375.

127. Ibid., p. 380.

128. Ibid., p. 358.

129. Ibid., p. 357.

130. Ibid., pp. 376–80.

131. Dr. Gross later moved to Philadelphia where he had an eminent career in surgery at Jefferson Medical College.

132. Seale Harris, pp. 104, 110.

133. Emmett B. Carmichael, "Nathan Bozeman," *Ala. J. Med. Sci.* 6 (1969): 234.

134. Ibid., p. 235.

135. Seale Harris, pp. 96, 271; and L. L. Hill, "Beacon Lights in Alabama," *J.M.A. Ala.* 46 (Sept. 1976): 20.

136. Hill, p. 17.

137. Ibid.

138. Ibid.

139. Taylor, "Report on Surgery," pp. 88–90; and L. H. Anderson, "Report on Surgery," *Trans.* (1852), pp. 38–49.

140. John J. Pullen, "Gentlemen, *This* Is Not Humbug," *Amer. Heritage* 30 (Aug./Sept. 1979): 81–96. Sulfuric ether was first used by Dr. Crawford W. Long of Jefferson, Georgia, in 1842. He removed a small tumor from the cheek of one James M. Venable while the patient was under the influence of ether.

Dr. William T. G. Morton and Dr. Horace Wells (both dentists) in 1845 administered nitrous oxide to a patient before Dr. John C. Warren's (Boston's famous surgeon) medical class. On October 16, 1846, Dr. Warren with Dr. Morton serving as the anesthetist gave a public demonstration of the use of ether anesthesia. (Pullen, pp. 84, 90.)

141. Seale Harris, pp. 79–80.

142. Ibid., pp. 80–81.

143. Ibid., p. 81.

144. Ibid.

145. Pullen, pp. 81–82.

146. Ibid., pp. 82, 95–96.

147. Wooten, p. 77.

148. A copy of charges from the Art Lewis' Modest Museum, Selma, Alabama, is in the author's possession.

Chapter 2

*Development of Hospitals**

Begun first and foremost to relieve suffering and distress, hospitals in the early territories found themselves adjusting their roles to suit the military, civilian, religious, or secular influences of the moment. When Alabama was young, the job of caring for the sick most often fell to the military authority of the colonial powers. In earliest Mobile, that power was France.

France first attempted to provide medical care for the Louisiana settlement when medical facilities everywhere were faced with victims of epidemics, with the sick from all walks of life, and with transients who might carry disease.[1] Fort Louis de la Mobile, and later the port city of Mobile, were particularly susceptible to such disasters. The first recorded yellow fever epidemic, for instance, arrived with the ship, the *Pélican*, in 1704, before Bienville's colony had moved to the present site of Mobile (1711).[2]

The French built Hospital Royal in the settlement of Mobile very early, and the King of France sent one "Docteur des Laurier," a surgeon, to manage it. By 1760, city maps show Hospital Royal located at the southeast corner of what is now Dauphin and Conception streets.

Three years later, Mobile was under the British flag. At that time the hospital seemed to have fallen into disuse because in 1766 the Assembly of West Florida petitioned the Commissioners of Trade and Plantations to supply £1,500 for the construction of hospitals at Mobile and Pensacola.[3] The British governor, Major Robert Farmar, was thus able to continue operation of Hospital Royal as a British hospital until the Spanish came into power in 1781. When the Spanish arrived, the hospital at Conception and Dauphin was renamed King's Hospital; and it remained King's Hospital even after the United States acquired it in

*Undoubtedly, there were many privately owned and operated small hospitals in Alabama, but few records remain, and space limitations mean that some worthy institutions have been omitted.

1814. Sometime later, the hospital was moved to the northwest corner of St. Louis and Royal streets.

Mobile General Hospital—1830
Mobile, Alabama

Hospitals in Mobile, like other institutions, were subject to numerous pressures: cultural, religious, political, and economic; and as governments changed, so did medical facilities.[4] Since 1819, the hospital once known as King's Hospital has been known as City Hospital, County Hospital, Port Hospital, Mobile General Hospital, and the University of South Alabama Medical Center Hospital and Clinics.

The city hospital idea has had a long and rich tradition in Mobile, and the physicians associated with it have been prominent and capable. Dr. Solomon Mordecai (1793–1869) was one of Mobile's first well-known physicians. He came to the city in 1824 and was active in the affairs of City Hospital. Dr. Thomas L. Carthy was the first director of the hospital; Dr. B. R. Hogan was his assistant.

From the time of the United States' acquisition, Mobile grew rapidly, and the city government was increasingly aware of the need for a larger and better-equipped hospital. By 1830, Mobile had opened the doors to a new hospital, one which was considered to be of the finest architectural craftsmanship, and one which boasted the latest in equipment. The first superintendent in this "new" City Hospital was Dr. Willis Roberts. How long Dr. Roberts served as superintendent is not known. Dr. Wolsingham Mather succeeded Dr. Hogan as assistant director in the spring of 1833.

Dr. Roberts had been instrumental in first securing women attendants at the hospital. A letter addressed to the mayor and board of aldermen of the city—dated May 3, 1831, and signed by Dr. Willis Roberts—outlines his plan for the women's attendant or nursing service at City Hospital. It appears reasonable to assume that Dr. Roberts's idea of an organized women's nursing profession antedates Florence Nightingale's by some twenty-four years. Unfortunately, the city fathers failed to appreciate this opportunity, and it was not until 1841 that Mrs. Sarah Debois was installed as the hospital's first matron. She was a capable individual and served with distinction until 1846.

The next known superintendent was Dr. Robert A. Walker in 1855; Dr. C. H. Mastin was listed as "physician and surgeon in charge" the same year.

In 1853, in spite of a yellow fever epidemic, the city built its first addition to the hospital: a wing for black patients. In 1859, construction began on the Medical College of Alabama a short distance from the

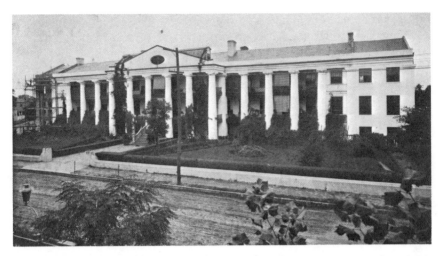

City Hospital, Medical College of Alabama in Mobile (1908) (Courtesy of the Heustis Medical Museum, Mobile, Alabama)

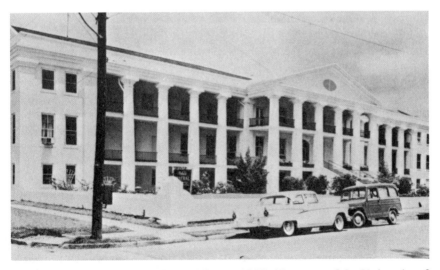

Mobile General Hospital, Mobile, Alabama (1958) (Courtesy of the University of South Alabama Medical Center Hospital and Clinics, Mobile, Alabama)

hospital. The school opened a year later, with City Hospital as its clinical teaching facility. Dr. G. A. Ketchum, who was once a medical student employed in the hospital, became one of its most outstanding physicians. In 1860, Dr. Ketchum became Professor of Theory and Practice of Medicine on the faculty of the newly opened Medical College.

Other physicians who served with distinction at this time were Drs. Jon Booth, H. Childers, Joseph Tucker, H. T. Cox, Aaron Lopez, D. K. Mandeville, A. Mancier, R. Miller, R. H. Sims, and a Dr. White.

In the spring of 1861, when every available man, physician, and nurse had answered the call to arms, the Sisters of Charity agreed to manage the hospital. Sister Gabriella was the first superintendent, accepting control of the hospital only as an emergency measure. Over a century later, the sisters were still ministering to the sick in Mobile General. In May of 1865, while Mobile was occupied by federal troops, a terrific explosion occurred at Marshall's Warehouse, on Lipscomb and Commerce streets, where munitions had been stored. The hospital was equal to the emergency.

In 1879, the city of Mobile was declared bankrupt and forced to give up its charter. The city was then called the "Port of Mobile," and in 1880, the hospital was renamed Port Hospital. The Sisters of Charity were accused of misappropriation of funds at the time and were dismissed from the hospital. Although the sisters were later completely exonerated, Port Hospital operated some fifteen years under the supervision of the nearby Medical College—without the sisters. It was through the efforts of Dr. Silas Tam that, in 1895, the services of the Sisters of Charity were again secured.

The city was rechartered in 1887. The hospital was again called City Hospital in 1888. In 1894, the yellow fever epidemic overtaxed the capacity of the hospital, and patients had to be quartered in tents at the rear of the hospital.

The city gave the Sisters of Charity permission to initiate a program to train student nurses in 1907, and by 1908, there were six nursing students enrolled. The curriculum for the nursing school was formalized, and the school began its affiliation with Spring Hill College in 1936. In 1943, a new and modern nursing school was built.

In spite of enlargements to the hospital in 1853, 1907, and 1908, the original building appears today much as it did in 1831. In 1912, the wing built in 1853 to house black patients was replaced by a brick building, which, until recently, was the clinic and private room section of the hospital.

The next major change came in 1917 when a pharmacy, operating rooms, emergency rooms, and additional patient areas were added. In 1923, Mobile's citizens voted a bond issue to finance wards for black patients, porches, an operating room, ambulance station, laundry and boiler rooms. The Holcombe Mental Unit, a holding and treatment center for mentally ill patients, was built with county and federal funds in 1951.

In 1932, the State Legislature passed an act requiring the county and city to divide the cost of operating the hospital. City Hospital operated under this financial arrangement until 1955, when legislation required all cities in Mobile County to contribute to the hospital on a per capita basis. This same legislation created the Mobile County Hospital Board. The hospital was renamed Mobile County Hospital.

The Sisters of Charity requested that they be relieved of operating the facility in 1959. Again the hospital was renamed: this time as Mobile General Hospital.

The University of South Alabama acquired Mobile General Hospital in 1970. It became the main clinical facility for the University and in April, 1975, became the University of South Alabama Medical Center Hospital and Clinics.

This, the oldest of the hospitals in Alabama, has served the citizens of Mobile with distinction since 1704. Its record of service and devotion to suffering mankind stands as a tribute difficult to equal. It truly is an "Ageless Servant of Humanity."

Marine Hospital (United States Public Health Service)—1837 Mobile, Alabama

The Marine Hospital building in Mobile, occupied since about 1837, is the oldest building used as a Marine hospital in the United States.[5] Construction began as early as 1834 and was completed at the end of 1837. The United States Government purchased the building from the city of Mobile, its original owner, in 1841. From 1841 to the outbreak of the Civil War, the building was used to treat members of the Merchant Marine. During the Civil War, until the surrender of Mobile in 1865, it was used as a Confederate hospital, and then for federal troops. The building was then leased by the secretary of the Treasury to private parties who contracted to operate it as a Marine hospital until September 1, 1875, when it reverted to the Marine Hospital Service. It continued under this service until it closed in 1952.

After reopening December 5, 1956, it was operated as the Sixth District Tuberculosis Hospital (later known as the Frank S. Keeler Memorial Hospital) until July 1, 1974. Following renovation, the building has housed the Mobile County Health Department. It was named to the National Register of Historic Places in 1974.

Providence Hospital—1854
Mobile, Alabama

Providence Hospital was founded August 15, 1854.[6] At that time, a Board of Providence Infirmary Trustees was formed. The Daughters of Charity of Saint Vincent de Paul actually took over the operation of the hospital on May 1, 1855, under the guidance of Sister Hilory Branner. Official existence of the hospital dates from February 1, 1858, when a charter was obtained from the General Assembly. From a small, 60-bed facility, Providence Hospital has grown to a 400-bed hospital and is still run by the Daughters of Charity.

Freedman's Hospital—1869
Talladega, Alabama

During the reconstruction period, a hospital for the recently freed, sick, and infirm slaves of Alabama was established in Talladega and supported by state funds.[7]

The secretary of the Board of Trustees of Freedman's Hospital, Joseph H. Johnson (1832–1893; superintendent of the School for Deaf, Dumb, and Blind, 1852–1893), signed the first annual report to the governor, the Honorable William H. Smith (governor of Alabama, 1868–November, 1870) on November 5, 1869. G. T. McAfee was president of the board, and George P. Plowman was another member. A second report dated January, 1871, was signed by W. H. Thornton as secretary of the board. All these men were citizens of Talladega and served without remuneration.

State appropriations for Freedman's Hospital—intended to cover all expenditures, such as those for food, clothing, and attendants—were: $4,019.98 in 1869, $5,767.03 in 1870, $4,098.01 in 1871, and $3,383.63 in 1872. These funds, however, provided only the bare necessities, and Talladega had to raise money—whether by taxes or by donations is not known—to provide supplies. There were complaints that the burden of this hospital was "too great a tax on the town," and in January, 1876, the Freedman's Hospital was discontinued.

Hillman Hospital—1888
Birmingham, Alabama

After a number of attempts in the 1870s and early 1880s to organize a hospital for the indigent sick in Birmingham, the Society of the United Charities, which had been organized in January, 1884, resolved to build and maintain such a hospital.[8] The Hospital of the United Charities was incorporated by the General Assembly in April, 1887.

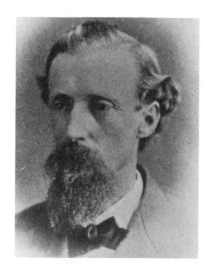

Joseph Henry Johnson, M.D., 1832–1893
(Courtesy of the Alabama Institute for
Deaf and Blind, Talladega, Alabama)

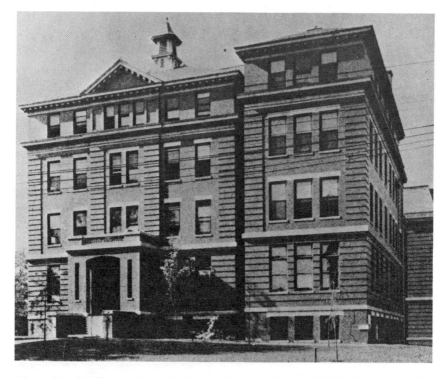

The original Hillman Hospital, Birmingham, Alabama (1903) (Courtesy of the
Alabama Museum of the Health Sciences, Lister Hill Library, Medical Center,
The University of Alabama in Birmingham)

Mr. T. T. Hillman, president of the Tennessee Coal, Iron and Railroad Company gave $20,000 in bonds as a trust, the interest from which was to be used to erect and support a charity hospital. On April 18, 1887, a well-known city physician, Dr. Joseph R. Smith, deeded a lot in Smithfield (Graymont) to the society for the hospital; and the city and county committed a monthly sum to the hospital, which, together with the income from the Hillman bonds, gave a monthly income of approximately $275. Other citizens conspicuous in promotional and fund-raising activities were Dr. R. W. Rowland, Dr. William Berry, W. T. Underwood, Capt. J. C. Henley, C. P. Williamson, Robert Jemison, Jr., and J. W. Cameron.* Dr. Locke Chew, one of the city's young physicians, was chairman of the committee. This committee drew up the plans for the hospital that were later accepted by the society. Individuals and businesses from all parts of the city helped outfit the hospital.

The Ladies of the United Charities met in September, 1888, at Saint John's Methodist Church and organized both a hospital board and a smaller board, which would begin a temporary hospital. Mrs. John Martin was elected president.[9] Between the first and second meetings, the Board of Managers rented a floor of the Hughes Building on Avenue B and 20th Street South for $1,000 a year. The Hospital of the United Charities opened October 23, 1888, with twenty-five beds. Miss Evalina McRae, a nurse trained at Old Blockley Hospital in Philadelphia, was employed as supervisor. On January 9, 1889, the *Age-Herald* reported that the Board of Managers had elected a professional staff for the hospital for one year: Drs. E. H. Sholl, W. H. Johnston, Charles Whelan, T. L. Robertson, Charles Drennen, and J. W. Sears. The surgeons appointed were Drs. H. P. Cochrane, W. Locke Chew, George L. Brown, B. L. Wyman, and J. B. Luckie. The specialists appointed were Drs. R. D. Webb—eye and ear, and Dr. S. L. Ledbetter—eye, nose, and throat. A physician and surgeon, selected to rotate every two months, were to have complete charge of the patients admitted to the institution.

The first report of the Board of Managers, quoted in part below, was dated January 9, 1889, and signed by Mrs. John Martin as president.

> For the support of the hospital we received from the county commissioners $150 and from the city $25. An appeal has recently been made by us to the mayor and aldermen for a larger appropriation. . . . From these

---

*The Men's Committee of Board of Managers included William Berney, W. T. Underwood, C. P. Williamson, Robert Jemison, Jr., T. T. Hillman, Samuel Ullman, Dr. A. W. Bolan, and Dr. Joseph R. Smith. The Board of Lady Managers included Mrs. John M. Martin, Mrs. J. W. Pierce, Mrs. T. H. Molton, Mrs. George C. Ball, Mrs. J. F. Johnston, Mrs. J. W. Collins, Mrs. I. Y. Sage, Mrs. T. T. Hillman, Mrs. T. O. Smith, Mrs. Samuel Ullman, and Miss Nancy Cahalan.

appropriations and the generous donations of our citizens we received an amount sufficient to justify us in renting a building at once and in proceeding to furnish it. This building has twenty-three rooms and is located on South Twentieth Street between Avenues A and B. . . . We found it necessary to have quite an amount of plumbing done, which has been our largest expenditure. We have six charity wards, one for white men and one for white women; one ward [each] for [black men and women] and a ward [each] for [white and black] children. These wards are all neatly furnished with nice iron beds, with necessary furnishings to make them comfortable and clean. A table for medicines, etc., is provided for every two beds, also comfortable chairs. Through the kindness of certain ladies of our city, we have three pay wards, more expensively and handsomely furnished. The Typographical Union has also a small ward nicely furnished for its members, with twin beds, etc., and pays a certain sum monthly for its support. These various wards give a total of twenty-eight beds. The building, however, furnished a capacity for fifty beds, and we will probably find it necessary to add these before spring. The operating room is provided with most of the necessary appointments, including a substantial and handsome operating table, a case for surgical instruments, bandages, etc., a medical closet and an eye box. We are now having a room prepared for Dr. Webb and Dr. Ledbetter for their especial clinic. . . . For the internal management of the institution we have employed the following: As matron, chief nurse and housekeeper, Miss Evalina McRae, who has as assistant nurses, Miss Story and Mrs. Wilson, assistant housekeeper, Mrs. Watson, also one cook and one orderly. Misses McRae and Story are graduates of the Philadelphia [Nurses] Training School and come to us with the highest credentials from the surgeons of Blockley Hospital of that city. The hospital was opened for the reception of patients on the 23rd of October [1888] since which time we have received and treated 53 patients, 46 white, 6 [black] and 1 child. There are now remaining in the hospital 15 patients, whites 14, [black] 1.

There have been seven major operations: One successful cataract, one laparotomy for gunshot wound, one removal of fragments of bone from the brain, radical cure of hernia and removal of shot.

. . .It is often necessary that an autopsy should be made, [it is] exceedingly improper that it should be held in the woods. It has been recommended by our staff of physicians that a room be provided without the building for this purpose.[10]

Approximately six weeks after the little hospital began, its facilities and personnel were severely strained by the tragic Hawes riot of December 8, 1888.[11] In a few brief minutes of gunfire, eleven were left dead or dying, and twenty-five young men had been seriously wounded. Seven were taken to the newly opened Charity Hospital. The sudden load appeared almost too much for the small staff of the fledgling hospital, and members of the Board of Managers were pressed into service along with the regular nursing staff.

The tragedy served to stimulate interest in the new hospital and probably added impetus to the drive for a new facility. Another calamity struck the medical community in the winter of 1889: Dr. W. Locke Chew, who had presented the plans for the new hospital, was shot and killed after a meeting of the Jefferson County Medical Society. Dr. J. D. S. Davis was charged with the murder but was later acquitted. Finally, a new hospital, planned and financed by the Society of the United Charities, was built during the summer of 1890 on the lot in Smithfield.

The hospital's difficulties seemed to multiply. Miss McRae was dismissed as head nurse because of internal dissension. A Dr. Kitchens was chosen superintendent on January 21, 1891, and Miss Story was appointed head nurse, housekeeper, and head of the training school at a salary of fifty dollars a month. Miss Amy Smith of Lakeside Hospital in Cleveland, Ohio—a Canadian by birth—was superintendent housekeeper at $900 a year. The county and city agreed to defray the expenses of the hospital.

Throughout 1892 and 1893, the physicians and surgeons disagreed with the authority of the lady managers; and the dissension culminated in the resignation of the entire medical and surgical staff in the fall of 1893.[12] However, new physicians were appointed, and work continued without interruption. The dispute had far-reaching effects, with the city and county withdrawing its support in an effort to force the Society of the United Charities and Board of Managers to give up the hospital. The hospital was forced to announce that it would close for lack of funds and that its remaining patients were to be transferred to the almshouse at Velma Station in Woodlawn. The modern red brick hospital, costing approximately $28,000, appeared to have a dismal future.

David J. Fox, Mayor of Birmingham, 1892–1894, is quoted as saying, "We cannot take the management of the hospital away from the ladies. They built it!"[13] And even though a reorganization was accomplished, with the hospital administration remaining in the hands of the lady managers, it was to no avail. The panic of 1893, with the battle for free silver, was on. The little town of Birmingham was hard hit. On August 1, 1893, the First National Bank failed—a month before the beleaguered little hospital was forced to close. A notice in the *Age-Herald* of September 3, 1893, stated that the charity hospital had closed its doors.

On September 7, 1893, the city council announced an appropriation of $400 per month to support the Hospital of the United Charities. This, with the $100 obtained monthly from the Hillman bonds, was deemed sufficient to support the hospital, provided only the needy were admitted. The hospital was promptly reopened and continued in operation for another year.

Disaster struck again December 1, 1894, when the newly built hospital was completely destroyed by fire. The thirteen patients were removed without incident to the Birmingham Medical College, which was in the Lunsford Building at 209 North 21st Street.

The hospital was closed for a year but reopened in January or February, 1896, in a wing of the private hospital of Drs. Copeland and Berry, where it remained about three years. The opening was made possible by insurance money, interest on the Hillman bonds, and the sale of various pieces of real estate. Meanwhile, it was decided that the name Charity Hospital was objectionable to many and that it should be changed to Hillman Hospital in honor of its greatest benefactor.

The General Assembly, on February 11, 1897, incorporated and granted a new charter to the Board of Lady Managers and gave them authority to manage Hillman Hospital. They, in turn, appointed a board of businessmen called the Hillman Hospital Council to act as advisors. A lot on Eighth Avenue North, purchased for this purpose, was sold when a petition came from the neighbors objecting to the hospital.[14]

A lot on Fourth Avenue and 18th Street North, on which an old building stood, was occupied temporarily by the hospital, and patients were received there in January, 1900. The frame building had nine rooms, seven of which were for patients—five for white and two for blacks. Miss Annie Otto was matron and a Miss Narramore was nurse. Early in 1902, the Board of Lady Managers elected a smaller body, the Board of Control, to manage the daily affairs of the hospital. About this time, the board purchased property on Avenue F (Sixth Avenue) and 20th Street South for a new building, and the Birmingham Medical College bought the adjacent lot. Architects Charles F. and Harry B. Wheelock were employed to draw plans for the new hospital. The cornerstone was laid on July 12, 1902; the cornerstone for the Medical College was laid an hour later. The new hospital building, completed in July, 1903, was an impressive, fireproof brick structure four stories high. It still stands facing 20th Street as that part of the University Hospitals complex known as the Old Hillman Building.

At its completion, the hospital could accommodate ninety-eight patients and was among the most modern of the period. It had two operating rooms, an obstetrical ward, a pediatric ward, and four surgical and medical wards. There was a nurse's dormitory on the top floor and an "outdoor clinic" for ambulatory patients. Much of the equipment was furnished by private citizens. Among those in the long list of donors were Drs. Lewis Morris and J. D. S. Davis, who furnished the two operating rooms. Dr. J. C. LeGrande outfitted the obstetrical ward.

The staff, primarily faculty of the Birmingham Medical College, included many area physicians. During the school year, the hospital was under the control of the Medical College, and its physicians were used to teach the medical students. The Hillman Training School for Nurses was also affiliated with the hospital and in 1903 graduated seven nurses. Miss Nannie Hamilton was both head of the school and superintendent of nurses for the hospital.

From the very beginning, the hospital found itself in financial difficulties. Funds raised in 1903 and 1904 fell far short of the amount needed, and these were years that Birmingham was experiencing tremendous growth. The mounting deficit forced the management first to consider turning away all new patients and finally to seek support from the local government. In 1904, both the city of Birmingham and the Board of Commissioners of Jefferson County were petitioned for regular annual appropriations. In exchange for financial support, the Lady Managers offered, in the *Age-Herald* of February 8, 1904, to make the hospital strictly a charity institution. The petition was denied. It was not until 1907, after the Lady Managers offered the hospital as a gift, that Jefferson County agreed to underwrite the operation of the Hillman Hospital.

Jefferson County took over the hospital on May 7, 1907, and agreed to pay the outstanding debt of $9,000 on hospital property, to continue to use it strictly as a charity hospital and never to relinquish its control to any religious sect or denomination.

The Medical College continued its association with the hospital and a year later, in return for instructing the nurses, was accorded the right to appoint staff members to the hospital. The school formalized this privilege in a ninety-nine–year contract with the Jefferson County Board of Commissioners.

To adapt the hospital to its new role, certain changes were made: an autopsy room and laundry were constructed in the basement; two clinical wards for treatment of patients, together with offices, were opened on the first floor; a ward for forty white patients on the second floor and a similar one for black patients on the third floor were opened. A Miss Bradford was to continue in her position as superintendent.

In 1912, a $100,000 bond was approved by the citizens of Jefferson County to alleviate overcrowded conditions at the hospital. Half of this sum was used to purchase adjoining property. The remainder was used to remodel the old hospital and build a new wing. Hospital capacity was increased to 140 beds, but the equipment remained inadequate. It was not until later, when a committee from the Board of Revenue of Jefferson County visited similar institutions around the country that the county agreed to equip the hospital properly. Dr. E. P. Hogan (1872–1964) was appointed superintendent and held this position for nineteen years. During this time, he directed the house staff training program.[15] Miss Lucille Dugan was made superintendent of nurses.

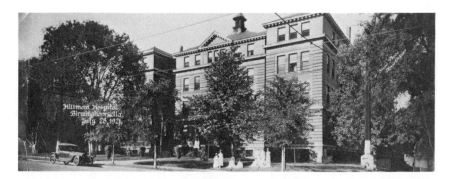

Hillman Hospital, Birmingham, 1921 (Courtesy of the Alabama Museum of the Health Sciences, Lister Hill Library, Medical Center, The University of Alabama in Birmingham)

The "outdoor clinic," operated by the Medical College until its closing in 1915, became the responsibility of Hillman Hospital. In 1918, when the Hillman Hospital staff adopted the minimum standards of the American College of Surgeons, quality of care and efficiency of service for indigent patients increased. Six residents and twelve interns served on the staff, and a dental clinic was organized for resident patients.

It was not long before the Hillman's old nemesis, overcrowding, struck again. The need was apparent to others. Dr. William Mayo, a visitor to the city in 1922, suggested to Dr. Hogan: "Let the people know about the conditions [here] and they will provide up-to-date, fireproof, adequate buildings with ample funds for equipment and maintenance."[16]

In 1924, a $400,000 bond issue was approved for constructing a 200-bed hospital annex and a nurses' home.[17] Construction began almost immediately, but it took more than four years to complete. The new annex opened on January 15, 1929, and the nurses' home on April 1, 1929. The latter had rooms for 100 nurses and 14 interns.

The fact that the depression forced the hospital to care for hundreds of additional sick, indigent men and women can be seen most dramatically in the increase in its budget: from $186,000 in 1928 to $452,000 in 1929. Although expenditures dropped to $360,000 a year later, the Jefferson County Board of Revenue believed at the time that the only way to decrease costs was to increase administrative efficiency.

In January, 1931, Dr. Hogan was replaced by Dr. R. F. Lovelady, who was to serve full time at an annual salary of $5,500. By 1934, Dr. Lovelady had been removed, and Dr. N. W. Wood, a Los Angeles hospital administrator, had been appointed in his place. Dr. Wood was succeeded by Dr. J. W. MacQueen after two years.

Seven members of the hospital staff, headed by Dr. J. S. McLester, had been appointed as an advisory board, but this board acted in more than an advisory capacity. In 1934, the County Commission actually delegated all its administrative power over the hospital to the advisory board.

The County Board of Commissioners became concerned about the increasing cost of operation of the hospital and turned to the city of Birmingham for financial support, pointing out that two-thirds of the patients came from the city proper. Finally, in 1939, the city agreed to pay 16 percent of the cost of operating the hospital.

For some time many Birmingham physicians felt the city needed a hospital designed especially for patients who were not financially able to go to a private hospital and yet did not qualify for the charity service. The Public Works Administration came to the rescue in 1938, when it announced a $900,000 grant and a $1.1 million loan for the purpose of building a "minimum charge" hospital at which everyone would pay according to his means. Dr. Harry Lee Jackson, a prominent surgeon of Birmingham and one of the prime movers for the new hospital, was named medical advisor. The construction began immediately and was completed in the fall of 1940. The new Jefferson Hospital, as it was named, was built adjacent to the Hillman Hospital and had sixteen stories and a capacity for 575 patients. On the fifteenth and sixteenth floors, living space was provided for 150 nurses and 25 interns and residents. The fifth floor was designed exclusively for a maternity ward, and the seventh floor had eight operating rooms. There were also three emergency operating rooms, three obstetrical delivery rooms, and clinical laboratories. One floor was devoted entirely to communicable diseases.

A $200,000 loan was made from local investment firms for initial operating expenses. Dr. Charles H. Young was named temporary director, and the hospital was scheduled to open on December 1, 1940. However, a dispute between the Jefferson County Civil Service Board, the County Commission, and the hospital as to who would make hospital appointments resulted in the inability of the hospital to begin operation. This was finally resolved February 1, 1941, and the first patients were admitted. The new hospital was acclaimed "the South's finest hospital— that rose like a prayer for healing." (See Chapter 3, "Efforts in Medical Education.")

In 1943, the question arose as to where to locate the proposed University of Alabama four-year medical school. Birmingham officials were quick to point out the advantages of their new Jefferson-Hillman Hospital (the two hospitals were combined in order not to duplicate staffs in 1943). They called attention to its size, wealth of clinical material, and four as yet incomplete floors which could readily be converted into classrooms. In addition, there was the possibility of options to purchase much of the adjoining property. This offer was difficult to counter, and when the Jefferson County Commission agreed that the medical school would have the exclusive right to appoint hospital staff members, Birmingham was selected as the site for the new proposed Medical College of Alabama.

The Medical Center became a reality when the University of Alabama School of Medicine moved to Birmingham from Tuscaloosa in 1945. A contract between Jefferson County and the University of Alabama was drawn in which Jefferson-Hillman Hospital was given outright to the University on December 20, 1944. An annual appropriation was to be continued payable to the hospital for the care of indigent patients. In return, the University of Alabama assumed the outstanding debt on the hospital; however, Governor Chauncey Sparks (governor of Alabama, 1943–1947) paid a portion of this debt from his contingency fund.

At first the plan was to use the old Hillman Hospital as an administration building for the hospital–medical school complex and to acquire by condemnation the three remaining blocks between 18th and 20th streets and Sixth and Eighth avenues. This was part of a $25 million plan that would have added several specialized hospitals and the City-County Board of Health to the Medical Center. There were even rumors that the Old Hillman Building would be torn down while the newer Hillman Annex would be used for classrooms. The Lady Managers of the Hillman Hospital, who had continued to meet regularly, immediately protested. On the occasion of their relinquishing the management of the hospital in 1907, they had been promised that the Hillman would remain a charity hospital. It was not until an agreement was reached to retain the name of the Hillman Hospital that the complete management of the hospital complex was finally taken over by the university.

The name of the hospital complex remained the Jefferson-Hillman Hospital until, by action of the Board of Trustees of the University of Alabama, it was changed to The University Hospital and Hillman Clinics in 1955. In 1965, it became The University of Alabama Hospitals and Clinics. Today it is owned by the state of Alabama and includes University Hospital, the Diabetes Research and Education Building, and Spain Rehabilitation Center.

Watkins Infirmary—1892
Montgomery, Alabama

Dr. Isaac Lafayette Watkins was born in Clayton, Alabama, in 1854.[18] In that small town lived a Dr. Winn, a very cultured and erudite man. One day Dr. Winn was approached by a tall and skinny country boy. The youth asked to be allowed to read medicine under him, as he wished to become a doctor. The skeptical Dr. Winn inquired if he knew Latin, knowing that he did not. Of course, the boy replied that he did not know Latin. When told that to be a doctor one had to know that subject, the boy asked that he be given time to learn. Dr. Winn thought that he had seen the last of him. To his surprise, a year later, Isaac Watkins returned with his Latin teacher, who informed the doctor that the boy knew as much Latin as he did. After reading medicine under Dr. Winn, the lad went first to New York to study and later to Europe. He graduated from Bellevue, New York, in 1878 and was licensed to practice by the Bullock County Board. He first practiced in Union Springs, Alabama, and later moved to Montgomery, Alabama. His office in Montgomery was first on Madison Street, then later in the First National Bank Building.

Wishing to own his own hospital, but having no capital, he was again fortunate. A Mr. Pinckard loaned him the money to buy three houses in the Oak Park area. These were remodeled, and he was soon busy with patients because of his distinguished work in gynecology.

Within a year, the hospital burned. While it was burning, a young girl from South Alabama got off the streetcar near the hospital. She was on her way to Dr. Watkins's office, but instead, she helped move the patients across the street to homes of neighbors for shelter and care. Observing her ability to aid the sick, Dr. Watkins asked if she would be interested in the nursing profession. He hired her on the spot. Her name was Mary Barfield, and she was an indefatigable nurse. She later ran the Watkins Infirmary, often assisting in operations and giving anesthetics.

In the journal *Alabama Medical and Surgical Age*, 1892, an advertisement appeared for: "An Infirmary for Women at Montgomery, Alabama, owned and operated by I. L. Watkins, M. D." The Montgomery City Directory, 1895, listed Dr. Watkins's office at 34 Dexter Avenue and the Highland Park Sanatorium on Forest Avenue. But perhaps most city inhabitants remembered the hospital as Watkins Sanatorium (Infirmary).

Dr. T. Brannon Hubbard, who took his patients to Watkins Infirmary and assisted in surgery, purchased the hospital in 1912 after Dr. Watkins became ill. Dr. Watkins lived for only a few weeks after the sale. Dr. Watkins was an active member of the state and county medical societies. He held many offices and presented a number of papers to the societies.

King Memorial Hospital—1896
Selma, Alabama

On December 6, 1896, Dr. Goldsby King (1860–1920), a prominent physician of Selma, opened the first private hospital in that city, known at first as the King Sanatorium and Rest Home.[19] It operated as the Goldsby King Hospital until Dr. King's death April 5, 1920. After his death, the hospital was purchased by Drs. Philip Ball Moss, A. S. Marcus, and Ira C. Skinner. It was designated the King Memorial Hospital and operated as such until 1953. In 1956, the hospital was reopened as the Dunn Rest Home.

Laura Croom Hill Infirmary—1897
Montgomery, Alabama

The Laura Croom Hill Infirmary (also known as the Hill Infirmary) was established in 1897 by Dr. Luther Leonidas Hill and his brother, Dr. Robert Sommerville Hill (1870–1952).[20] It was named for their mother, Laura Croom Hill, who was the wife of the Reverend Luther L. Hill of Montgomery. Dr. Robert Hill specialized in gynecology, and Dr. Luther L. Hill was the general surgeon. Dr. John Anderson served as the anesthetist. The hospital, located in a remodeled house, also served as a training school for nurses; the nurses' home was next door to the hospital. The hospital closed in 1932. Both the Drs. Hill were very prominent physicians in Alabama.

Saint Vincent's Hospital—1899
Birmingham, Alabama

At the invitation of the Reverend Patrick A. O'Reilly, pastor of Saint Paul's Roman Catholic Church, a meeting of interested citizens of Birmingham occurred June 8, 1898, in the Temperance Hall of Saint Paul's Church to consider the establishment of another hospital to serve Jefferson County and the city of Birmingham.[21] As a result, the Sisters of Charity Hospital Association was organized for the purpose of building a Catholic hospital. Those involved, in addition to Reverend O'Reilly, were Dr. B. L. Wyman, H. H. Sinege, W. P. McCrossin, J. M. McCartin, Allen J. Krebbs, Robert Jemison, Jr., B. Steiner, and the Most Reverend Bishop Edward Patrick Allen, Diocese of Mobile. Others were the Reverend Father R. A. Lennon, superior of the Order of the Daughters of Charity; Sisters Benedicta and Magdeline, who undertook the organization of a temporary hospital; and Sisters Placida, Patricia, and Antonia, who participated in its operation.

Originally, and as a temporary measure, the home of Mr. H. F. DeBardeleben, on the corner of 15th Street and Avenue B in Fountain Heights, was converted into a hospital. On March 13, 1899, ground-breaking ceremonies took place for the first permanent building at 2701 Ninth Circle South. The location, selected by Mother Mariana, superior general of the Daughters of Charity in the United States, became known

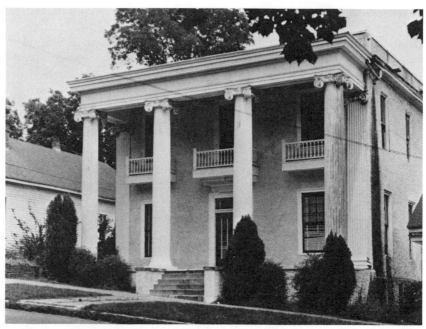

Laura Croom Hill Infirmary, Montgomery, Alabama (1877) (Courtesy of the Alabama State Department of Archives and History)

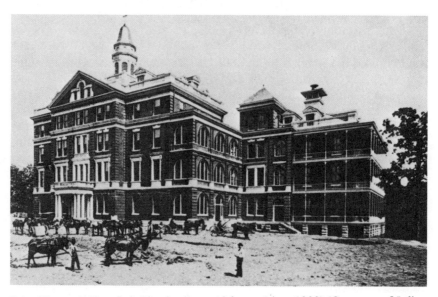

Saint Vincent's Hospital, Birmingham, Alabama (circa 1900) (Courtesy of Julius Linn, Jr., M.D.)

as Mount Saint Vincent. The first permanent home of the hospital was opened on Thanksgiving Day in 1900. The first administrator of the new hospital was Sister Chrysoston Moynahan. The first hospital-based X-ray equipment in Birmingham was installed here.

In May, 1972, the new Saint Vincent's Hospital complex was completed. The new complex, still located at 27th Street and Ninth Court South, replaced the original structure that had opened in 1900. In 1972, the complex had a capacity of 296 beds. As of 1980, the hospital has a 305-bed capacity.

The Daughters of Charity of Saint Vincent de Paul are in charge of the administration of the hospital. The hospital operates as a voluntary, nonprofit corporation under the Board of Trustees of the Order and a Lay Advisory Board of community leaders.

Harrison Sanitorium—1900
Talladega, Alabama

In 1900, the J. M. Lewis home in the Highlands of Talladega was rented by Dr. William Groce Harrison (1871–1955), a graduate of the University of Maryland Medical School, and his father, Dr. John Tinsley Harrison (1834–1915).[22] The Lewis home was opened as a private hospital. This building later became the Nurses Home of Citizens Hospital. Dr. Harrison's hospital was the first of its kind for the citizens of Talladega. Staff privileges were open to other physicians of the town.

These quarters were not sufficiently large for the hospital; so the Drs. Harrison, in 1901, purchased the Manning house on South Street. They enlarged this building and converted it into a more modern hospital. The patient capacity, however, was never large. The sanatorium closed March 1, 1905, and Dr. W. G. Harrison moved to Birmingham, where he entered a specialized practice in ear, nose, and throat. Dr. J. T. Harrison remained in Talladega and resumed his private practice.

Saint Margaret's Hospital—1901
Montgomery, Alabama

Early in 1901, the Reverend Dennis Savage, pastor of Saint Peter's Church in Montgomery, began negotiations with Father R. A. Lennon of Baltimore concerning the feasibility of building a modern hospital to serve Montgomery.[23] Father Lennon was the superior of the Daughters of Charity who had recently opened Saint Vincent's Hospital in Birmingham.

Father Lennon assured Father Savage that the sisters would build a hospital there which would cost no less than $50,000, provided the citizens of Montgomery would contribute $10,000 to help purchase a site suitable for this purpose. Within a short time, more than the required $10,000 was in hand. An advisory board was appointed and consisted of J. M. Falkner, E. A. Graham, James P. Ferrell, Tennent Lomax, Frank P. Glass, R. E. Steiner, E. B. Joseph, Phares Coleman, James McIntyre, Alex Rice, William B. Jones, Thomas H. Carr, A. A. Wiley, Leon Weil, J. C. Haas, John P. Kohn, W. W. Screws, and Dr. J. B. Gaston. Sister Chrysoston Moynahan, the administrator of Saint Vincent's Hospital in Birmingham, was appointed by Father Lennon to purchase a site for the new hospital. She was assisted by John P. Kohn. The site selected for the new hospital was located on Adams Avenue between Jackson and Ripley streets. Ground breaking took place on April 3, 1902. The cornerstone was laid by the Most Reverend E. P. Allen, bishop of Mobile, on May 20, 1902, and the hospital was dedicated to Saint Margaret of Scotland. Two sisters, Sister Margaret and Sister Scholastica, arrived on June 9, 1902.

On this site was the mansion of former Governor Thomas Hill Watts, which was used by the nuns as a residence. The ballroom was converted into a chapel. The mansion had to be torn down in February, 1957, to make room for further expansion of the hospital.

The hospital opened on September 23, 1903, and cost $150,000. It was incorporated by the state of Alabama on October 15, 1903, with Sister Scholastica Kehoe, Sister Vincent Trexler, and Sister Agnes Darwin as its trustees. The staff of physicians was organized on August 10, 1905. Dr. L. L. Hill performed the first surgical operation in the new hospital.

Garner Hospital—1907
Anniston, Alabama

The original hospital was a twenty-five–bed facility organized by Drs. E. M. Sellers and W. D. Sellers in 1907 as the Sellers Hospital.[24] In 1908, two nurses, Oma Dickert and Olga Landt, opened Anniston Hospital which became Saint Luke's Hospital in 1912 after an effort to consolidate with Sellers Hospital failed. In 1921, Sellers Hospital burned and was replaced with a fifty-bed facility that opened in 1923.

In 1929, the city of Anniston bought Sellers Hospital and the Saint Luke's Hospital property. In 1930, the city opened Garner Hospital, a sixty-bed facility in the Sellers Hospital buildings. The hospital was named after Robert E. Garner, who left a bequest of $25,000 to be used toward the purchase of the property. A nursing home occupies the Sellers Hospital buildings today.

South Highlands Hospital—1910
Birmingham, Alabama

South Highlands Hospital was founded in 1910 by Dr. Edmond Mortimer Prince and his associates, Dr. David Sanders Moore, and Dr. Joseph Grover Moore.[25] At that time, it was known as South Highlands Infirmary and had a sixty-bed capacity. The infirmary was located at 1127 South 12th Street. The purpose of this hospital was to give the community a much-needed additional hospital facility. The South Highlands Infirmary School of Nursing opened at the same time the infirmary opened in October, 1910.[26]

As Birmingham grew, so did the hospital. In 1971, it became known as South Highlands Hospital. Today, it is a 219–bed facility and a nonprofit organization under a Board of Trustees. It has the latest equipment and facilities, but its goals and ideals are the same as in 1910—"rendering maximum service to its patients in a sympathetic and cooperative manner."

The Mobile Infirmary—1910
Mobile, Alabama

The Mobile Infirmary is a voluntary, nonprofit community hospital.[27] From 1896 until the institution opened on October 21, 1910, a group of devoted women raised funds by holding bazaars and social functions. This group was known as the Mobile Infirmary Association. They purchased the site for the original building on Springhill Avenue. The first hospital consisted of thirty-two rooms and four wards and was financed with a private bond issue. Two million dollars was raised through the joint cooperation of the Jewish, Protestant, and Greek churches, and civic-minded citizens. In June, 1947, the present site was purchased. Federal aid for construction was granted under the Hill-Burton Act. The dedication of the 285-bed facility was held on January 19, 1952. In 1956, with the aid of a $155,000 Ford Foundation Grant, additional beds were added. In 1963, another major addition was completed. A bequest of Mr. E. A. Roberts made possible the addition of fifty specialized beds in 1969. The hospital now has a total of 535 beds. The affairs of the Mobile Infirmary Association are managed by a twenty-one–member Board of Trustees; twelve members are designated as denominational trustees and represent the various religious denominations with the exception of the Roman Catholics. All other trustees are designated as trustees at large.

The Children's Hospital of Alabama—1911
Birmingham, Alabama

In 1911, Holy Innocents Hospital was founded by the ladies of the Episcopal Diocese in Birmingham.[28] Prominent ladies served as officers with the responsibility for fund raising. In the early years, funds for the hospital were raised through a large number of small monthly private subscriptions plus a supplemental subsidy from Jefferson County. The hospital, for the care of the "sick, maimed or crippled child," opened March, 1912. At that time, the hospital had a bed capacity of twenty-five and provided free care to children under fourteen who were referred by social agencies or approved by an admissions committee. The physicians of Birmingham volunteered their services.

In May, 1914, the name was changed to the Children's Hospital of Alabama. It was and still is a private, nonprofit hospital that admits indigent and part-pay patients and is run by a voluntary board of trustees.

Children's Hospital sees more than 100,000 patients yearly from all over the Southeastern United States. There are specialized units—the Burn Center, Cancer Clinic, Adolescent Clinic, Teen-Tot Clinic, and the Kidney Unit. At present, a new eight-story tower is under construction and will open in the fall of 1982.

Vaughan Memorial Hospital—1911
Selma, Alabama

Vaughan Memorial Hospital came into being in an old building that had served as an orphanage, as a courthouse, and as a school.[29] The original building was constructed prior to 1848 by the Selma Fraternal Lodge No. 27 of the Free and Accepted Masons for use as a school for orphans of indigent Masons; presumably it was for both boys and girls. The school was called "The Central Alabama Masonic Institute." Its operation was short lived, and it closed due to financial difficulties. On May 16, 1866, Dallas County acquired the Institute from the city of Selma in order to use the building as the Dallas County Courthouse.

The building was purchased from Dallas County by the trustees of Mr. Henry White Vaughan's estate on August 8, 1904, in order to establish a hospital in memory of Mr. Vaughan's father, Dr. Samuel Watkins Vaughan. Mr. Vaughan left a bequest of $10,000 for this purpose. The hospital was to be known as Vaughan Memorial Hospital.

In 1905, Dr. Francis Goodwin DuBose, a prominent physician of Selma, had opened a hospital known as the DuBose Sanitorium on Lapsley Street. Sometime later the buildings that comprised the sanitorium burned. In 1911, Dr. DuBose and his associates agreed to operate Vaughan Memorial Hospital. The hospital was proprietarily operated by the staff physicians whose offices were in the hospital itself.

The hospital closed in 1960, and a new building was constructed at its present location on New Orrville Road. The new hospital, New Vaughan Memorial Hospital, is a nonprofit corporation and has an open medical staff. The old building was later purchased by the city of Selma and renovated for use as the Selma Historic and Civic Building.

John A. Andrew Memorial Hospital—1912
Tuskegee Institute—Tuskegee, Alabama

The John A. Andrew Memorial Hospital is owned, controlled, and operated by Tuskegee Institute.[30] This hospital is a 175–bed, short-term, general hospital, which originally was founded for dispensing medical care to Tuskegee Institute's students, faculty, and staff on an outpatient basis.

In 1912, the first section of the hospital was erected with student labor at a cost of $55,000. Mrs. Elizabeth Mason of Boston gave funds for construction of this building as a memorial to her grandfather, the Honorable John Albion Andrew, war governor of Massachusetts from 1861 to 1866. Three additions (1929, 1940, and 1946) have increased the capacity and scope of the hospital services.

Talladega Infirmary—1912
Talladega, Alabama

In 1912, Dr. B. B. Simms and Dr. S. W. Welch purchased the Lanier home on the west side of South Court Street.[31] They converted it into a fourteen-bed hospital, the Talladega Infirmary. Associated with Drs. Simms and Welch was Dr. Lawson Thornton, who, in 1913, moved first to Birmingham and then to Atlanta where he became an outstanding orthopedic surgeon. Miss Bertha McElderry, graduate of Johns Hopkins School of Nursing, served as superintendent of the hospital.

During World War I, approximately twenty-five soldiers were cared for in this hospital. They were sent from the overcrowded army hospital at Fort McClellan. The hospital originally operated under a Board of Directors, with Dr. S. W. Welch serving as acting chairman. Later, A. G. Storey was chairman. The hospital had an open staff for the physicians of Talladega. In 1920, the hospital was sold to Dr. C. W. C. Moore.

Dr. Moore named the hospital the Mary Elizabeth Hospital for his two daughters. He added twelve beds to the hospital and opened a small training school for nurses with a capacity for six nurses.

Although the hospital operated with an open staff, no other physicians were financially associated with it. There were no provisions for charity patients. The Mary Elizabeth Hospital closed in 1925.

Lloyd Noland Hospital—1912
Fairfield, Alabama

In 1912, Dr. Lloyd Noland accepted the post of superintendent of Tennessee Coal and Iron's health department in Fairfield.[32] Here he led the first extensive experiment in industrial medicine in the South. His health and sanitation program was a milestone in the progress against infectious disease in Alabama. (See Chapter 5, "Medical Practice after the Civil War.")

During World War I, the United States Steel Company, under the direction of Dr. Noland, began the Employees' Hospital of the Tennessee Coal, Iron and Railroad Company. The hospital was completed in 1919. Dr. Noland became medical director of this 350–bed hospital and remained its director until his death in 1949. The hospital was later named for him.

Carraway Methodist Medical Center—1916
Birmingham, Alabama

The original facility, established in 1916 as the Norwood Hospital, consisted of a thirty-five–bed hospital on the corner of 25th Street and 16th Avenue North in Birmingham.[33] It was organized initially by Dr. C. N. Carraway and five other men as a stockholding group.

The property was deeded in trust to the First Methodist Church of Birmingham in December, 1936. In 1947, the North Alabama Methodist Conference voted to accept the property. At that time, the name of the facility was changed to the Carraway Methodist Hospital.

Additions to the hospital have been made, and each addition has been named for the presiding bishop of the North Alabama Methodist Conference. At present, the hospital will serve 419 inpatients.

In May, 1971, a new corporation was formed and named the Carraway Methodist Medical Center. The North Alabama Annual Conference of the Methodist Church elects the Board of Trustees for staggered terms of three years, with the resident bishop serving as chairman of the board. The Board of Directors is elected by the trustees. Dr. Ben Carraway, son of Dr. C. N. Carraway, is the present chairman of the board.

Birmingham Baptist Hospital—1921
Birmingham, Alabama

The Birmingham Infirmary, located at 702–712 Tuscaloosa Avenue, West End, was owned originally by Dr. W. C. Gewin.[34] In November, 1921, it was purchased by the Birmingham Baptist Association. It consisted of a former residence to which an east wing had been added. The original Board of Trustees included Dr. J. R. Hobbs, chairman, David M. Gardner, secretary, and J. A. Coker, treasurer. The Birmingham Baptist Hospital was incorporated on December 21, 1921. Dr. J. M. Long was the first superintendent, and Miss Dorothea Ely was superintendent of nurses. In July, 1922, the staff of the hospital was organized with Dr. J. D. Heacock as first president. In 1925, a nurses' residence was constructed at 610 Seventh Street, SW. In 1930, the Birmingham Baptist Hospital leased the fifty-bed Gorgas Hospital on Highland Avenue. In 1934, this hospital and the nearby Seale Harris residence were purchased by the Birmingham Baptist Association. On September 19, 1936, the Birmingham Baptist Hospital reorganized under bankruptcy and operated under the jurisdiction of the federal court until 1941. In April, 1949, the three hospitals were deeded to the Alabama State Baptist Convention as a gift from the Birmingham Baptist Association. Less than a year later (November, 1949), they were deeded back to the Birmingham Baptist Association.

Throughout the 1950s, plans for the expansion and construction of new facilities were underway. The hospital facilities on Highland Avenue were sold. The original Birmingham Baptist Hospital was completely renovated and remodeled and was opened April, 1966, as Baptist Medical Center—Princeton (West End Hospital) with a 427-bed capacity.

In December, 1966, Baptist Medical Center—Montclair opened as a 485-bed hospital. Multimillion dollar expansion programs began in January, 1980, at both Montclair and Princeton and should be completed in late 1982.

Good Samaritan Hospital—1922
Selma, Alabama

A hospital established for black patients opened in Selma in 1922, under the direction of Mrs. Mamie Morris, who remained administrator until ill health forced her retirement.[35] She died on March 22, 1951. The original property was purchased from Mr. H. S. Sullivan by the Alabama Baptist Hospital Board on March 8, 1922, for the sum of $5,000 and remodeled as a hospital.

Known as the Good Samaritan Hospital, the facility operated as an annex to the Selma Baptist Hospital. Selma Baptist opened in 1921 when it was purchased and operated by the medical staff.

In 1943, the original buildings owned by the Baptist Good Samaritan Hospital Association were purchased by the Fathers of Saint Edmund under the leadership of Father Francis Casey, S.S.E., first director of the Edmundite Southern Missions.

Much was accomplished during the following years. In May, 1946, the original Good Samaritan became the second general hospital in Alabama and the fourth in the United States for blacks to receive approval from the American Hospital Association.

In 1947, a fireproof, seventy-eight-bed convalescent unit was opened, and ten years later, a twenty-six-bed skilled nursing home was added. The hospital continues to function under the auspices of the Edmundite Southern Missions and the Sisters of Saint Joseph.

Eliza Coffee Memorial Hospital—1922
Florence, Alabama

The Eliza Coffee Memorial Hospital, a thirty-bed facility, was established by the city of Florence in 1922 and was made possible by a gift from Mrs. Camilla Madding Coffee in memory of her daughter.[36] In 1938, the city of Florence and Lauderdale County joined together to construct and operate a modern sixty-bed hospital at its present location on Alabama Street. The original name of the hospital was retained.

Since 1943, the hospital has increased its bed capacity to 296 beds, including 39 psychiatric beds operated as a comprehensive mental health center. In 1952, the Mitchell-Hollingsworth Annex, a convalescent and nursing home operated by the hospital, was made possible through a gift from Mr. and Mrs. Jewett T. Flagg and the J. T. Flagg Knitting Company. This supplemental facility now has 202 beds.

Huntsville Hospital, Inc.—1926
Huntsville, Alabama

The Huntsville Hospital, Inc., was built in 1925–1926.[37] It was opened for patients in June, 1926. The original hospital, which had been in operation since 1904, was known as the Huntsville Infirmary, and was a private, nonprofit institution regulated by a self-perpetuating Board of Trustees. In June, 1961, the facility was deeded to the city of Huntsville. Presently, it operates under a Board of Control, four members of which are appointed by the city council and two by the Madison County Commissioners. It presently has a 460-bed capacity.

Northeast Alabama Regional Medical Center—1944
Anniston, Alabama

World War II saw construction of the Anniston Memorial Hospital by the United States Government's Federal Works Administration.[38] Public funds contributed by Calhoun County citizens were also used for this hospital's construction. The new hospital was named Anniston Memorial Hospital in honor of servicemen who lost their lives in World War II.

Anniston Memorial Hospital opened in 1944 with 100 beds. Soon after its opening, the city of Anniston bought the facility for $326,000. A 48-bed addition was finished in 1953, and a four-story south tower in 1962, making the hospital a 300-bed facility.

In 1972, the Alabama Department of Public Health designated the hospital as a regional medical center. In mid-1974, the Anniston City Council transferred ownership of the hospital to a board composed of representatives of several local cities. It was renamed the Northeast Alabama Regional Medical Center.

Southeast Alabama Medical Center—1957
Dothan, Alabama

The Southeast Alabama Medical Center in Dothan, Alabama, opened for admission of patients on September 9, 1957.[39] It was originally named Southeast Alabama General Hospital and was an 111-bed facility. The hospital was made possible by a general tax on the citizens of Houston County, July 22, 1949.

In the more than twenty years that have passed since the opening of the hospital, many additions and improvements have been made. By April, 1981, the hospital had a bed capacity of 400.

Medical Center Hospital—1971
Selma, Alabama

The Selma Medical Center Hospital was first known as the Selma Baptist Hospital and was opened in 1921.[40] The Union Street Hospital of Selma, an institution founded by Drs. Samuel G. Gay and John P. Furniss, was in existence shortly after the turn of the century until 1921. At that time, the staff physicians collaborated with the Alabama Baptist to build Selma Baptist Hospital. The Alabama Baptist Convention originally owned and operated the hospital and eventually sold the hospital to a group of twenty physicians in Selma. In August, 1968, the Selma Baptist Hospital was sold to the Hospital Corporation of America. The Selma Medical Center Hospital, Inc., was opened by the Hospital Corporation on July 20, 1971. The new facility is a 150-bed ultramodern hospital located on a thirty-acre site adjacent to U.S. Highway 80 West. The hospital is a general medical and surgical, short-term hospital. While it is owned by the Hospital Corporation of America, it is operated by the Board of Trustees of the hospital, which is composed of the administrator and a group of six or more staff physicians.

Notes

1. John Duffy, ed., *The Rudolph Matas History of Medicine in Louisiana* (Baton Rouge: Louisiana State University Press, 1958), 1: 82.

2. Peter J. Hamilton, *Colonial Mobile, A Historical Study* (New York: Houghton, Mifflin & Co.; Cambridge: Riverside Press, 1897), pp. 52, 55.

3. L. D. S. Harrell, "Colonial Medical Practice in British West Florida, 1763–1781," *Bull. Hist. Med.* 41 (1967): 544.

4. Francois Ludger Diard, ed., *The Tablet* 2 (Mobile, Ala.: n.p., April 1961): 1–8. Copy in the author's possession.

5. Marie Bankhead Owen, *The Story of Alabama: A History of the State* (New York: Lewis Historical Pub. Co., Inc., 1949), 2: 570; Natalie Crozier, "New Life Planned for Keeler Memorial Hospital," *Mobile Register*, 12 June 1974, sect. A; and "Old Marine Hospital Now Historic Place," *Mobile Press*, 9 July 1974.

6. Providence Hospital, "Providence Hospital, Mobile, Alabama," 17 April 1971, dedication brochure in the author's possession.

7. E. Grace Jemison, *Historic Tales of Talladega* (Montgomery, Ala.: Paragon Press, 1959), pp. 308–09.

8. Howard L. Holley and Eugenia Blount Dabney, "The History of the Hillman Hospital, The Hospital of the United Charities, Part 1," *De Hist. Med.* 5 (Jan. 1961): 9–16; and Howard L. Holley and Velimir Luketic, "The History of the Hillman Hospital, Part 2," *Ala. J. Med. Sci.* 6 (1969): 228–32.

9. Helen Bethea, *The Hillman Hospital—A Story of the Growth and Development of the First Hospital in Birmingham: 1888–1907* ([Birmingham]: n.p., 1928).

10. The report was printed in the *Age-Herald* of January 9, 1889, and is included in the January minutes of the Board of Managers in the Jefferson–Hillman Hospital Papers, Alabama Museum of the Health Sciences.

11. Richard R. Hawes was accused of murdering his wife and two children. He was apprehended and held in jail, but a lynch mob attempted to seize him. The sheriff resisted, and a gun battle ensued.

12. Minutes of the Board of Managers of Hillman Hospital, September 1, 1893. Jefferson–Hillman Hospital Papers, Alabama Museum of the Health Sciences.

13. *Age-Herald*, 31 August 1893, as quoted in Holley and Dabney, p. 14.

14. The original petition is included in the Jefferson–Hillman Hospital Papers, Alabama Museum of the Health Sciences.

15. Robert S. Hogan, "Edgar Poe Hogan—Physician, Surgeon and Public Servant," *Ala. J. Med. Sci.* 2 (1965): 99–100.

16. Edgar Poe Hogan, a circular sent to citizens of Birmingham, as quoted in Holley and Luketic, p. 230.

17. The new Hillman Hospital is administrative offices for the University Hospitals. The nurses' home is now the Roy R. Kracke Clinical Services Building.

18. Watkins Infirmary, letter and information compiled by Mrs. Lela Legare, and Dr. T. Brannon Hubbard of Montgomery. Mrs. Legare is a columnist for the *Montgomery Advertiser.*

19. Thomas McAdory Owen, *History of Alabama and Dictionary of Alabama Biography* (Chicago: S. J. Clarke Publishing Co., 1921), 3: 980; and Eleanor R. Falkenberry, TS, Selma, Ala., 30 April 1980, copy in the author's possession.

20. Lela Legare, TS on Dr. R. S. Hill, and a personal interview with Mrs. Carney Laslie, Senator Lister Hill's sister, n.d., in the author's possession.

21. St. Vincent's Hospital, "Saint Vincent's Hospital; The Hospital Reputation Built," 27 May 1972, dedication ceremonies brochure in the author's possession.

22. Jemison, pp. 309–10.

23. St. Margaret's Hospital, "St. Margaret's Hospital Quarterly," (Montgomery: n.p., March 1977) 1, no. 2; "A 'Splendid Public Hospital,' " *The Montgomery Advertiser*, 11 April 1977; St. Margaret's Hospital patient information brochure, (Montgomery: n.p., 1977); "St. Margaret's Hospital: A Brief History," (Montgomery: n.p., [after 1976]); "St. Margaret's Celebrates 75th Year," *The Montgomery Advertiser/Alabama Journal*, 3 April 1977, sect. D, p. 3. Material collected by Michael L. Tapley, director of Public Relations for Saint Margaret's Hospital, 3 June 1977; now in the author's possession.

24. "Two Doctors Organized City's First Hospital," *The Anniston Star*, 27 February 1977, sect. 2B.

25. Tinzie Hicks, R.N., director of Personnel, South Highlands Hospital, collection of promotional materials, 20 September 1972; South Highlands Hospital, anniversary brochure, October 1978; "Inside South Highlands" anniversary publication, which includes reprints from a local newspaper of 10 October 1910; letter received from Ms. Nancy Matthews, coordinator of Public Relations, South Highlands Hospital, 6 February 1980; all material in the author's possession.

26. South Highlands Hospital, South Highlands Hospital Papers, Alabama Museum of the Health Sciences.

27. Mobile Infirmary, "Mobile Infirmary, Mobile, Alabama," (n.p.: n.p., [probably 1970–1976]), patient information brochure in the author's possession.

28. Letter received from Marianne B. Sharbel, director of Public Information, The Children's Hospital, Birmingham, Alabama, 28 October 1980; and Edward S. Lamonte, "The Mercy Home and Private Charities in Early Birmingham," *J. B'ham Hist. Soc.* 5 (July 1978): 15.

29. Letter received from R. C. Stapler, administrator, New Vaughan Memorial Hospital, Inc., Selma, Ala., 24 January 1973; and letter with TS included from Eleanor Falkenberry, Selma, Ala., December 1980.

30. Letter received from Howard W. Kenney, M.D., medical director, Tuskegee Institute, Tuskegee, Ala., 28 August 1969; includes a reprint of E. H. Dibble, Jr., L. A. Rabb, and R. B. Ballard, "John A. Andrew Memorial Hospital," *J. Nat. Med. Assoc.* 53 (March 1961): 103–18; in the author's possession.

31. Jemison, p. 310.

32. E. Bryce Robinson, Jr., "Lloyd Noland and T.C.I.," *De Hist. Med.* 4 (Aug. 1959): 3–24. Tennessee Coal and Iron was purchased in 1907 by the United States Steel Company.

33. T. Doron, director of Public Relations, Carraway Methodist Medical Center, TS, "Carraway Methodist Medical Center," 15 September 1972, copy in the author's possession.

34. Janie Lott, publications director for Baptist Medical Centers, TS, "Baptist Medical Centers: Short Historical Sketch," 21 September 1972, copy in the author's possession.

35. Correspondence from Father Paul A. Morin, S.S.E., Good Samaritan Hospital, 2 November 1972; includes a memorandum from a Mr. Wright to Father Crowley of 21 August 1967 that attempts to date correctly the establishment of the Good Samaritan Hospital. Father Morin also included his own typescript, "Good Samaritan Hospital," and *Good Samaritan Hospital Newsletter* 1 (1964): no. 1, copy in the author's possession.

36. "A Short History of Eliza Coffee Memorial Hospital," Florence, Ala., TS, n.d., in the author's possession.

37. Huntsville Hospital, "Huntsville Hospital" (Cleveland, Tenn.: Hospital Publications, 1972); brochure in the author's possession.

38. "Two Doctors Organized City's First Hospital," *The Anniston Star*, 27 February 1977, sect. 2B.

39. Southeast Alabama General Hospital, "Things in General," 2 (Sept. 1974), no. 13; Southeast Alabama Medical Center, "The Future Medical Center," (Dothan, Ala.: n.p., November 1976); correspondence and material from Jack Parsons, assistant administrator of Southeast Alabama Medical Center, Dothan, Ala., 14 June 1977, in the author's possession; and "Medical Center Observes 23rd Anniversary," *SAMC Newsletter* 2 (Sept./Oct. 1980): 2, 5, in the author's possession.

40. Letter from J. L. Armour, administrator, Medical Center Hospital, Selma, Ala., 20 September 1972.

Chapter 3

Efforts in Medical Education

Rapid extension of the southern frontier after 1800 had succeeded in opening new country where popular culture, in general, and medical standards, in particular, were inevitably low. This was due not only to the presence of irregular practitioners with their various systems of health care, but also to poor training received by the majority of regular practitioners. Medical schools and other professional institutions developed relatively late in the South.[1] During the early nineteenth century, Southerners who desired formal medical training had to go north where there were good schools in Philadelphia, New York, and Lexington, Kentucky. Study abroad was also desirable when the student could afford the expense, and it is surprising how many early Alabama physicians had such training.

As a result, most regular physicians in the South were trained by the preceptor system—that is, reading medicine with a reputable practicing physician. The terms were of variable length and quality, and there is little evidence that after such training, the physicians made any attempt to keep up with new developments and ideas in medicine. There were few books, most of which were out of date, and still fewer medical periodicals. Communication and mail delivery were not well developed, and even when a journal was available, physicians often could not afford the subscription price. The practice of medicine in most frontier towns was far from lucrative.

As the population increased, the growth of the larger cities with their professional leaders made possible the establishment of medical schools. The Medical College of South Carolina was established at Charleston in 1824. A medical department was organized at the University of Virginia shortly thereafter. In 1832, a medical college was organized in Augusta, Georgia. Medical schools were also founded in New Orleans in 1835 and in Richmond in 1838. These pioneer schools adopted standards then prevalent in the better northern schools. The curriculum usually involved a four or five months' course of lectures plus extensive preceptorial requirements. With assistance from some state and local governments, the schools prospered and both their standards and enrollments steadily increased until 1861.[2]

Unfortunately, these schools were unable to meet the growing demand for physicians in the South. Because of poor transportation, each isolated frontier community needed its own resident medical practitioner. To meet this demand, a new group of medical schools, whose standards ranged from bad to worse, opened along with the older schools. Without exception they bore the so-called proprietary label. Even university-connected schools were under the complete control of faculties who shared any profits made either by the schools from student fees or from the increased practice engendered by being on the faculty of the medical school. No agency existed to regulate medical school standards, and abuses were frequent. Almost any man with an elementary education could take a course of lectures for one or two winters, pass an examination, and achieve the right to practice medicine under state law. Laboratory and clinical work was ignored, and since preceptor training had been gradually abandoned, physicians could be turned out in less than a year.[3] Indeed, as late as 1900, there were individuals practicing medicine who did not have the requirements for entrance to a good liberal arts college. Dr. Oliver Wendell Holmes of *Breakfast-Table* fame critically referred to some of these schools as "inferior schools wrongly located."[4] His remarks brought on a flurry of angry denials, and although he should have included a number of northern schools as well, he was substantially correct. Particularly corrupt, both in the North and the South, were the so-called diploma mills, which charged large fees and graduated physicians with little or no training.

Alabama had its share of this ill-trained crop, a situation extremely galling to reputable physicians of the state who were faced with trouble both from the excesses of the irregular practitioners and from their ill-trained brethren. As a result, they did everything in their power to improve the situation. They backed the Licensure Act of 1823 and, later, in 1847, created the Medical Association of the State of Alabama, which, it was hoped, would bring together all physicians in the state and enable them to exchange ideas and improve their general knowledge of medicine.[5] Both attempts failed to improve the standards of the medical profession perceptibly. The physicians then came to believe that only a good medical school could improve the situation.

The first charter for a medical school in Alabama was granted by the General Assembly in 1845 to the trustees of the "Alabama Medical

University."[6] The school was to be at Wetumpka, and the trustees would have the right to elect the faculty and grant diplomas. Two courses of lectures were to be offered, but a student could fulfill his requirements by attending one of the courses at another "respectable medical college." In 1846, the charter was amended, permitting the trustees to establish the school at any suitable place in Alabama. This effort failed to materialize. Another charter was granted in 1849 establishing the "Alabama Medical College" at Montgomery.[7] The trustees, several of whom were prominent Montgomery physicians, could appoint the faculty and hold property not in excess of $50,000. Trustees and faculty were jointly authorized to grant diplomas, make college rules, and fill faculty and trustee vacancies that might occur. The twenty-one-year charter was renewed in 1873 despite the fact that no school had been established. By the 1890s, most of the trustees had died leaving no quorum for business. These two attempts to found a medical school in Alabama were failures.

The Graefenberg Medical Institute

The Graefenberg Medical Institute, a proprietary school that epitomized the sort of practices and principles that so disturbed the state's more reputable practitioners, was established in Dadeville in 1852.[8] Its founder, Philip Madison Shepard, a characteristic frontier personality, was born in 1812 in Columbia County, Georgia. When Shepard was thirteen, his father died, and for the next five years he single-handedly supported his mother, brother, and four sisters. Lacking time to go to school, he studied alone after finishing his work in the fields. His mother remarried when he was nineteen, thus enabling him to study medicine with a local practitioner, Dr. John B. Boon. Dr. Shepard stayed with this physician for eighteen months and was preparing to start practicing on his own when he obtained sufficient funds to attend the Georgia Medical College at Augusta. After a four-month term, he received his degree and began practice at Social Circle, Georgia. In the fall he returned to school, receiving a second degree in 1835. The next year he married, sired a son, and moved to Lafayette, Alabama, where he practiced for the next eight years. Dr. Shepard established a small medical school, which he designated "Students Institute." Its primary purpose was to prepare young men for admission to medical school. In 1845 he moved again, this time to Wetumpka, where in addition to his practice, he apparently did some anatomical dissecting, staged medical debates with colleagues, and prepared some twenty young men for college by lecturing on his "favorite topics, Anatomy, Philosophy, Botany and Chemistry."[9] In the latter part of 1846, he moved to Dadeville, a recently

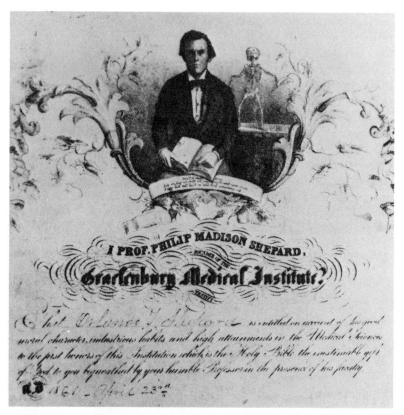

The Diploma of the Graefenberg Medical Institute with likeness of Philip
Madison Shepard, M.D., 1812–1861 (Courtesy of the Alabama Museum of the
Health Sciences, Lister Hill Library, Medical Center, The University of Alabama
in Birmingham)

incorporated community in the Piedmont Section of Tallapoosa County,
where he bought land, built a house, started farming, and developed an
extensive medical practice.

Events leading to the establishment of the school began during the
summer of 1851 when Dr. Shepard ran an advertisement in *The Advertiser and State Gazette* of Montgomery, announcing the opening of the
"Graefenberg Infirmary and Hydropathic Establishment."[10] Later, the

General Assembly chartered the "Graefenberg Medical Institute of the State of Alabama," stating that "the graduates of this Institute were entitled to all the privileges accorded graduates of leading Medical Colleges."[11] Shepard was installed as "proprietor and professor"; his half-brother, W. Banks, was appointed president of the Board of Trustees; another half-brother, J. T. Banks, and a cousin of Mrs. Shepard, M. L. Fielder, were named trustees. Dr. James I. Shackleford and William M. A. Mitchell rounded out the board, as Dr. Shepard had apparently exhausted his supply of relatives. Dr. Shepard's multifarious activities also included proprietorship of the Winston Male College, a school with a military department, state-supplied muskets, and a cannon; and the Octavia Walton Lee Vert Normal College for Young Ladies.[12]

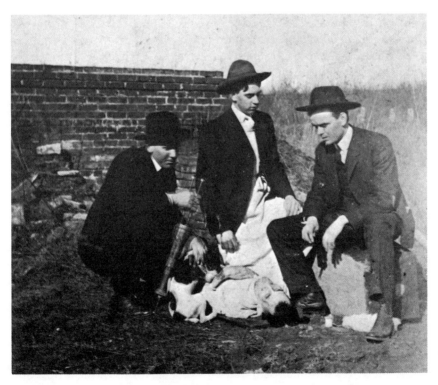

Grave robbing (Courtesy of the Alabama Museum of the Health Sciences, Lister Hill Library, Medical Center, The University of Alabama in Birmingham)

Facilities of the Graefenberg Medical Institute included an Anatomical Museum, which contained many specimens, a good library, some 1,000 plates as "large as life," chemical and surgical apparatus, a herbarium with drawings "truly attractive," and a fine cabinet of minerals, along with an auditorium and classrooms for the other schools. The institute filled a large three-story building. Skeletons that dangled from rods were available for instruction. The cadavers for dissection were largely procured by grave robbing, execution of criminals, and by shipments from Montgomery and New Orleans.[13] These were stored in metal-lined vats. Herbs filled the school garden and medicines filled the school pharmacy, substantiating the proprietor's claim that "Allopathy, Hydropathy, Homeopathy, and Botany would be taught scientifically."[14]

Teaching, primarily lectures and quizzes, was supplemented by bedside instruction held in the six cottages of the Graefenberg Infirmary and Hydropathic Establishment. Shepard frequently took his students to see patients in their homes. Bible study was stressed. Dr. Shepard was eager to advertise the simple, religious, healthy life of his students. He alone did most of the teaching until 1855 when his eighteen-year-old son, John, graduated. Within three years, John held three professorships simultaneously and shared one with his father. When a younger son, Philip Madison, Jr., graduated in 1858, he was allowed to share two professorships with his father. In 1860, at the age of seventeen, a third son, Orlando Tyler, became Professor of Obstetrics and Diseases of Women and Children. The family business would have absorbed another Shepard but for an act of God: the fourth child was a girl. The daughter, Louisa, received the same training as her brothers and won a medical degree, but she did not join the faculty. Popular sentiment was decisively opposed to female medical professors.[15]

The school offered two sessions per year, one from May to October and the other from November to March. Tuition was sixty dollars, but bargain rates were available, especially for summer students. Students lived in an annex of Dr. Shepard's home and ate with the family. The good doctor apparently had no entrance requirements, and, as was the custom, graduation followed after one session. By far the most grueling experience for students was final examinations, which were open to the public. Examinations were administered by the Board of Trustees, lasted three days and three nights, and often consisted of more than 5,000 questions.[16] During the nine years of the school's existence, some fifty students suffered this ordeal and received Shepard's "Fine Quality" diploma.

Dr. Shepard accidentally cut himself while performing an autopsy and died of septicemia. Shepard's death and the Civil War closed the school in 1861. The influence of his school proved to be rather feeble. Although several prominent physicians from the Dadeville area were on the Institute's Board of Trustees, neither the board nor Shepard was ever mentioned in the *Transactions of the Medical Association of the State of Alabama*. In 1873, the building burned, destroying the library, museum, and school records. When, in 1860, Shepard had attempted to change the institute's name to "Alabama Medical University" in order to solicit state financial aid, the venture failed. By then physicians of the state had turned toward Mobile, where a well-equipped and well-staffed medical school had recently opened.

The Medical College of Alabama

The new school, organized by a group of prominent Mobile physicians, had leadership of a different character. Mainstays of the school for the next fifty years were Dr. Josiah C. Nott, Dr. William H. Anderson, and Dr. George A. Ketchum.

Dr. William Anderson's (1820–1887) credentials were impressive. A graduate of William and Mary College, he took a course of private lessons in medicine, and in 1842, after a year at the University of Virginia, received his M.D. degree. He practiced for a year and then became a resident at the Baltimore Almshouse Hospital. In 1844, he attended a lecture course in Philadelphia, and in 1845, he was in New York taking a year-long course of lectures at the University of the City of New York and visiting Bellevue Hospital daily with a private tutor. Dr. Anderson went to Europe in 1846 visiting London, Edinburgh, Berlin, and Paris. In Paris, he took an eight-month course with Claude Bernard (1813–1878), the famed physiologist. In 1849, he settled in Mobile, practicing until his death in 1887.[17]

Dr. George A. Ketchum was a native of Mobile, read medicine with Dr. F. A. Ross, and served as resident medical student at the City Hospital for two years. In 1844–1845, he took a lecture course at the Medical College of South Carolina at Charleston and then interned at Old Blockley in Philadelphia. Later in 1845, he entered the University of Pennsylvania, took two lecture courses, wrote a thesis, and received an M.D. degree. After returning to Mobile, he was elected in 1848 physician-in-chief of the City Hospital. For several years he was in partnership with Anderson, and together with Nott and Anderson he founded a highly successful private infirmary for blacks. In 1847, Ketchum played a leading role in organizing the Medical Association of the State of Alabama.[18]

Dr. Josiah C. Nott was active in the public health movement in Alabama, and his biographical sketch is included in Chapter 12. Dr. Nott

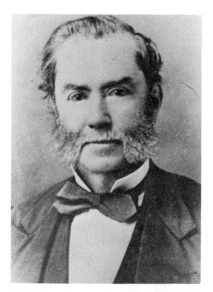

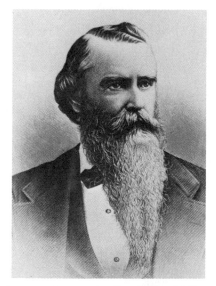

William Henry Anderson, M.D., 1820–1887, Dean 1859–1861, 1868–1885 (Courtesy of the Alabama Museum of the Health Sciences, Lister Hill Library, Medical Center, The University of Alabama in Birmingham)

George Augustus Ketchum, M.D., 1825–1906, Dean 1885–1906 (Courtesy of the Alabama Museum of the Health Sciences, Lister Hill Library, Medical Center, The University of Alabama in Birmingham)

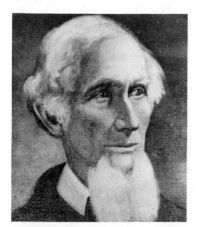

Josiah Clark Nott, M.D., 1804–1873 (Courtesy of the Alabama Museum of the Health Sciences, Lister Hill Library, Medical Center, The University of Alabama in Birmingham)

was the chief advocate for a medical school in Mobile. He wrote of his plans in a letter to a Mobile friend dated August 17, 1870:

> My idea always has been to have a school as near free as possible and to have the course of instruction more complete. If it had not been for the war my plan was to work on, amass all the funds we could and have the College so endowed as to have the professors *paid*, and independent of the classes—We shall never have any medical education in this country, as long as the pay depends entirely on the size of the class, and the schools are made matters of private speculation. The professors ought to be paid— ought to be compelled to devote more time to instruction, the course should be 7 months—should extend over 3 or 4 years—should commence with elementary branches, as Anatomy, Chemistry, etc., and there should be frequent examinations, as the classes advance, so as to keep boys always up to their work.
> . . . if the South had continued peaceful and prosperous, this scheme I think could have been worked out . . .[19]

The beginning, indeed, held promise. Largely through Nott's efforts, a charter was obtained in 1856 for the "Alabama Medical College at Mobile."[20] But the General Assembly failed to provide funds, and the charter expired while Nott taught anatomy at the University of Louisiana. Returning to Mobile in 1859 after two years in Louisiana, he obtained another charter for a medical school from the Probate Court of Mobile County and managed to raise some $25,000 from the citizens of Mobile (other sources state this sum to have been $50,000). Plans were laid, rooms were rented, and the school was to open in the fall, but as the sectional differences between the North and the South steadily increased in the years prior to 1861, the medical profession was inevitably drawn into the controversy.

The South closed its ranks in defense of slavery and states rights, and professional men of all fields were forced to choose sides. The emergence of what has been termed "states' rights medicine" became inevitable.[21] The proponents of this concept argued that medicine as it was practiced in the South was distinctly different and separate from that of the North. They also claimed that there were fundamental, anatomical, and physiological differences between the white and black races, which necessitated differences in the treatment of the two groups. Certainly, the diet and living conditions of the blacks as compared to the whites accounted for some variation in the clinical pictures of many illnesses. Also, most medical authorities had long recognized that climate does affect the clinical manifestations of disease. Therefore, there was at least some theoretical basis for Southern physicians to argue that medicine as it was practiced in the South was different.

Professional as well as political individuals gave strong support to these views. The concept that there was a necessity for a distinct southern medical practice was partly responsible for the development of a number of southern medical schools in the 1850s. Dr. Nott, the leading organizer of the medical college in Mobile, was a strong proponent of racial differences, particularly in the anthropological and possibly in physiological functions.[22] Certainly, the founding of the Medical College of Alabama in Mobile was based at least in part on this premise. The prevailing political climate unquestionably influenced the General Assembly in 1860 to appropriate funds for the college's use.

The Medical College of Alabama was given a separate, self-perpetuating Board of Trustees and $50,000 with which to purchase a lot and erect a building.* In return, the college was expected to give a free tuition scholarship to one indigent student from each county.

That summer, after the architectural design of the building was decided upon and construction was begun, Dr. Nott left for Europe to purchase equipment. Although he visited every major medical center in Europe—London, Edinburgh, Munich, Vienna, Paris, and Berlin—most of the preparations, specimens, and equipment came from Paris, the foremost medical center in Europe. Dr. Nott returned to Mobile early in October with a collection of equipment equalled by no other institution in the United States. This collection was to be one of the most important assets of the Mobile Medical School.

The first Board of Trustees was composed of Newton St. John, J. C. Dubose, Robert A. Baker, William D. Dunn, A. R. Manning, Duke W. Goodman, H. T. Smith, C. R. Foot, Murray F. Smith, Samuel G. Battle, Theophilus L. Toulmin, John Little Smith, Charles Lebaron, N. H. Brown, and John Forsyth.[23]

The school opened its doors on November 14, 1859, with Dr. Nott as Professor of Surgery; Dr. Anderson, dean and Professor of Physiology and Pathology; Dr. Ketchum, Professor of Principles and Practice of Medicine; Dr. F. A. Ross, Professor of Materia Medica, Therapeutics, and Clinical Medicine; Dr. F. E. Gordon, Professor of Obstetrics and Diseases of Women and Children; Dr. J. F. Heustis, Professor of Anatomy; Drs. Goronwy Owen and A. P. Hall, demonstrators of Anatomy; and Dr. W. J. Taylor of Philadelphia, Professor of Chemistry. Within a year, W. J. Taylor had been replaced by Dr. J. W. Mallet, one of the leading chemists in the South. Dr. Nott stressed training in the "elementary" branches, as is evidenced by Mallet's appointment and the presence of three instructors of anatomy. Nor were the clinical branches

---

*In 1859, the General Assembly recognized the college as the Medical Department of the University of Alabama.

neglected. The catalog for the first session repeatedly emphasized the wealth of clinical material found in Mobile, a city of some 35,000 people.[24]

One hundred and eleven matriculants registered for the first session. Entrance requirements for this session apparently consisted of at least one year of preparatory reading with a reputable physician. To receive a degree, a student had to attend "two full courses of lectures in this institution," but attendance at another institution or "four years of reputable practice" could substitute for one of the courses of lectures. Each session was four months long. Degree candidates had to complete satisfactorily all the subjects taught at the school, and "to write an acceptable thesis, [either in English, Latin, French, or German] on some subject connected with medicine."

Fifteen of the 111 students won degrees after the first session. About 120 were expected to attend the next session. At graduation, the new building was near completion. It was three stories high with two lecture rooms, pathology, anatomy, and chemistry laboratories, a well-equipped museum and library, offices, cloak rooms, and examination rooms. Dr. Nott looked to the future with confidence and visions of an enrollment of 200 to 300 students, plus an endowment large enough to pay professors to teach full time.[25]

The dream was shattered by the Civil War. Both faculty and students answered the call to arms, and the school closed its doors in 1861. Mobile fell to federal troops in April of 1865, and the school's building was occupied by federal troops and later made into a black school by the Freedman's Bureau. It was not until 1868 that the Medical College faculty regained possession and reopened the school. The task appeared hopeless. There was no money and no chance that the destitute state government could help. The building was dilapidated, many of the valuable specimens damaged or stolen, and the ranks of the faculty decimated.

A description of the Medical College at Mobile during reconstruction has been preserved in a report by N. B. Cloud, superintendent of Public Instruction, to Governor William H. Smith on November 10, 1869. Cloud described the Medical College as "this noble institution with its several and large appointments, such as its rare and magnificent museum, its cabinets of natural history and geology and chemical apparatus for facilitating the acquisition of medical knowledge."[26] In this same report, he stated that he inspected the college building and described it as follows: ". . . spacious and conveniently arranged lecture rooms, museums, the chemical laboratory, the spacious and beautifully filled cabinet of specimens in materia medica, and last but not least interesting, the finely arranged dissecting rooms."[27]

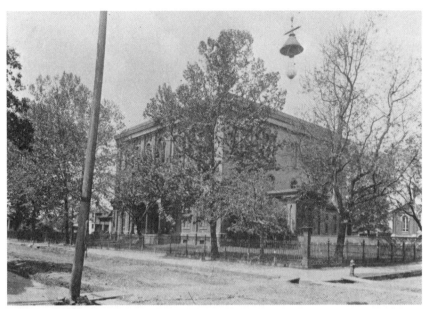

Medical College of Alabama, Mobile (1890) (Courtesy of the Alabama Museum of the Health Sciences, Lister Hill Library, Medical Center, The University of Alabama in Birmingham)

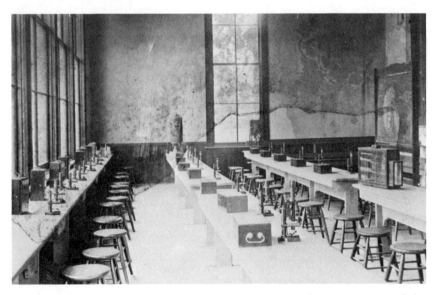

Chemistry Laboratory (circa 1900) (Courtesy of the Alabama Museum of the Health Sciences, Lister Hill Library, Medical Center, The University of Alabama in Birmingham)

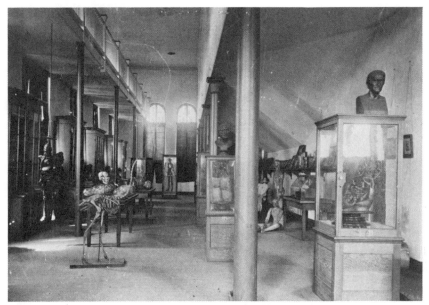

Anatomical Museum (1890) (Courtesy of the Alabama Museum of the Health Sciences, Lister Hill Library, Medical Center, The University of Alabama in Birmingham)

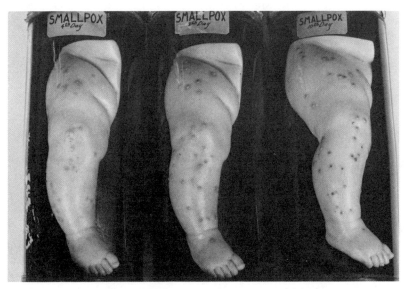

French Wax Models (Smallpox) purchased by Dr. Nott in 1860. (Courtesy of the Department of Pathology, University of Alabama School of Medicine, The University of Alabama in Birmingham)

Mr. Cloud further noted with much regret the condition he found the Medical College to be in at that time: "the dilapidated condition of the walls, plastering, etc., endangering seriously the injury and waste of many of the rare and valuable specimens in the museums which have been collected in Europe and deposited here at a cost of $70,000.00."[28] He suggested that a sufficient appropriation be made to repair the college building and to replenish the lost apparatus, especially in the chemistry department. The reconstruction legislature had just repealed the law that gave the Medical College at Mobile its only state revenue; therefore, the Medical College was denied any state funds.

Drs. William H. Anderson, George A. Ketchum, and James F. Heustis remained at the Medical College of Alabama after its reopening in 1868, but Gordon was dead and Mallet left to become Professor of Chemistry at the University of Virginia. Failing health forced both Ross and Nott into retirement: Dr. Nott moved to Baltimore and New York away from the heat and humidity of Mobile summers. New faculty members included Dr. J. T. Gilmore in Surgery, Dr. Jerome Cochran in Chemistry, Dr. E. P. Gaines in Clinical Medicine, Dr. Robinson Miller and then Dr. Goronwy Owen in Obstetrics, and Dr. E. H. Fournier in Materia Medica and Therapeutics. Dr. Anderson remained dean until 1885 when he was succeeded by Dr. Ketchum.

During the three years following the war while the school was closed, students returning from the war and wishing to study medicine were forced to look to other institutions for instruction. When the Mobile school did reopen, part of its uphill fight was to win back lost patronage.[29] In 1868–1869, there were only twenty-three matriculants, of whom only four graduated. In order to attract students the following year, the faculty announced a "free system of lectures," which required students to pay only a twenty-five-dollar matriculation fee, a ten-dollar anatomy fee, and a thirty dollar graduation fee. Rumbles of disapproval resonated from some members of the State Medical Association who said the "free system" would attract the ill-prepared and those interested in "squeezing dollars from disease."[30]

But there was little else the Medical College could do. The South lay prostrate; only a few could afford prewar tuition. Medical schools in Louisville and Nashville had been forced to cut fees, and Mobile had been forced to follow. Dr. Jerome Cochran defended the low fees for another reason. He felt that formal education was so important that it should be made more available. Speaking before the State Medical Association in 1870, he said medical schools were powerless to improve the level of education under laws allowing poorly trained physicians to practice.[31] As long as physicians did not face stringent licensing laws, they would take training at those institutions that charged the lowest fees and required the least work. Dr. Anderson examined the problem in 1881 while asking the State Association to help raise the medical school's entrance requirements and extend the length of the medical course:

> Under the present system it will not do to trust altogether the medical colleges to require a literary degree, or to make preliminary examinations before permitting students to matriculate. There are few colleges that will honestly carry out their promise. . . . The temptation to get in students both for pecuniary gain and the éclat of large classes, is too great not to be yielded to.[32]

Through Dr. Cochran's efforts, the state's second Medical Practice Act passed in 1877. It placed medical licensure under the jurisdiction of the Medical Association and authorized the boards of censors of the state and county associations to act as medical examiners. Although it was not until 1907 that the sole right to license was given to the State Board of Censors, standards of medical education in Alabama improved tremendously. During this period, however, the General Assembly steadfastly refused pleas for funds to aid medical education. Between 1868 and 1907, the state authorized less than $20,000, most of which was for repair of the Mobile school building.[33] Fees, still the school's principal financial source, were reinstated at fifty dollars in 1877 and increased to seventy-five dollars in 1881.[34]

With limited funds, the faculty maintained and improved the school as best it could. For the time being, little could be done about hiring a full-time faculty or buying much-needed modern equipment to improve instruction in the basic sciences. Instructors continued spending most of their time on private practice while teaching by didactic lectures, recitations, and demonstrations that the students merely observed. Only in anatomy were sufficient materials available to give students a thorough grounding.

Clinical branches received more attention. In the early days, clinical instruction was generally held in the private infirmaries of the faculty members. Later, in 1872, the Medical College took over the medical, surgical, and obstetrical wards of Mobile City Hospital. Three years later, the city dispensary was moved to the college building and put under faculty control. In 1879, the faculty gained control of the rest of City Hospital. The new arrangement provided that several students would be selected annually to fill the positions of apothecary and ward masters, and to do other duties as might be required by the attending physicians and surgeons. These students were given an excellent field for practical study, and in return for their services, they were furnished rooms in the hospital building and were boarded at the expense of the hospital department.[35] This practice was later extended to the Mobile and Providence Infirmaries and remained in effect until the Mobile school closed in 1920.[36]

Additional improvements took the form of new courses of study. In 1872, the school added a course in hygiene and medical jurisprudence under Dr. Cochran. In 1878, Dr. William Sanders became instructor of eye and ear diseases and four years later became instructor of histology. That same year genitourinary surgery was added with Dr. T. S. Seales as professor. About that time, a department of pharmacy apparently was opened, inasmuch as the 1879 catalog announced two pharmacy graduates for that year. The 1885 catalog announced establishment of a Chair of Pharmacy and regular pharmacy degrees, receivable "by paying for the ticket in Practical Pharmacy ($10.00) and for the diploma."[37]

Quality instruction and longer sessions also came to Mobile's medical school. The school completed installing the three-year course in 1893, thereby implementing guidelines set up by the Southern Medical College Association. The school joined the American Medical College Association in 1884 and complied with an extension of the length of sessions from four to five months. The following year daily "quizzes" were given after midterm. Announcements said they "will be so arranged as not to interfere with any lecture or other duty, and will be of great interest, especially to those who contemplate applying for graduation."[38] The quizzes formed part of a campaign to get voluntary adoption of a graded course covering three years. The catalog of 1886 stated:

> Whilst this extended term is not obligatory, its adoption by the students is urged as the best means of acquiring a thorough medical education, and insuring a successful final examination . . . and will avoid the necessity of a year's preliminary reading, so often aimless and unprofitable to the student.[39]

Even transfer students had to pass examinations in anatomy, physiology, chemistry, and materia medica before they could enroll at the Medical College of Alabama.

The 1896 catalog announced preliminary requirements for all matriculants: a letter of recommendation from a reputable physician under whom the applicant had studied and a certificate from a legally constituted high school or a superintendent of education.[40] These preliminary requirements did not apply to graduates of colleges of pharmacy, dentistry, veterinary medicine, homeopathy, and eclectic medicine or matriculants of recognized medical colleges who had completed the "elementary branches of medicine, including chemistry and biology." Laboratory training in normal and pathological anatomy, bacteriology, chemistry, and operative surgery were added to a curriculum now expanded to three sessions of six months each.

The curriculum was divided among the three years as follows: first year, anatomy—didactic and practical physiology; chemistry—didactic and practical laboratory course; materia medica and therapeutics; obstetrics, surgery, and anatomy and diseases of the eye and ear; hygiene and medical jurisprudence; and a laboratory course in histology. The second year included all the above with the addition of theory and practice of medicine, diseases of women and children, medical and surgical clinics, minor surgery, physical diagnosis, and microscopical pathology. The third year, the students took a laboratory course in pathology and bacteriology; a laboratory course in operative surgery, bandaging, and dressing; practical physical diagnosis; obstetrical operations; surgery; diseases of the eye and ear; medical and surgical clinics; theory and practice of medicine; obstetrics and diseases of women and children; hygiene and medical jurisprudence; minor surgery; chemistry and dermatology.

Despite these innovations, the Alabama school barely kept pace with developments that were then revolutionizing medical education in the United States. Influenced by spectacular advances made in Europe during the last half of the nineteenth century, many American medical schools abandoned the lecture-recitation-demonstration method of instruction in favor of an expanded role for laboratory and clinical work. Textbooks contained most of the material previously covered by lectures, so professors wanted students to spend most of their time in laboratories (the first two years) and on wards (the last years).

Such a rigorous course of instruction required students to have a thorough background in the basic sciences (college level chemistry, biology, and physics), and it required that medical schools provide well-equipped laboratories. It also meant that medical schools should have control of a teaching hospital and a faculty devoted exclusively to teaching. Funding for such facilities was expensive. In 1910, Dr. Abraham Flexner estimated minimum operating cost for a medical school of 250 students at $100,000–$150,000 per year.[41] Few schools, especially those depending on student fees for their funds, could afford such expenditures. Many poorer schools, caught between rising costs and decreasing enrollments induced by higher entrance requirements, were forced to close. The process was accelerated when, in 1904, the Council on Medical Education of the American Medical Association began classifying medical schools according to recommended standards: Class A+—acceptable; Class A—needs minor improvements; Class B—needs major improvements; Class C—needs complete reorganization.

The publication of Abraham Flexner's survey of medical education for the Carnegie Foundation, *Medical Education in United States and Canada*, appeared in 1910. Flexner's survey was to have a profound effect on medical education in Alabama as well as in the United States. His critical look at medical schools across the country was responsible for closing some schools and improving the rest.

The Medical College of Alabama, always with inadequate funds, now faced constantly rising standards of medical education. Again, the faculty did as much as possible with the limited funds available. In 1893, the school had three sessions of six months each. In 1900, the board added a fourth session, and each session was lengthened to seven months. Beginning in 1902, 80 percent attendance at lectures was required as a prerequisite for promotion to the next session.[42]

Laboratory work attained new status. A new Department of Microscopy (including histology, pathology, and bacteriology), Nervous and Mental Diseases opened in 1897 with Dr. E. D. Bondurant (1862–1950) as head of the department. He later became the school's fourth dean.

An amphitheater for clinical instruction was constructed in 1893–1894, and in 1902, a new chemical laboratory went up, the old one passing to the Department of Pharmacy.[43] Financing for such improvements came largely from increased tuition fees ($100 per session, $125 for the fourth year) and newly imposed laboratory fees. The years 1893–1910 saw attendance range from 150 to 200. The faculty had grown substantially because of the new specialized subjects. Twenty-four faculty members are mentioned in the 1897 catalog. Sizable sums were spent for equipment. Purchases for the 1895 session included: Thoma's Microtome, with freezing apparatus; Koch's Steam Sterilizer; Hot Air Sterilizer; Warm Stage and Vegetable Apparatus.[44] But the faculty realized early that without outside help it could never have the full-time instructors whose presence on a medical school staff had become essential to the status of a good medical school. So the Medical College cultivated the University of Alabama. Catalogs of the two schools appeared as one for the first time in 1896. The Medical College also approached the state for funds, but it was not until 1907 that the State Legislature, in return for investing the University Board of Trustees with complete control of the Medical College, granted the school $45,000 for the repair and addition to buildings and $5,000 annually for maintenance.[45]

It was not quite what the medical faculty wanted, since in the exchange independence was swapped for security, but the Medical College was starved for funds. With money granted by the legislature, the Medical College erected a dispensary building housing a darkroom, amphitheater, pharmacy, and several special rooms. The main building was remodeled and fitted with histology and pathology laboratories, each with twenty-four microscopes for fifty students; a newly equipped anatomy dissecting room with tables for 100 students; a bacteriology labora-

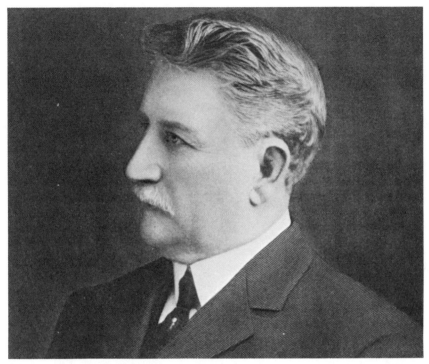

Rhett Goode, M.D., 1852–1911, Dean 1906–1912 (Courtesy of the Alabama State Department of Archives and History)

tory furnished with incubators; and a chemistry laboratory with space for 100 students.[46] The library also grew. One donation included 1,000 books bequeathed by Dr. George Ketchum, who died in 1906. Dr. Ketchum had served the school for forty-seven years as Professor of Practice and Theory of Medicine and as dean from 1885 until he was succeeded by Dr. Rhett Goode (1852–1911) in 1906.

New equipment meant increased time was spent in both laboratory instruction and clinical instruction.[47] This paved the way for introduction of courses suggested by the Council on Medical Education: anatomy, physics, chemistry (organic, inorganic, and physiologic), pharmacology, biology, embryology, histology, bacteriology, and pathology during the first two years; and therapeutics, pathology, internal medicine (including physical diagnosis, pediatrics, nervous and mental diseases), surgery (including surgical anatomy and operative surgery on the cadaver), obstetrics, gynecology, laryngology, rhinology, ophthalmology, dermatology, hygiene, and medical jurisprudence during the last two years. Legislation in 1907 had further consequences. Since the college was now a part of the University of Alabama, the first two years could be taken at the main campus in Tuscaloosa. Entrance requirements were the same as those of the university: three years of Latin; two of Greek, French, or German; three of English; two of history; three of mathematics; and one of electives.[48]

But changes were too late and too little. Early in 1909, Abraham Flexner (1866–1959) visited Mobile, the first stop on a nationwide inspection tour for the Carnegie Foundation. He issued a condemnation. Dr. Flexner had just come from studying the organization of Johns Hopkins Medical School, at that time the best in the United States and later a model for reforming medical schools across the country. Naturally, he was disappointed with Mobile.[49] Flexner said that the laboratories were too small and poorly equipped, the museum and library out of date, and the entrance requirements too low. He suggested that more money was needed to acquire a full-time faculty. Physicians, however, who inspected the school for the Council on Medical Education were impressed by the devotion of the faculty, by recent improvements, and by the possibility, suggested by 1907 appropriations, that the State Legislature might fully support the college. They continued the school's Class A rating.[50] Legislative support was problematical, since the Medical College of Alabama was not the only medical school in the state looking for governmental financial support. (See the Birmingham Medical College.)

Southern University

In 1871, the Southern University of Greensboro, Alabama, had opened a medical department staffed by five local physicians: Drs. F. M. Peterson, Professor of Materia Medica and Obstetrics; T. C. Osborn, Professor of Principles and Practice of Medicine and Medical Jurisprudence; R. Inge, Professor of Anatomy; T. O. Summers, Professor of Physiology and Chemistry; and J. O. Osborn, Professor of Principles and Practice of Surgery. Instruction was largely by lecture. Some dissecting took place in anatomy although the faculty could not persuade the trustees to build a separate dissecting room.[51] The school apparently did not operate a hospital, and it is not known what arrangements were made for the students to see patients.[52]

A graduate had to study medicine "for at least three years, under suitable instruction" and attend two full courses at Southern or attend one course at Southern and furnish proof of either four years' reputable practice or attendance at another medical institution.[53] Between 1872 and 1875, there were six graduates, most of them studying medicine in conjunction with some other subject offered at Southern.[54] After 1875, it is not known if there were any graduates. Although Southern University continued to list the medical department in its catalogs until 1880, there were apparently no classes. This was at a time when Southern University was desperately struggling to raise funds for its own needs and was simply unable to expend the large sums needed to support a medical school.

Montezuma University

In 1896, another medical school opened in Bessemer, Alabama, as a part of Montezuma University.[55] This coeducational institution was founded by J. A. B. Lovett, a minister who held a Ph.D. degree. The institution offered a course of study ranging from kindergarten through grammar school, high school, and college.[56] The schools of commerce, pedagogy, pharmacy, law, music, art, and education were all housed in a building that was the former Montezuma Hotel, hence the name of the school. Henry F. DeBardeleben, a Birmingham industrialist, brought the structure from New Orleans where it had served as the Mexican Pavilion at the New Orleans Exposition. The building contained several lecture rooms, a chemical laboratory, and an operating room. An anatomy room was in a separate building. Some of these rooms were reequipped for the 1898–1899 session.[57] The main building also housed students for twelve dollars each per month.

The first faculty was made up of seventeen professors and lecturers among whom were J. A. B. Lovett, president and Professor of Chemistry, Toxicology and Forensic Medicine; Drs. J. C. Carson, dean and Professor of Gynecology; E. P. Lacy, second dean and Professor of Surgery; and W. H. Johnston, dean of the School of Pharmacy and Professor of Materia Medica and Therapeutics. Although catalogs pointed out the practical experience to be gained from the numerous patients of Jefferson County's industrial area, most instruction was by "the recitation and the lecture methods [with] the recitation method [being] given the prominence its merits demand."[58] The school did not have control over a hospital, and applied work seems to have consisted of "practical operations upon the cadaver [or] lower animals." Senior students did assist instructors of surgery during operations on private patients and performed some urinalyses.

Both entrance and graduation requirements were low. However, after 1898, the entrance requirements were similar to those of the Medical College of Alabama. Matriculants for the first session were required to present a certificate of prior attendance before starting the second session, meanwhile taking courses in other departments of the University. How students managed this since the catalog stated "the lectures and clinical instruction will occupy all of the student's time," was not explained. To graduate, a student was required to attend three lecture courses of not less than six months each in three separate years. During the three-year period, the student "must have dissected in two courses of clinical instruction," and attended lectures in chemistry, operative surgery, bacteriology, and histology.[59] The catalogs detailed nothing about twelve other medical subjects offered by the college. How many students attended Montezuma University Medical College is not known, but three graduated in 1896 and five in 1897. Then just before the third session began, the main building burned. The insurance was insufficient to replace the building, and although Dr. Lovett struggled for several years to start the school again, he was unsuccessful.

Birmingham Medical College

A third medical school in the state, which was to rival the Mobile school for state funds, was organized in the rapidly developing Jefferson County. The Birmingham Medical College was a proprietary school owned by nine Birmingham physicians. Among them were the surgeons J. D. S. and W. E. B. Davis; Drs. W. H. Johnston, president of the Medical Association of the State of Alabama in 1896; B. L. Wyman, past secretary of the state association; R. M. Cunningham, director of the Tennessee Coal, Iron and Railroad Company's hospitals; J. C. LeGrande (1854–1906), editor of the *Alabama Medical and Surgical Age*; and B. G. Copeland, owner of one of the most successful infirmaries in Birmingham. These men, according to a charter issued in 1897 by the General Assembly, controlled the school's curriculum, entrance requirements, granting of degrees, and as stockholders were entitled to a 6 percent return on their investment.[60] The stock was not inheritable or collectable for debt and, upon death of a shareholder, reverted to the company. The remaining physicians then had the right to reissue the stock but only to a local physician willing to become a member of the faculty and to open his infirmary for clinical instruction.[61]

The school opened October 1, 1894, at the old Lunsford Hotel at 209 and 211 North Twenty-first Street in Birmingham, a building shared

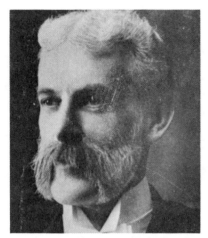

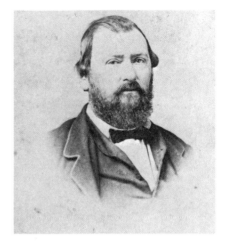

John Clark LeGrande, M.D.,
1854–1906 (Courtesy of the Alabama
Museum of the Health Sciences,
Lister Hill Library, Medical Center,
The University of Alabama
in Birmingham)

George Summers Brown, M.D.,
1860–1913
(Courtesy of Dr. Julius Linn, Jr.)

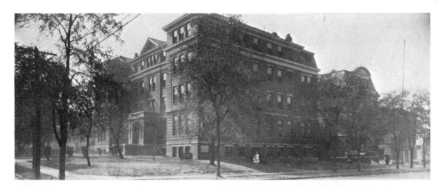

Hillman Hospital with the Birmingham Medical College to the right (Courtesy of
the Alabama Museum of the Health Sciences, Lister Hill Library, Medical
Center, The University of Alabama in Birmingham)

with the Birmingham Dental College (an institution that in 1910 joined the Birmingham Medical College to form the Birmingham Medical, Dental and Pharmaceutical College). The building was five stories tall, carpeted throughout, and had electric lighting. It contained offices, reception rooms, and two large lecture rooms, plus clinical, microscopic and histological laboratories. It also housed a free dispensary, open daily from noon to 1:00 P.M., where clinical instruction was given. For the rest of the clinical material, the college depended on the city charity hospital, two infirmaries owned by members of the faculty, and clinics in the surrounding villages.[62]

As a member of the Southern Medical College Association, the Birmingham Medical College had the same entrance requirements as the Medical College of Alabama in Mobile: an apprenticeship with a reputable physician and a diploma from a high school or a certificate from a superintendent of education. To graduate, the student had to be twenty-one years of age, of good character, and must have attended three lecture courses of six months each. The last course had to be taken at the Birmingham school. The subjects taught were: principles and practice of medicine and clinical medicine (Dr. W. H. Johnston); materia medica and therapeutics and diseases of children (Dr. H. N. Rosser); physiology (Dr. J. H. McCarty); principles and practice of surgery and clinical surgery (Dr. J. D. S. Davis); gynecology and abdominal surgery (Dr. W. E. B. Davis); practical anatomy and clinical surgery (Dr. B. G. Copeland); chemistry and toxicology (J. A. B. Lovett); oral surgery and special pathology (Dr. T. M. Allen); microscopy, bacteriology, and normal and pathological histology (Dr. Cunningham Wilson); eye, ear, and throat (Dr. L. G. Woodson); physical diagnosis and clinical medicine (Dr. R. M. Cunningham); and obstetrics (Dr. George S. Brown); hygiene and medical jurisprudence (Dr. J. C. LeGrande); and neurology (Dr. E. D. Bondurant).[63] Only bacteriology and pathological histology had a prerequisite, and that was normal histology. The rest of the courses were taught to first-, second-, and third-year students. The only stipulation was that anatomy and physical diagnosis were to be undertaken for two terms and that clinical microscopy was to be studied in the third year. Since the courses were not graded, professors had to make sure they were reaching poorly prepared students, who frequently kept the level and quality of instruction at a low level.[64]

The descriptions of the courses of study listed in the college catalog suggested that great value was placed on practical work. Physical diagnosis and clinical medicine were taught so that students would "examine cases for themselves under the direction of the Professor." The catalog said that in gynecology "special prominence will be given to clinical instruction," but again most instruction was in the form of lectures, as evidenced by a list of courses for the 1899–1900 session.[65] At that time, Birmingham Medical College was changing to a four-year course. Under the new system, the first two years were separated from the last two years with more qualified students taking more specialized courses. Although all courses were fully graded by 1910, the method of instruction remained the same, mostly lectures. This is the outline for the fourth year of the Birmingham Medical College for 1899–1900:

Theory and Practice of Medicine—two lectures and one recitation per week; Clinical Medicine—two clinical lectures and bedside instruction; Physical Diagnosis—one lecture and practical work at the hospital; General Surgery—two lectures and one recitation; Clinical Surgery—two clinical lectures and operative surgery in sections; Minor Surgery and Fracture Dressing—one lecture and one practical demonstration; Genito-Urinary Surgery—one clinical lecture; Obstetrics—two lectures, one recitation and one practical instruction under supervision; Gynecology and Abdominal Surgery—two lectures and one clinic; Diseases of Children—one clinical lecture; Neurology—two lectures; Ear, Eye, Nose and Throat—two lectures and one clinic; Clinical Microscopy—two hours in the laboratory.[66]

Laboratory branches suffered especially from the lack of practical work; physiology and materia medica had no assigned laboratory time, while histology and clinical microscopy had only two hours each per day. Only in anatomy with twelve hours and in chemistry with four hours was there sufficient practical instruction.

In spite of weaknesses, the Birmingham school was successful. It filled a need in North Alabama, and enrollment climbed from thirty-two in 1894 to ninety-four in 1902.[67] The outstanding surgery department was led by the Davis brothers, who gained national reputations for their experimental surgery on dogs.[68] By 1900, the quarters at 209 and 211 North Twenty-first Street were crowded; and like the Medical College in Mobile, the Birmingham school faced pressures to improve its facilities and instruction. Steps in this direction had begun in 1899 when the number of sessions was increased to four, and when neurology, hygiene, and medical jurisprudence were added to the curriculum. A year later, dermatology was also added to the list of courses.[69]

In 1902, the faculty increased the stock of the company from $15,000 to $75,000 and built a modern four-story building on a lot at Avenue F and Twentieth Street South. The school now had three large amphitheaters seating 250 each, and the chemistry, bacteriology, and histology-pathology laboratories were expanded. The entire top floor was assigned to the anatomy department. The school also had offices, a lounge, and reading areas for students.[70] During the school year 1903, clinical facilities expanded rapidly with acquisition of staff control of the adjoining Hillman Hospital and its ninety-eight beds. In 1908, the arrangement was extended for ninety-nine years, with the faculty maintaining complete control of the hospital staff in return for providing two medical student scholarships annually and for providing nursing instruction.[71]

As in the case of the Medical College of Alabama in Mobile, these improvements did not satisfy Abraham Flexner. He condemned the lax enforcement of entrance requirements; small and poorly equipped laboratories, library, and museum; and the lack of full-time instructors.[72] This time the Council on Medical Education of the American Medical Association agreed with Flexner. In August, 1910, it classified the Birmingham Medical College as a Class B school.[73] Dr. W. P. Colwell, secretary of the council, suggested the following measures: steady improvement of entrance requirements until they equalled those of the University of Alabama; lengthening each session from twenty-eight to thirty weeks; keeping attendance records; graded courses; requiring students to pass all courses in one year before advancing to the next one; adding physiology, physiological chemistry, and pharmacology laboratories; and, above all, employment of five or six full-time instructors of the laboratory sciences.[74] In the opinion of the council, no defect was as serious as the proprietary status of the Birmingham school, for as such it could not ask for the outside help necessary to finance the recommended changes. Dr. Colwell suggested that Birmingham seek affiliation with the University of Alabama and start a local fund-raising campaign.

Eager to regain the school's Class A status, the faculty set out to institute reform. By judicious use of student fees ($21,471.60 in 1910–1911 and $25,485.15 in 1911–1912), the college building was renovated. Laboratories, library, and museum were set up in time for the 1910–1911 session.[75] In 1911, a special pathology building was opened, complete with amphitheater and laboratory where students could perform laboratory work on assigned patients. A year later, Jefferson County voted a $100,000 bond issue for enlargement of the Hillman Hospital, and in 1913, a regularly scheduled outpatient dispensary began operation. The faculty also took steps to enforce entrance and attendance requirements. Clinical and laboratory work came to dominate the instruction, and the four yearly sessions became separate and distinct. All courses became fully graded by 1908.[76]

The school launched a local fund-raising campaign, and in 1911, the State Legislature was asked to give Birmingham Medical College half the $5,000 annual grant of the Medical College of Alabama at Mobile. In 1912, the Birmingham Medical School was handed over to an independent board of trustees, and the University of Alabama was approached concerning a possible takeover of the Birmingham Medical College. These maneuverings understandably influenced the Mobile school, which felt its existence threatened. There was a danger of an unsavory regional political fight, but Dr. George Denny, president of the University of Alabama, arranged a compromise that transformed the Birmingham Medical College into the Graduate School of Medicine of the University of Alabama.[77]

The Birmingham property, valued at $60,000, was given to the University and undergraduate instruction ceased with the graduation of the class of 1915. The faculty of the Birmingham Medical College resigned, and most of them accepted reappointment in the graduate school. The new school aimed at both training specialized physicians and keeping local general practitioners abreast of the latest medical developments.[78] Therefore, any graduate of an accepted medical college or a licensed physician could attend, and the curriculum was arranged so that a physician would be away from his practice as short a time as possible. Sessions of nine months were subdivided into three-month and six-week periods. Courses were in such general areas as medicine and physical diagnosis (Course A), surgery (Course B), and the basic sciences (Course C). There were also courses specifically designed for local practitioners who were unable to take time away from their private practices. A special Course E in general pathology met from 7:30 A.M. to 9:30 A.M. twice a week for six months.

The graduate school opened September, 1913, but records are not available as to how many students attended sessions or if there were any graduates. In 1912, all graduates of the Birmingham Medical College became alumni of the University and received diplomas upon payment of the usual fee.[79] In that same year, a bill providing funds to operate the graduate school was vetoed by Governor Charles Henderson (governor of Alabama, 1915–1919), a balance-sheet conservative.[80] The wound was fatal. The University was unable to keep its part of the agreement, and after graduation of the Class of 1915, the Graduate School of Medicine in Birmingham closed its doors. The property, which reverted to the physicians who originally owned the college, served for a time as a high school building, then as an outpatient building, and later as the nurses' residence of the Hillman Hospital.

With the failure of the Birmingham Medical College, the Medical Department of the University of Alabama in Mobile (The Medical College of Alabama) was the only medical school in Alabama; but this school also had difficulties. Just as in the case of the Birmingham school, the state refused to supply funds necessary to operate a Class A school in Mobile. In Mobile, however, the school managed to survive on the limited funds available. There were even small improvements. New specimens were purchased for the museum, and the library began to subscribe to a number of foreign and domestic journals. A comparative anatomy building was erected in 1911, and the hours of the Medical School Dispensary were lengthened. In 1912, each of the laboratory sciences was assigned separate laboratories; and after decreasing the salaries of other professors (several were not paid at all), the instructors of anatomy, physiology, chemistry, pathology, histology, bacteriology, physiological chemistry, and pharmacology became full-time teachers.[81] Laboratory work and bedside instruction finally became the predominant methods of instruction.

During this time, entrance requirements steadily rose. In 1910, a greater effort was made to enforce the requirement, adopted in 1907, of fourteen units of high school work. Two years later, the school eliminated the practice of allowing students to present high school certificates at the beginning of the second year in medical school. In 1914, a year of college with courses in chemistry, biology, physics, and foreign language was required. A year later, the school required two years of college to conform to a similar requirement of the State Medical Licensing Board.[82] Unfortunately, as requirements rose, enrollment fell. In 1909, the entering class numbered forty-three, and a year later it numbered twenty-seven. In 1915, when a full college load was required for the first time, the number dropped to nine. For a school that depended almost exclusively on student fees for its operating funds, this proved disastrous. The faculty, under the leadership of Dean Tucker Frazer (1859–1920), struggled valiantly; but the end became only a matter of time.[83]

The situation was made no easier by the practice of playing politics with the funding from the State Legislature for the Medical Department of the University of Alabama in Mobile.

Birmingham had never given up hope. Flexner had recommended it as the best possible location for a medical school. Birmingham continued to take a lively interest in the State Legislature's discussions of the Mobile school's annual budget request. In 1915, Dr. E. P. Hogan, former secretary of the Birmingham Medical College who had been elected to the State Legislature, cosponsored a bill providing that, if it became impossible to maintain a Class A school in Mobile, the medical school would be moved to Birmingham. Dr. Hogan got only half a loaf, for the bill passed without specifying a new location.[84] Lack of a location clause was very much to the taste of Dr. George Denny, who hoped that eventually all departments of the University of Alabama would be housed in Tuscaloosa.[85] He publicly maintained that the University had a moral obligation to keep the medical school in Mobile, and he endeavored, at least on the surface, to raise the funds it required. In 1919, however, he requested that the AMA Council on Medical Education

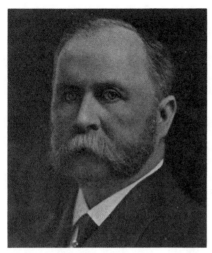

Tucker Henderson Frazer, M.D., 1859–1920, Dean 1916–1920 (Courtesy of the Heustis Medical Museum, Mobile, Alabama)

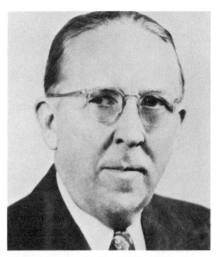

Clyde Brooks, M.D., 1881–1962, Dean 1920–1928 (Courtesy of the Alabama Museum of the Health Sciences, Lister Hill Library, Medical Center, The University of Alabama in Birmingham)

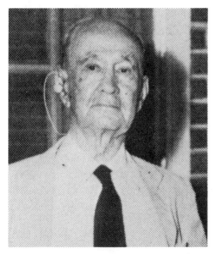

Daniel Thompson McCall, M.D., 1869–1955, Dean 1920. Dean Frazer died in office and was succeeded by Dr. McCall. (Courtesy of the Heustis Medical Museum, Mobile, Alabama)

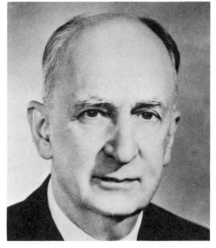

Stuart Graves, M.D., 1879–1954, Dean 1928–1945 (Courtesy of the Alabama Museum of the Health Sciences, Lister Hill Library, Medical Center, The University of Alabama in Birmingham)

reevaluate the school in Mobile in an attempt to have the entire Medical College moved to Tuscaloosa. This proved to be a fatal blow.

Result of the inspection was foregone. Dr. H. D. Arnold of Harvard, who headed the group surveying the school, stated:

> Even more serious, in my opinion, than the lack of financial resources and physical equipment and the limitation of clinical opportunities, is the lack of appreciation on the part of the school authorities of what modern medical education should be. I say this regretfully—with full appreciation of the genuine devotion and loyalty of these men to the school and the personal sacrifices made by many in its behalf. Their fundamental conception, however, is too near to that of the old-time medical school. . . . It is clear that the authorities have tried, with the limited means at command, to meet the advanced requirements as stated on paper.
>
> Under the circumstances it would seem wiser for the University of Alabama to abandon the attempt to conduct a four-year medical school, and to confine its efforts in undergraduate medical education for the present to the development of a really first class medical school which gives the training of the first two years of the medical course.[86]

The trustees of the University implemented the recommendation. Dr. Jack P. Montgomery, Professor of Organic Chemistry, was commissioned to transfer two boxcar loads of chemicals, equipment, and anatomical models to Tuscaloosa from Mobile. These were temporarily stored in two United States Army barracks and in 1922 were moved to the newly constructed Josiah Clark Nott Hall. Dean Clyde Brooks (1881–1962) served simultaneously as Professor of Physiology, Physiological Chemistry and Pharmacology. Much of the instruction was done by assistants who had finished only two or more years of medical school.[87] About fifty freshmen matriculated each year, a number that was increased to sixty in 1928. Most of these took the so-called combined course, which lasted four years and enabled them to earn the bachelor of science degree as well as attend the first two years of the medical course. In this way, a student could get both B.S. and M.D. degrees in six years. He simply transferred to another institution for the two years of clinical work. The school quickly regained its Class A status, but this success did not satisfy many physicians in the state.

The Four-Year Medical College in Birmingham

Col. Hopson Owen Murfee (1874–1942) is the unsung architect of what has come to be one of the outstanding medical centers in the nation.[88] It all began in 1936 when he organized a private citizens' committee to promote better medical facilities for Alabama, among which would be a four-year medical school. Murfee was convinced that health care in Alabama was lagging and that preventive medicine would keep more people healthy and reduce the need for hospitalization. There were prominent names of the time connected with the Alabama Citizens' Committee for the State Hospitals and the Public Health. (See Chapter 13, "The History of the Mental Health Movement in Alabama" for the committee members.)

Colonel Murfee, the founder, executive secretary, and director of the Citizens' Committee, worked without pay or public office and almost single-handedly made the people aware, as never before, of the health needs of the state.

Colonel Murfee was a prominent citizen of Prattville, Alabama, who spent a lifetime in educational work. He held an A.B. and M.A. from the University of Virginia. The University of Alabama conferred an LL.D. on him in 1913. He served as an instructor of mathematics at the University of Virginia and was later a fellow in physics at the University of Chicago. While there, he was a research assistant on the famous physics team of Drs. R. A. Milligan and A. A. Michaelson. Later, he became professor of physics and eventually succeeded his father as president of Marion Military Institute, Marion, Alabama, and served from 1905 to 1918.

Colonel Murfee and his committee's first target was the mental institutions of the state. Murfee obtained a million dollar appropriation for the state mental hospitals, and once this was secured, he turned the committee's attention to the need for establishment of a state medical center. His concept of the center included facilities for education, research, statewide health service, prevention of disease, and conservation of health.

Murfee visited some of the outstanding hospitals and health facilities in the nation to garner the best thinking on this subject. Specifically, he wanted more information concerning the necessary procedures for replacing the two-year medical school in Tuscaloosa with a four-year facility. He was also concerned with the question of whether the school would remain on the Tuscaloosa campus or be moved to a larger city. Many prominent medical educators in the country responded.[89]

Agitation for a four-year school began almost immediately after the closing of the Mobile school. In 1928, Dr. J. D. S. Davis, president of the Medical Association of the State of Alabama, suggested that the association appoint a committee to discuss with the president and trustees of the University the possibility of opening a four-year school.[90] That same year, Dr. Stuart Graves (1879–1954), newly appointed dean of the Medical Department of the University of Alabama, toured the state speaking before county medical societies about the need for a four-year medical school. In 1938, through Dr. Graves's efforts, two committees were organized, one made up of alumni of the University and the other of members of the State Medical Association. Drs. W. D. Partlow, J. P. Collier, E. V. Caldwell, and S. A. Gordon were appointed to a standing committee by the Alumni Association of the Medical Department. The committee's objective, like that of Colonel Murfee, was a four-year medical college. Dr. W. D. Partlow, superintendent of the Alabama Hospitals for the Insane, was the chairman of both committees.

Later, the work of the alumni committee was taken over by the Medical Association of the State, and Drs. S. L. Ledbetter, B. F. Austin, John H. Blue, Emmett B. Frazer, P. P. Salter, and A. M. Walker were added to the committee. The work of these men, together with Dr. Graves's unrelenting efforts, was largely responsible for producing the political interest and public desire that resulted in the creation of the four-year medical college of Alabama. In 1942 at the Medical Association's meeting in Montgomery, President J. M. Mason pushed the campaign toward a successful end when he appealed to the association "to bring to bear its great influence in obtaining a four-year school."[91] Colonel Murfee died in 1942 at age sixty-eight, too soon to see the tangible results of his efforts, which were to come six months later.

By 1943, Governor Chauncey Sparks had been won over and, in his inaugural address, he recommended establishment of a four-year medical school.[92] The State Legislature responded with Act No. 89, which established "The Medical College of Alabama," through appropriation of $1 million for buildings and equipment and $366,750 for annual maintenance. An additional $25,000 was provided for the use of the building commission.

A modern four-year medical college was now assured. On March 14, 1944, Governor Sparks appointed the Advisory Board for the proposed school. The Advisory Board consisted of Dr. W. M. Salter of Anniston for a five-year term, Dr. James S. McLester of Birmingham for four years, Dr. J. Mac Bell of Mobile for three years, Dr. W. D. Partlow of Tuscaloosa for two years, and Dr. Harry Lee Jackson of Birmingham for one year. Also Dr. Stuart Graves, dean of the School of Medicine, was appointed an *ex-officio* member by the governor.[93]

The Building Commission was also appointed by Governor Sparks to select a location for the school. On August 17, 1943, the governor appointed the following to the Building Commission: Dr. W. D. Partlow of Tuscaloosa, B. Lonnie Noojin of Gadsden, Dr. T. J. Jones of Marion, James C. Lee, Sr., of Birmingham, Dr. Fred Wilkinson of Montgomery, A. F. Delchamps of Mobile, Dr. C. L. Salter of Talladega, H. A. Berg of Birmingham, and Gordon Madison, Esq., of Tuscaloosa.[94] The governor served as chairman. This committee had the arduous and important task of choosing the best place to establish the four-year medical college.

The commission was divided into two subcommittees: the Building Committee and the Contract Committee. The Building Committee was composed of A. F. Delchamps, Lonnie Noojin, and Dr. W. D. Partlow (chairman). Gordon Madison, Esq., James C. Lee, Sr., and Dr. C. L. Salter made up the Contract Committee. The cities of Mobile, Tuscaloosa, and Birmingham were the front-runners for the location of the medical college. Finally, on February 16, 1944, after a long and careful study and after many public hearings, the committee adopted a resolution locating the college in Birmingham. No other city could rival the offer made to the University of the Jefferson–Hillman Hospital complex.

. Mr. Oscar Wells was chairman of the Citizens Committee of Birmingham. This committee raised $150,000 to purchase a block of property to be given to the new center.[95] Victor H. Hanson, W. D. Moore, Walter E. Henley, Jesse Yeates, Herbert C. Stockham, W. J. Christian, James E. Mills, Robert Gregg, Joseph H. Loveman, Charles E. Oakes, Ed L. Norton, George A. Mattison, Jr., Robert Meyer, Frank E. Spain, and L. E. Foster were members of the Citizens Committee. The following physicians assisted the Citizens Committee: Drs. James S. McLester, John D. Sherrill, C. N. Carraway, D. S. Moore, Harry Lee Jackson, Walter F. Scott, E. C. Ray, C. J. Colquitt, C. B. Bray, and Stanley Tullsen.[96]

Dr. Roy Rachford Kracke was appointed dean of the Medical College of Alabama on August 1, 1944. The first freshman class was admitted on October 8, 1945. Clinical instruction had started earlier, many students having transferred from Tuscaloosa to Birmingham for their last two years, and the first class graduated on October 25, 1946.[97]

The Early Development of the University of Alabama
School of Medicine

There were four factors that entered into the medical school's progress and its contributions to the development of an outstanding medical center. These factors were faculty, space, money, and students. The original faculty was made up of the existing faculty of the former two-year school in Tuscaloosa and of more than seventy-five leading Birmingham physicians who served on a part-time basis. The following physicians served as division chiefs in 1944: Dr. James S. McLester, chief of Medicine; Dr. J. M. Mason, chief of Surgery; Dr. James R. Garber, chief of Obstetrics; Dr. Alfred A. Walker, chief of Pediatrics; Dr. John Sherrill, chief of Orthopedics; Dr. W. N. Jones, chief of Gynecology; Dr. Gilbert E. Fisher, chief of Otolaryngology and Bronchoscopy; Dr. D.

Baker, chief of Pathology; Dr. Walter Scott, chief of Urology; Dr. George Denison, chief of Public Health and Preventive Medicine; Dr. J. W. MacQueen, chief of Hospital Administration; Dr. Charles M. Goss, chief of Anatomy; Dr. John M. Bruhn, chief of Physiology; Dr. Robert Teague, chief of Pharmacology; Dr. Ralph McBurney, chief of Bacteriology and Laboratory Diagnosis; and Dr. Emmett B. Carmichael, chief of Biochemistry. Dr. Kracke emphasized his good fortune in acquiring a faculty of such quality during war conditions and said,

> The fact that we are able to open the Medical College of Alabama at this critical time when the country is at war and more than 60,000 physicians are away in the military service is due in part to the willingness and spirit of self-sacrifice on the part of our practicing physicians who are willing to devote much of their valuable time to the instruction of young doctors.[98]

On June 3, 1945, the medical school added the following physicians to its staff: Drs. R. O. Noojin, Professor of Dermatology and Syphilology; Louis L. Freidman, director of the Outpatient Clinic; John Carangelo, Assistant Professor of Obstetrics; Robert Guthrie, part-time instructor in Surgery; William H. Riser, Jr., Assistant Professor of Pathology; Joseph Donald, Assistant Professor of Surgery; Edgar Givhan, Jr., Assistant Professor of Medicine; J. Garber Galbraith, Assistant Professor of Neurosurgery; James S. McLester, Professor of Medicine; Seale Harris, Professor Emeritus of Medicine; and Stuart Graves, dean emeritus. Miss Virginia Baxley became the registrar, and Paul Schatz was the business manager.[99]

Deans of the University of Alabama
School of Medicine

Mobile*

William Henry Anderson	1859–1861
William Henry Anderson	1868–1885
George Augustus Ketchum	1885–1906
Rhett Goode	1906–1912
Eugene DuBose Bondurant	1912–1916
Tucker Henderson Frazer	1916–1920
Daniel Thompson McCall	1920

Tuscaloosa

Clyde Brooks	1920–1928
Stuart Graves	1928–1945

---

*The Mobile school was originally The Medical College of Alabama from 1859 to 1920. In 1897, the Mobile school became affiliated with the University of Alabama and in 1920 was moved to Tuscaloosa as a two-year medical school.

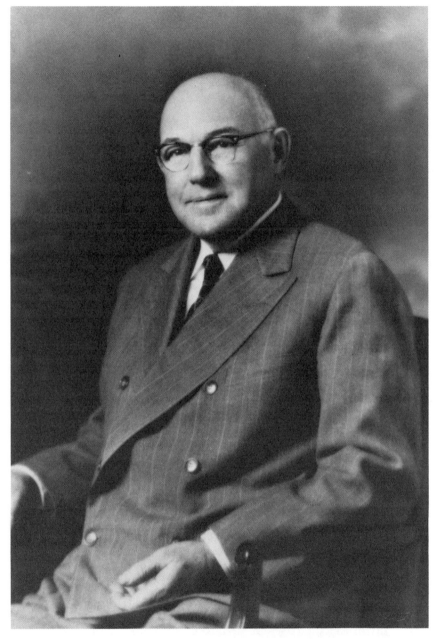

James Johnson Durrett, M.D., 1889–1974, Dean 1951–1955 (Courtesy of Mrs. James J. Durrett and Dr. James Joseph Durrett)

Birmingham

Roy Rachford Kracke	1944–1950
Tinsley Randolph Harrison	1950–1951 (acting dean)
James J. Durrett	1951–1955
Robert C. Berson	1955–1962
Samuel Richardson Hill, Jr.	1962–1968
Clifton K. Meador	1968–1973
James A. Pittman, Jr.	1973–

The Medical Center Today

In 1945, the School of Medicine had been moved to Birmingham from the University campus at Tuscaloosa and became a four-year school. This was the beginning of what later became the Medical Center. That same year, the State Legislature created the School of Dentistry, but its first class was not enrolled until 1948. In 1966, the University of Alabama School of Nursing was moved to Birmingham from the Tuscaloosa campus; and in 1969, the School of Optometry opened.[100] In 1969, the State Legislature established the School of Community and Allied Health Resources to include the School of Health Services Administration, which had been established in 1966. Today this is the School of Community and Allied Health.

The University of Alabama Hospitals, according to the school's catalog of 1979–1980, is the heart of the Medical Center and provides

- professional, technical and human concern services for patients and their families from every county in Alabama and beyond. With exceptional facilities for diagnosis and the specialized care involved in acute general medical and surgical services, the Medical Center is ranked among the finest regional centers for comprehensive health care.

The University of Alabama System, composed of The University of Alabama, Tuscaloosa, The University of Alabama in Birmingham, and The University of Alabama in Huntsville, was created in 1969. The Medical College of Alabama, located in Birmingham, became known as the University of Alabama School of Medicine in 1969.

The State Legislature recognized a need for coordinating the medical education programs throughout the state, especially within the newly formed system, and mandated a study for such a plan. The resulting program, adopted by the Board of Trustees in 1972, was called the University of Alabama System Medical Education Program (UASMEP), encompassing the University's medical education and residency programs, but specifically excluded nursing. In 1979, the Board of Trustees of The University of Alabama placed all medical education under the auspices of the University of Alabama School of Medicine.

In the undergraduate medical education program, the first two "basic science" years are taught on the main campus of the University of Alabama School of Medicine in Birmingham; the last two "clinical years" are divided among the main campus and the two branch campuses of the School of Medicine at The University of Alabama in Huntsville and The University of Alabama (Tuscaloosa). The three campuses interact in numerous ways to provide this education, most specifically in the elective and residency programs available to the students.

Outstanding Medical Educators at The University of Alabama in Birmingham

Roy Rachford Kracke

The opening of the new four-year medical school in 1945 attracted a number of outstanding scientists and teachers to the state. Among these was Dr. Roy Rachford Kracke (1897–1950), a widely known hematologist.[101]

He was born in Hartselle, Alabama, and received his M.D. degree from Rush Medical College, University of Chicago. After graduation, he joined the faculty of the School of Medicine, Emory University, where he served until 1944 as Professor of Pathology, Bacteriology and Laboratory Diagnosis. Dr. Kracke was the author of the textbook entitled *Diseases of the Blood and Atlas of Hematology* and also editor of the *Textbook of Clinical Pathology*.*

In 1934, Dr. Kracke was awarded a certificate of honor from the American Medical Association for his research on the relationship of the drug aminopyrine to the occurrence of agranulocytosis in young women. Also in 1934, he was awarded the Ward Burdick gold medal from the American Society of Clinical Pathologists. In 1935, he was awarded the Hardeman Cup for Medical Research by the Medical Association of Georgia. The University of Chattanooga conferred on him the honorary degree of LL.D. in 1946.

Dr. Kracke resigned his position at Emory University to become the dean of the newly opened four-year medical school in Birmingham, Alabama on August 1, 1944. Under his leadership the new medical school made great strides.

Diseases of the Blood and Atlas of Hematology was published by J. B. Lippincott Company, Philadelphia, 1941, and the *Textbook of Clinical Pathology* was published by Williams and Wilkins, Baltimore, 1940. Dr. Kracke also was author of *Color Atlas of Hematology* which was published by J. B. Lippincott Company, Philadelphia, 1947.

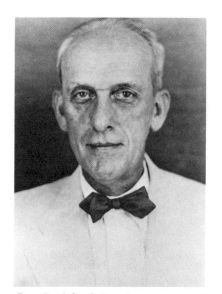

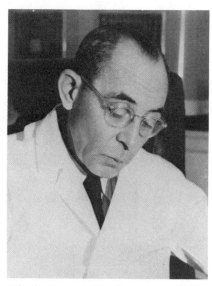

Roy Rachford Kracke, M.D., 1897–1950, Dean 1944–1950 (Courtesy of the Alabama Museum of the Health Sciences, Lister Hill Library, Medical Center, The University of Alabama in Birmingham)

Tinsley Randolph Harrison, M.D., 1900–1978 (Courtesy of the Alabama Museum of the Health Sciences, Lister Hill Library, Medical Center, The University of Alabama in Birmingham)

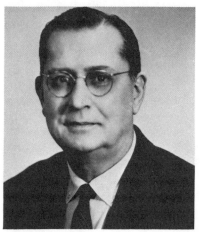

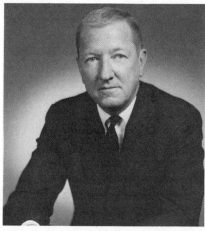

Champ Lyons, M.D., 1907–1965 (Courtesy of the Alabama Museum of the Health Sciences, Lister Hill Library, Medical Center, The University of Alabama in Birmingham)

Walter Benedict Frommeyer, M.D., 1916–1979 (Courtesy of Mrs. Walter B. Frommeyer)

Tinsley Randolph Harrison

Dr. Tinsley Randolph Harrison (1900-1978) was one of the great teachers of medical students and a cardiologist of international fame.[102] He was born near Talladega, Alabama, son of an Alabama physician, Dr. W. G. Harrison, the grandson of an Alabama physician and of four additional grandfathers in succession who had been physicians.

He was educated at the medical school at Johns Hopkins University, where he received the M.D. degree with distinction in 1922. His graduate training was at Johns Hopkins and the Peter Bent Brigham hospitals. He served as chief resident in Medicine at Vanderbilt at the same time that Dr. Alfred Blalock (1899–1964), who later became a world renowned cardiac surgeon, was chief resident in Surgery. He then studied in Vienna, Austria, and in Freiburg and Breisgau, Germany.

As Assistant Professor of Medicine at Vanderbilt University Medical School from 1928 to 1932 and as Associate Professor from 1932 to 1941, Dr. Harrison was known for his outstanding scientific studies on cardiovascular physiology and disease. His book entitled *Failure of the Circulation* was a landmark in clarifying the mechanisms of the symptoms of heart failure.* He was a pioneer in clinical investigation.

Dr. Harrison served as the first full-time professor and chairman of departments of medicine at three schools in three states: at the new schools of Bowman Gray in Winston-Salem in 1941, at Southwestern Medical School in Dallas in 1944, and at the Medical College of Alabama in Birmingham in 1950. At each of these schools, he is remembered for his ability to excite and inspire students and members of the faculty.

Dr. Harrison was the first Distinguished Professor and the first Distinguished Faculty Lecturer at The University of Alabama in Birmingham Medical Center. Also, he was the second Distinguished Physician in the United States Veterans' Administration; the winner of the Kober Medal, the highest award to an internist in the United States, given by the Association of American Physicians; and was the Billings Lecturer for the American Medical Association. Dr. Harrison was the recipient of silver and gold awards from the American Heart Association, the Honor Award of the American Medical Writers' Association, the Distinguished Service Award of the American Medical Association, a Fellowship in the American Academy of Arts and Sciences, the Honorary Doctor of Science Degree from the University of Alabama, a Mastership and Distinguished Teacher Award of the American College of Physicians, and membership in the Alabama Academy of Honor.

Harrison's textbook, *Principles of Internal Medicine*, became a classic in medical literature in the 1950s–1980s. It is now in its ninth edition and

---

Failure of the Circulation was published by Williams and Wilkins, Baltimore, 1939.

available in nine languages.* He was also coauthor of a book on ischemic heart disease and the author of a book on the future of health care in the United States.** His service at the new medical school in Birmingham, both as chairman of the Department of Medicine and as acting dean, furnished a solid foundation on which the University's Medical Center grew to its present position of international prestige. Dr. Harrison served as acting dean of the Medical College of Alabama after Dr. Kracke's death in June of 1950, and until Dr. James J. Durrett became dean in 1951.

Dr. Harrison wrote words of dedication for the medical profession which have been widely reproduced and have become an enduring beacon to the profession:

> No greater opportunity, responsibility, or obligation can fall to the lot of a human being than to become a physician. In the care of suffering he needs technical skill, scientific knowledge and human understanding. He who uses these with courage, with humility and with wisdom will provide a unique service for his fellowman, and will build an enduring edifice of character within himself. The physician should ask of his destiny no more than this, he should be content with no less!

Champ Lyons

Dr. Champ Lyons (1907–1965) was a native of Lancaster, Pennsylvania, but spent most of his life in Mobile.[103] He attended Harvard Medical School where he held the James Jackson Cabot Research Fellowship in Physiology. He graduated *cum laude* in 1931, and following his internship and residency at Massachusetts General Hospital, he studied in London under the auspices of the Mosely Traveling Fellowship in Surgery in 1936–1937.

He was the first full-time Professor of Surgery and chairman of the Department of Surgery at the Medical Center at The University of Alabama in Birmingham. He was a Fellow of the American College of Surgeons and a member of many prestigious associations and societies, including the Society of University Surgeons. He was a founding member of the Southern Society for Clinical Investigation.

During Dr. Lyons's tour of duty in the United States Army in World War II, he was widely recognized for his work in the surgical investiga-

---

Principles of Internal Medicine was originally published by Blakiston, Philadelphia, 1950. The ninth edition is published by McGraw-Hill, New York, 1980.

**Dr. Harrison was the author of *Your Future Health Care* and coauthor of *Principles and Problems of Ischemic Heart Disease. Your Future Health Care* was published by Warren H. Green, Inc., St. Louis, Missouri, 1974; and *Principles and Problems of Ischemic Heart Disease* was published by Year Book Medical Publishers, Inc., Chicago, 1968.

tion of penicillin therapy, for which he received the Legion of Merit Award.

He served as chairman of the section on surgery of the American Medical Association and chairman of the Board of Regents of the National Library of Medicine. Dr. Lyons served in many consultant capacities to the secretary of war and to the surgeon general of the United States Army.

The University of Alabama in Birmingham named Dr. Lyons Distinguished Professor of the University in 1964, and awarded him the honorary degree of D.Sc. in 1965. His colleagues at the University of Alabama Medical Center chose him as Distinguished Faculty Lecturer for the year 1964–1965.

At the time of his death on October 24, 1965, Dr. Lyons was Kerner Professor of Surgery and chairman of the Department of Surgery, University of Alabama School of Medicine.

Walter Benedict Frommeyer

Dr. Walter Benedict Frommeyer's (1916–1979) contributions to medicine and medical education in Alabama and the United States were outstanding.[104] He served as associate dean of the Medical School (1954–1957) and chairman of the Department of Medicine at The University of Alabama in Birmingham (1957–1968). Concurrently, he also served as physician-in-chief at the University Hospital and Hillman Clinic. He is best remembered for his dedication to teaching and his innovations during his long service on the national scene in medical education.

Many honors were bestowed on Dr. Frommeyer. He was a Distinguished Faculty Lecturer, a Distinguished Professor of the University, and a member of the Alabama Academy of Honor. He served as governor of the American College of Physicians for Alabama, then as regent, and finally as president (1973–1974). He was awarded the Alfred Stengel Award for his outstanding service to the American College of Physicians. He also served as president of the American Heart Association (1968–1969) and as vice-chairman of the American Board of Internal Medicine.

Dr. Frommeyer was born in Cincinnati, Ohio. He attended the University of Cincinnati Medical School and received his M.D. degree in 1942. He served in the United States Army in World War II. After the war, he spent a year at Harvard Medical School as a research fellow and as an assistant in medicine. Upon completion of this fellowship, he came to Birmingham, Alabama in 1949.

The University of South Alabama College of Medicine

The first medical school in the state of Alabama was founded by Dr. Josiah C. Nott in Mobile in 1859.[105] Mobile was the site of the Medical College of Alabama until 1920. The next four-year state medical school was established in Birmingham in 1945. Some years later, the city of Mobile decided to ask the University of South Alabama to develop a new state medical college. In 1961, a special act of the State Legislature established the Mobile County Foundation for Higher Public Education for the purpose of developing a state-supported university in Mobile County. In 1963, the University of South Alabama was formally authorized by the State Legislature to develop a medical college. In 1969, the State Legislature passed a resolution stating its desire to establish a second four-year medical school to be located at the University of South Alabama in Mobile. This was to be dependent on a favorable assessment by the Association of American Medical Colleges and the American Medical Association and a statement of support by the Medical Society of Mobile County. Plans for construction of the building now comprising the University of South Alabama College of Medicine were announced in 1971 supported by a State Bond Issue. In January, 1973, the first medical class was admitted, and on June 6, 1976, the first class of twenty students graduated. Mobile General Hospital, which was acquired by the University of South Alabama in 1970, is used as its main clinical facility. Mobile General Hospital became the University of South Alabama Medical Center Hospital and Clinics in April, 1975.

Deans of the University of South Alabama
College of Medicine

Robert M. Bucher, M.D.	1971–1974
Arthur J. Donovan	1974–1976 (acting dean and vice-president for Health Affairs)
Alan M. Seigal, M.D.	1976
Robert A. Kreisberg, M.D.	1976–1980 (acting dean)
Clyde G. Huggins, Ph.D.	1980 (acting dean)
Stanley E. Crawford, M.D.	1980–

Native Alabamians Who Have Had Distinguished Careers in Medical Education

John Allan Wyeth

Dr. John Allan Wyeth (1845–1922) was born in Marshall County, Alabama, and received his M.D. degree from the University of Louisville in 1869.[106] He also graduated from Bellevue Medical College in 1873. In 1874, he was appointed Professor in Anatomy at the Bellevue Hospital Medical College. In 1878, he visited Europe to study in the great medical centers of London, Paris, and Berlin. In 1881, Dr. Wyeth founded the New York Polyclinic Medical School and Hospital, the first postgraduate medical school in America. He became Professor of Surgery and surgeon-in-chief and later was president of the institution. He was offered, but declined, the professorship of surgery at Tulane University. Dr. Wyeth was elected president of the American Medical Association and presided at its Fifty-Third Annual Session at Saratoga Springs, New York, in 1902.

He was a prolific writer. His literary efforts included numerous articles about his research, as well as his autobiography and experiences in the Civil War. *With Sabre and Scalpel,* published in 1914 by Harper and Brothers in New York, includes twelve of his poems. His book, *Life of General Nathan Bedford Forrest,* also published by Harper and Brothers in New York in 1899, received wide acclaim. Dr. Wyeth had entered the Confederate States Army at the age of fifteen as an irregular soldier. Later he became a regular line soldier.

Dr. Wyeth, one of America's outstanding surgeons, died on May 8, 1922. A bronze statue of Dr. Wyeth stands on the capitol grounds in Montgomery.

Charles Alexander Pope

Another distinguished national medical educator, Charles Alexander Pope (1818–1870), was born in Huntsville, Alabama.[107] He began his medical studies as an apprentice with Drs. Thomas Fearn and Albert Russell Erskine (1827–1903) of Huntsville.

Dr. Pope attended his first organized course of lectures in medicine at the Cincinnati Medical College from 1837 to 1838. He had been attracted to the school by Dr. Daniel Drake's reputation as an excellent teacher and lecturer. In 1839, he graduated with the M.D. degree from the School of Medicine of the University of Pennsylvania.

Soon after his graduation, Pope went to Europe for further study. He spent nearly eighteen months in Paris and afterwards visited the great continental medical schools, those of Great Britain and Ireland. After his return, Dr. Pope settled in St. Louis in 1841 where he became one of the founders of the Medical Department of St. Louis University. Dr. Pope was appointed Professor of Anatomy at that school and in 1847 became Professor of Surgery. Dr. Pope became dean of the faculty of the Medical Department at the age of 31. He held this position for fifteen years.

Robert Archibald Lambert

One of the outstanding physicians and humanitarians interested in the improvement of medical education for black students was Robert Archibald Lambert (1883–1960).[108] He was born in Wilcox County, Alabama, and graduated with an M.D. degree from Tulane University School of Medicine in 1907. In 1909, he was appointed Assistant Professor of Pathology at Columbia University after completing two years of postgraduate study in pathology at Johns Hopkins. From 1916 to 1917, Dr. Lambert accompanied the Rice Scientific Expedition to the Amazon regions of Brazil. He was acting head of the Department of Pathology, Columbia University, during World War I. He was director of laboratories for the Near East Relief Mission in Syria and Turkey from 1919 to 1920.

He joined the faculty of Yale University School of Medicine in 1919 as Assistant Professor of Pathology. From 1923 to 1925, he was Professor of Pathology and Anatomy, Faculdade de Medicine de São Paulo, Brazil. The Rockefeller Foundation sponsored this position. Also from 1926 to 1929, he was Professor of Pathology and director of the School of Tropical Medicine, University of Puerto Rico, under the auspices of Columbia University.

In 1928, he became associate director for the Medical Sciences at the Rockefeller Foundation. He held this position until 1948 when he retired. He first became associated with the Rockefeller Foundation in 1922. At that time, he was under foundation sponsorship and lectured at the University of San Salvador and surveyed medical education in Central America.

Dr. Lambert received many citations and honors. He received the Decoration of Chevalier de la Légion d'Honneur from the French Government and was nominated to the Methodist Hall of Fame in Philanthropy. He also received an appointment as Academico Honorario, University of San Salvador and was awarded the Dictorate Honoris Cause by the University of São Paulo, Brazil. In 1949, Tulane University conferred the LL.D. degree upon him. He served as a member of the Board of Visitors of Tulane University from 1953 to 1956.

Upon retirement, he returned to his home in Greensboro, Alabama. He served on the Southern Regional Education Board and was a consultant for the Pan-American Sanitary Bureau Regional Office of the World Health Organization in Washington. Because of his interest in furthering the education of blacks, he became a member of the Interim Committee of Meharry Medical College, Nashville, from 1951 to 1952.

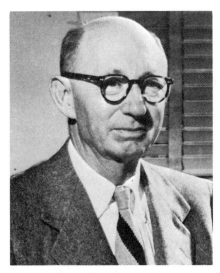

Robert Archibald Lambert, M.D.,
1883–1960 (Courtesy of the Alabama
Museum of the Health Sciences, Lister
Hill Library, Medical Center, The
University of Alabama in Birming-
ham)

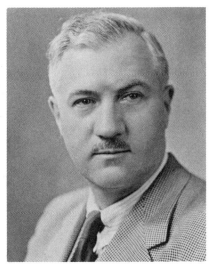

Allen Walker Blair, M.D., 1900–1948
(Courtesy of Canadian Cancer Society,
Saskatchewan Division)

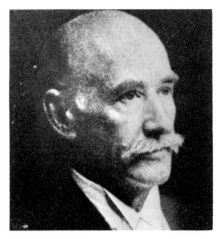

John Allan Wyeth, M.D., 1845–1922
(Courtesy of the Alabama Museum of
the Health Sciences, Lister Hill Library, Medical Center, The University
of Alabama in Birmingham)

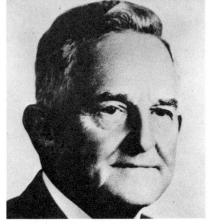

Lawrence Reynolds, M.D., 1889–1961
(Courtesy of the Alabama Museum of
the Health Sciences, Lister Hill Library, Medical Center, The University
of Alabama in Birmingham)

While on this committee, he served as acting president, vice-chairman, and chairman of the Board of Trustees.

Lawrence Reynolds

Dr. Lawrence Reynolds (1889–1961), a native of Ozark, Alabama, attended undergraduate school at the University of Alabama and received his M.D. degree from Johns Hopkins Medical School in 1916.[109] He became the first resident in Radiology at the Johns Hopkins Hospital. From 1917 to May, 1919, he served in France with the World War I American Expeditionary Forces. The next three years were spent in Boston as a roentgenologist at the Peter Bent Brigham Hospital and instructor in Roentgenology at the Harvard Medical School. In 1922, he joined the staff of the Harper Hospital in Detroit where he remained until his death.

Dr. Reynolds served as editor of the *American Journal of Roentgenology, Radium Therapy and Nuclear Medicine*. He received the Gold Medal Award of the Radiological Society of North America and was an honorary member of similar organizations in Germany, Italy, and Colombia, South America. He was awarded the Honorary Degree of Doctor of Laws by the University of Alabama and by Wayne State University.

Dr. Reynolds amassed one of the finest collections in this country of historical masterpieces of medical literature and presented these to the Medical College of Alabama in Birmingham in 1958. It is now housed in the Reynolds Historical Library within the Lister Hill Library of the Health Sciences at the Medical Center in Birmingham.

The inscription on the plaque of dedication marking the entrance to the library eloquently expresses Dr. Reynolds's philosophy, which prompted this truly exceptional gift:

Here are housed the books collected and
loved by
Lawrence Reynolds
Physician, scholar and philanthropist
The official dedication ceremony of the Reynolds
Library was held on February 2, 1958, but the more
meaningful dedication will come from you who
read these books.

Each time one of you reaps from the great minds of
the past the desire for finer achievement in your
profession and nobler development of your own character

The Reynolds Library will have been rededicated.
                    —Tinsley Randolph Harrison, M.D.

Prominent Physicians Associated with Medicine in Alabama

George T. Pack

Dr. George T. Pack (1898–1969), a native of Antrim, Ohio, received his M.D. degree in 1922 from Yale University.[110] In 1923, Dr. Pack was appointed Associate Professor of Pathology and Associate Dean of the University of Alabama School of Medicine in Tuscaloosa. After moving to New York (1926), he continued to maintain a professional relationship with the medical profession in Alabama.

Dr. Pack was interested in cancer, its treatment and its cure. He established one of the first tumor clinics at Yale University. Later, he practiced at Memorial Cancer Center in New York City. Dr. Pack founded The Pack Medical Group and The Pack Medical Foundation in order to continue his clinical investigations, to pursue his ideas concerning cancer education, and to treat the patient as a whole individual using the best methods available.

Writing about Dr. Pack, his colleague, Dr. Irvin M. Ariel, made the following statement: "He knew cancer as did few physicians of his day, and he was a true oncologist in that he carefully synchronized surgery, radiation therapy and chemotherapy for the maximum benefit for a given patient."

Allan Walker Blair

Allan Walker Blair, M.D. (1900–1948), a Canadian educated in Saskatchewan who received his M.D. degree at McGill University, served as Assistant Professor of Pathology and Bacteriology at the University of Alabama School of Medicine in Tuscaloosa (1929–1934).[111] During his tenure there, he determined to resolve the conflicting evidence that existed in the early 1930s regarding the poisonous nature of the bite of the black widow spider (female *Latrodectus mactans*).

On a Sunday morning in November, 1933, Dr. Blair allowed a black widow spider to bite him and meticulously recorded the subsequent development of excruciating pain, labored breathing, abdominal rigidity, weak thready pulse, hypotension, and leukocytosis. His findings are now recognized as classic for untreated black widow spider bites.

Conclusion

More than a century has passed since that Christmas Eve, 1823, in Cahaba when the General Assembly passed the first medical licensure act. For Alabama and her people, the years have not been easy. Progress in medicine, particularly in medical educational institutions, has been spasmodic and faltering; however, the present is good and the future appears bright. In expressing his hopes for the new medical college in Birmingham, William H. Brantley, Jr., said, "May this be such a college as would satisfy the dreams and ideals of those stalwart Alabama men who lived their lives for medicine and now are gone, John Bassett, Marion Sims, John Allan Wyeth, Jerome Cochran and William Crawford Gorgas."[112]

Notes

1. John Duffy, ed., *The Rudolph Matas History of Medicine in Louisiana* (Baton Rouge: Louisiana State University Press, 1962), 2: 56.

2. Ibid., p. 58.

3. Richard H. Shryock, *Medicine in America: Historical Essays* (Baltimore: Johns Hopkins Press, 1966), pp. 56–57.

4. Ibid., p. 61.

5. William H. Brantley, Jr., "Alabama Doctor," *Ala. Lawyer* 6 (1945): 248-55 (hereafter cited as Brantley, "Alabama Doctor").

6. Brantley, "Alabama Doctor," p. 261; and Howard L. Holley, "Medical Education in Alabama," *Ala. Rev.* 7 (1954): 248 (hereafter cited as Holley, "Medical Education"). Alex Berman, quoting several sources, states that the Alabama Medical Institute, Wetumpka, Alabama, received a state charter in 1844 and closed in 1845 after one session. The faculty was composed of seceding professors from the Southern Botanico Medical College (neo-Thomsonian) of Forsyth, Georgia. (Alex Berman, "Neo-Thomsonianism in the United States," *J. Hist. Med. & Allied Sci.* 11 [1956]: 133–55.)

7. Brantley, "Alabama Doctor," p. 261.

8. Roy H. Turner, "Graefenberg, The Shepard Family's Medical School," *Ann. Med. Hist.*, NS 5 (1933): 552.

9. The Graduates and Friends of the Graefenberg Medical Institute, *The Celebration of the Birthday and Life of Professor P. M. Shepard* (Dadeville, Ala.: n.p., 1859), pp. 15–16. Alabama Museum of the Health Sciences.

10. *Montgomery Advertiser and State Gazette*, 21 June 1851.

11. Acts of Alabama, 7 February 1852, p. 260.

12. Turner, pp. 552–53.

13. Ibid., pp. 554–55.

14. See Note No. 10.

15. Turner, p. 554.

16. Ibid., p. 553.

17. "William H. Anderson," *Representative Men of the South* (Philadelphia: Charles Robson, Co., 1880), pp. 136–43.

18. Emmett B. Carmichael, "George Augustus Ketchum—Teacher—Administrator—Physician," *Ala. J. Med. Sci.* 5 (1968): 511–14.

19. Josiah C. Nott, letter to unidentified doctor, 14 August 1870, Alabama Museum of the Health Sciences.

20. Brantley, "Alabama Doctor," p. 262.

21. Duffy, pp. 95–98.

22. J. C. Nott, "Thoughts on Acclimation and Adaptation of Races to Climates," *Amer. J. Med. Sci.* 32 (Oct. 1856): 320–34.

23. William H. Brantley, Jr., "An Alabama Medical Review," *Ala. J. Med. Sci.* 4 (1967): 193 (hereafter cited as Brantley, "Medical Review").

24. Stuart Graves, "Medical College of Alabama: Notes from Old Catalogs," 1859 catalog, pp. 1–4, Alabama Museum of the Health Sciences.

25. *Mobile Weekly Register*, 10 March 1860.

26. Brantley, "Medical Review," p. 193.

27. Ibid., pp. 193–94.

28. Ibid., p. 194.

29. Willis G. Clark, *History of Education in Alabama 1702–1889*, Bureau of Education Circular Information, no. 3, (Washington, D.C.: GPO, 1889), pp. 147–52.

30. "Address of Dr. Weatherly on Medical Education," *Trans.* (1871), pp. 32–45.

31. "Dr. Cochran's Address on Medical Education," *Trans.* (1870), pp. 176–77.

32. William H. Anderson, "The Annual Message of the President," *Trans.* (1881), pp. 28–29.

33. Brantley, "Alabama Doctor," p. 265.

34. Graves, 1877–1878 catalog, p. 7; 1881–1882 catalog, p. 8.

35. Ibid., 1879–1880 catalog, p. 7.

36. H. B. Dowling, interview with Velimir Luketic, Mobile, Ala., 9 July 1969.

37. Graves, 1885–1886 catalog, p. 10.

38. Ibid., 1886–1887 catalog, p. 11.

39. Ibid.

40. Ibid., 1896–1897 catalog, p. 16.

41. Abraham Flexner, *Medical Education in United States and Canada* (New York: D. B. Updike; Boston: Merrymount Press, 1910), pp. 126–42.

42. Graves, 1902–1903 catalog, p. 20.

43. Ibid., 1893–1894 catalog, p. 15; 1902–1903 catalog, pp. 19–20.

44. Ibid., 1895–1896 catalog, p. 15.

45. Brantley, "Alabama Doctor," p. 265.

46. Velimir Luketic, "Abraham Flexner and Medical Education in Alabama," *J.M.A. Ala.* 38 (1969): 701 (hereafter cited as Luketic, "Abraham Flexner").

47. University of Alabama, Bulletin, 1909–1910.

48. Luketic, "Abraham Flexner," p. 701.

49. Flexner, pp. 185–87.

50. Luketic, "Abraham Flexner," pp. 699–707.

51. J. H. Parks and O. C. Weaver, Jr., *Birmingham-Southern College, 1856–1956* (Nashville, Tenn.: Parthenon Press, 1957), p. 74; and Brantley, "Alabama Doctor," p. 265.

52. Holley, "Medical Education," p. 257.

53. Southern University, Catalogue, 1879, p. 28.

54. Ibid., 1874.

55. Brantley, "Alabama Doctor," p. 265.

56. Montezuma University Medical College, Catalogue, 1898–1899.

57. Ibid., 1898–1899.

58. Ibid., 1896–1897, p. 8.

59. Ibid., 1897–1898, p. 7.

60. Acts of Alabama, 16 February 1897, pp. 1186–89.

61. Velimir Luketic, "The Birmingham Medical College," *Ala. J. Med. Sci.* 6 (1969): 447 (hereafter cited as Luketic, "The Birmingham Medical College").

62. Ibid., p. 448.

63. Birmingham Medical College, Catalogue, 1894–1895, pp. 3–14.

64. Luketic, "The Birmingham Medical College," p. 449.

65. Birmingham Medical College, Catalogue, 1894–1895, p. 12; 1899–1900.

66. Luketic, "The Birmingham Medical College," p. 449.

67. Ibid., p. 450.

68. R. M. Moore, "The Davis Brothers of Birmingham and the Southern Surgical and Gynecological Association," *Trans. South. Surg. Assoc.* 74 (1962): 9–11.

69. Luketic, "The Birmingham Medical College," p. 450.

70. Birmingham Medical College, Catalogue, 1910–1911, p. 15.

71. Howard L. Holley and Velimir Luketic, "The History of the Hillman Hospital, Part 2," *Ala. J. Med. Sci.* 6 (1969): 228; and "Minutes of a Called Meeting of the Board of Directors of the Birmingham Medical College," 20 October 1909, Alabama Museum of the Health Sciences.

72. Flexner, pp. 186–87.

73. Luketic, "Abraham Flexner," p. 704.

74. N. P. Colwell, secretary, Council on Medical Education, letter to Dr. E. P. Hogan, secretary, Birmingham Medical College, 17 May 1910, Alabama Museum of the Health Sciences.

75. Birmingham Medical College, "Statistical Report," 1912.

76. Luketic, "The Birmingham Medical College," pp. 451–53.

77. *Birmingham Age-Herald*, 19 September 1912.

78. University of Alabama, Graduate School of Medicine, "First Announcement," 1 September 1913, Alabama Museum of the Health Sciences.

79. "Resolution of the Board of Trustees of the University of Alabama, 1912," Alabama Museum of the Health Sciences.

80. James F. Sulzby, Jr., *Birmingham Sketches: From 1871 Through 1921* (Birmingham: Birmingham Printing Co., 1945), pp. 89–90.

81. Emmett B. Frazer, interview with Velimir Luketic, Mobile, Ala., 9 July 1969.

82. Luketic, "Abraham Flexner," pp. 699–707.

83. Dean Frazer died in office and was succeeded by Dr. Dan McCall (1869–1955).

84. Edgar Poe Hogan, secretary, Birmingham Medical College, letter to Sidney J. Bowie, former trustee of Birmingham Medical College, 3 July 1915, Alabama Museum of the Health Sciences.

85. Ibid.

86. "T. M. Stevens vs. E. Thames," *In the Supreme Court of Alabama* (Montgomery, 1920). Cited in Holley, "Medical Education," p. 256.

87. Stuart Graves, "Medical College of Alabama, 1920–1945," Nott Memorial Program Exercises, Alabama Museum of the Health Sciences.

88. Boone Aiken, "Meet Man Who Put UAB on the Map of Medicine," *Birmingham News*, 30 October 1979, p. 31.

89. Hopson Owen Murfee, "An Alabama State Medical Center," *Ala. J. Med. Sci.* 13 (1976): 215–39.

90. J. D. S. Davis, "The President's Message," *Trans.* (1928), p. 21.

91. Brantley, "Medical Review," p. 204.

92. "In April, 1944, the State Medical Association meeting adopted the following resolution: Resolved, That as a token of gratitude to Dr. Partlow, 'the Father of the new Four-Year Medical School' the Medical Association of the State of Alabama adopt as one of its objectives for the year 1944–45, the raising of funds to employ one of the best artists of the nation to paint a portrait of our beloved Dr. W. D. Partlow, to be placed in the library of the Medical College of Alabama when it is re-established . . ."
Portraits of Dr. Partlow and Governor Chauncey Sparks now hang in the main library of The University of Alabama in Birmingham Medical Center. Katherine Vickery, *A History of Mental Health in Alabama* (Montgomery: Alabama Department of Mental Health, 1972 [?]), p. 186.

93. Brantley, pp. 194–95.

94. Ibid., p. 195.

95. Ibid., p. 206.

96. Robert Russell Kracke and William Gunter Kracke, "The University of Alabama Medical Center, The Past, The Present and The Future," *Ala. J. Med. Sci.* 4 (1967): 329.

97. Holley, "Medical Education," pp. 261–62. On June 4, 1945, instruction to twenty-two juniors began. J. D. L. Holmes, *A History of the University of Alabama Hospitals* (Birmingham: University of Alabama in Birmingham Print Shop, 1974), p. 66.

98. Kracke and Kracke, p. 318.

99. Ibid.

100. The Hillman Hospital Nurses' Training School was founded in 1903, and the Jefferson Hospital School of Nursing was founded in 1942. These were the forerunners of the present University of Alabama School of Nursing. B. M. Roberts, *A Determination of Medical Nursing and Health Professions* (Birmingham, Ala.: n.p., 1971), pp. 22–29.

101. Emmett B. Carmichael, "Roy Rachford Kracke," *Quart. Phi Beta Pi Med. Frat.* 45 (Nov. 1948): 157–60, 167–68.

102. James A. Pittman, Jr., "Tinsley Randolph Harrison, 1900–1979 [1978]," *Trans. Assoc. Amer. Phys.* 92 (1979): 30–32.

103. Lee Frommeyer and W. B. Frommeyer, Jr., M.D., personal communication, 1970.

104. Thomas N. James, "Walter B. Frommeyer, Jr., 1916–1979," *Forum on Medicine* 2 (March 1979): 230.

105. Mary Pritchett, administrative assistant II to Robert A. Kreisberg, M.D., dean, University of South Alabama College of Medicine, Mobile, Alabama, TS, 8 August 1979, copy in the author's possession.

106. Thomas McAdory Owen, *History of Alabama and Dictionary of Alabama Biography* (Chicago: S. J. Clarke Pub. Co., 1921), 4: 1813–14.

107. Emmett B. Carmichael, "Charles Alexander Pope," *Ann. Med. Hist.*, 3rd Ser. 2 (Sept. 1940): 422–31. On May 2, 1854, at the age of 34, Dr. Pope was elected president of the American Medical Association. In 1855, he was elected president of the Missouri State Medical Association. He was one of the founders of the St. Louis Academy of Science.

108. Emmett B. Carmichael, "Robert Archibald Lambert: Pathologist—Teacher—Physician," *J.M.A. Ala.* 32 (1963): 232–34.

109. Howard L. Holley, "Lawrence Reynolds, M.D., 1889–1961: An Appreciation," *J.M.A. Ala.* 31 (Dec. 1961): 210; and Lawrence Reynolds, "The Evolution of the Lawrence Reynolds Library," *De Hist. Med.* 5 (Oct. 1958): 12–15.

110. Irving M. Ariel, "George T. Pack, M.D., 1898–1969, A Tribute," *Amer. J. Roentgen., Radium Therapy & Nuclear Med.* 107 (1969): 443–46.

111. Frances Breslin and Robert E. Pieroni, "Dr. Blair and the Black Widow Spider," *J.M.A. Ala.* 51 (1981): 22, 58; and A. W. Blair, "Spider Poisoning: Experimental Study of the Effects of the Bite of the Female *Latrodectus mactans* in Man," *Arch. Int. Med.* 54 (1934): 831–43.

112. Brantley, "Medical Review," p. 195.

Chapter 4

The Role of Alabama in Confederate Medicine*

The medical practitioners of the South gave their lives and fortunes to their country, without any prospect of military or political fame or preferment. They searched the fields and forest for remedies; they improvised surgical implements from the common instruments of every day life; they marched with the armies, and watched by day and by night in the trenches. The Southern surgeons rescued the wounded on the battle-field, binding up the wounds, and preserving the shattered limbs of their countrymen; the Southern surgeons through four long years opposed their skill and untiring energies to the ravages of war and pestilence.[1]

Soon after the opening of the Civil War in the spring of 1861, large numbers of men from the Confederate States responded to President Jefferson Davis's call to arms. Patriotic fervor was at a peak, and many young men volunteered. Mobilization was rapid and the recruits were sent to poorly planned and constructed training camps, where instead of battle, many soldiers met illness and death. Communicable diseases were common and spread rapidly.

The medical problems that faced physicians of the Confederacy during the four years of civil war were as difficult and overwhelming as were the military problems. Only later would the discoveries of Pasteur and Lister free soldiers from their deadliest foe, infectious disease.

Throughout history, disease has been the chief cause of loss of life in armies. It accounted for at least two-thirds of the deaths in the Confederate Army.[2] Most deadly were typhoid, pneumonia, diarrhea, and

---

*Meeting in Montgomery in January, 1861, the Alabama Secession Convention was made up of 100 elected delegates of which ten were physicians. They were Lang C. Allen, Marion County; Joshua Prout Coman, Limestone County; James Wilson Crawford, Bibb County; Andrew Jackson Curtis, Choctaw County; James Madison Foster, Macon County; George Augustus Ketchum, Mobile County; Allan Kimball, Tallapoosa County; John Perkins Ralls, Cherokee County; George Rives, Sr., Autauga County; Joseph Silver, Baldwin County. Dr. Allen prepared for medicine but changed to industry (thread factory), and Dr. Silver was educated in medicine but became a planter.

dysentery. Other common and serious illnesses were tuberculosis, small-pox, scurvy, and malaria. Ignorance of the cause of disease, lack of sanitation, impure water, poor nutrition, and food improperly prepared and preserved, all contributed to widespread illness. Disease struck the recruits early, and its initial onslaughts proved devastating. Early in the war it was not uncommon for half or more of the men of a regiment to be incapacitated at one time by sickness.[3]

Prominent among the factors contributing to widespread illness was the policy of enlisting all men who volunteered. Almost anyone who could stand without support was allowed to enlist. It was not until the fall of 1862 that a program of physical examination for recruits was insti-tuted; but even then the enlistment of men with defects such as partial deafness, blindness in one eye, reducible hernia, and muscular rheuma-tism was still permitted. Although imperfect, these new physical stan-dards were a decided benefit. The 1864 Conscription Act, however, forced older men into the army who were particularly susceptible to disease.[4]

The so-called childhood diseases were especially prevalent, for there was very little endemic immunity in the population at large. Recruits came from rural areas where many had never attended public school and had neither been exposed to nor contracted illnesses such as measles and mumps. In reading state regimental histories, it is appalling to note how many of these young men died from measles and scarlet fever. However, these statistics may be misleading in that these infectious diseases were probably complicated by pneumonia. Later during the war, "hospital gangrene," a highly fatal streptococcus infection, became a principal hazard. The infectious nature of erysipelas and hospital gangrene was poorly understood, and where they occurred they took their deadly toll. Where these diseases were recognized as infectious, the mortality was contained.

Exposure to rain and cold was another factor contributing to disease. Many of the troops marched without raincoats and slept on the muddy ground without benefit of shelter. Scarcity of clothing and lack of blankets, combined with cold rains, inflicted indescribable misery, which was often aggravated by an inadequate wood supply for camp fires. The men either did not have sufficient time or were too fatigued to cut the wood. Pneumonia increased during the winter months and diminished in summer. Dr. Joseph Jones (1833–1896) stated that approximately one out of every six cases of pneumonia proved fatal. He estimated that 17 percent of the soldiers were stricken by this disease during a nineteen-month period in 1862 and 1863.[5] Bronchitis and pulmonary tubercu-losis were also common.

An inadequate diet contributed to the soldiers' poor health. Very seldom were there enough vegetables or fruit in camp rations, and available food was often neither appetizing nor wholesome. A standard practice in the early part of the Civil War was to fry flour flapjacks in bacon grease. The soldiers lived for months on flapjacks and fried fatback.

Although the Quartermaster Department made a valiant effort to feed the armies, it was often frustrated by unavailability and inadequate transportation of food supplies. The home front was not always efficient in supplying food, either due to breakdown in production or at times pure indifference. Foraging was allowed, but not always with the approval of the populace at large. Near the end of the war, with the transportation breakdown, the highly mobile armies had to survive on very poor rations, that is, parched corn, raw or poorly cooked pork, and a beverage resembling coffee made from roasted corn or acorns.

The filth of encampments could explain many epidemics. The lack of discipline by elected officers and the carelessness of the recruits were factors contributing to unsatisfactory conditions, but, most of all, ignorance served to defeat any earnest efforts of higher authorities to enforce sanitation. Latrines, or "sinks" as they were called by soldiers, were situated close to bivouacs, and there was a continued prevalent predisposition of the soldiers not to use those that were present.

On many occasions impure water played havoc with army health. The soldiers drank from rivers, creeks, badly situated springs, and even from muddy puddles of water. Troops frequently depended for their water supply on shallow holes dug about the camps, which were apt to be so close to latrines as to make contamination inevitable.

As the war went on, the deadlier ailments diminished in the Confederate soldier, but chronic diarrhea and dysentery progressively increased.[6] These were the most common of all the illnesses, and they led to the death of one out of every ten. Several factors, but mainly inadequate diet and exhaustion, made diarrhea and dysentery not only more prevalent but also more fatal.

Malaria was also a common disease in the rebel army. While the connection between mosquitoes and malaria was not known in the Civil War days, experience had taught that smoke smudges, dry camp sites, and other measures which gave relief from mosquitoes tended also to lessen malaria. Quinine was generally recognized as the remedy for malaria. Since it was imported from abroad, mainly from France, it became increasingly scarce as the war continued and as the Union naval blockade became more effective.

Smallpox occurred in 1862 in the Army of Northern Virginia. In order to combat the spread of smallpox in the Confederate Army, medical authorities adopted rigorous measures such as isolation and quarantines, and vaccination was required. However, there was no compulsory vaccination on entering the army.

Typhoid fever appeared early in the course of the war and was said to have caused one-fourth of the deaths from disease in the southern armies. Epidemics appeared in the wake of large-scale inductions of troops, most of whom came from rural areas. According to Dr. Joseph Jones, writing several years after Appomattox, "typhoid fever progressively diminished during the progress of the war, and disappeared almost entirely from the veteran armies."[7] Evidence drawn from Federal experience tends to prove his statement. The men had apparently developed immunity to the disease.

There was considerable disagreement as to whether "camp fever," which bedeviled the army, was typhoid or some vague newcomer. The authorities could not then arrive at a definite decision, but modern students are inclined to believe that paratyphoids, then unknown, were responsible.[8]

Medical science was in a process of transition everywhere, but medicine as practiced by physicians in the South before the war was considered to be as advanced as in any part of the nation. The number of medical colleges had increased steadily with some of the most competent medical men in the nation serving on the faculties of the southern schools. The standards were relatively high, and the enrollments showed an encouraging growth. Medical journals were circulated more widely, and professional societies were becoming commonplace.[9]

The germ theory had not yet been accepted by scientists, and the work of Pasteur would come later. Surgery was the dominant specialty in the armies: extraction of bullets and amputation of limbs were the most common procedures. Anesthesia—mainly chloroform—was a scarce commodity, and alcohol was commonly used as a substitute. Infection and shock associated with surgery were the major causes of mortality.

Medical practice during this period was primitive, with the "heroic" methods of treatment—purging and bleeding—still widely used. Besides calomel and jalap, such drugs as morphine (mostly tincture of opium), quinine, and digitalis were used when available. Local measures such as mustard plasters were still in use.

There was a shortage and maldistribution of physicians in Alabama, although the physicians available were reasonably well trained by the standards of the day. Most physicians had been educated in American medical schools, and some had received training in schools abroad. Certainly some were trained by apprenticeship, which was a common practice at that time.

The State of Alabama Department of Archives and History has preserved a list of 395 medical officers who served in Alabama regiments, Alabama Confederate hospitals and supply positions. A sampling of fifty-eight of these physicians reveals that fifty-six were graduates of a medical college. Twenty-one had graduated from the University of Pennsylvania Medical Department and twelve from Jefferson Medical College, both of which were located in Philadelphia and considered the best medical colleges in the country at that time. Three were graduates of the University of New York City, and the remaining twenty had graduated from southern medical schools. These were Transylvania (1817) in Kentucky, the Medical College of South Carolina (1824) at Charleston, the University of Virginia (1825) at Charlottesville, the Medical College of Louisiana (Tulane, 1834) at New Orleans, and the Medical College at Richmond (1838).

The Medical College of Alabama had opened in Mobile in 1859 with several outstanding men on its faculty, but the Medical College had had little time to influence the practice of medicine in Alabama. When war came, the school closed. Most of the faculty served in responsible positions in the Medical Department of the Confederate Army.

Organization of the Medical Department

The Medical Department of the Confederate States Army was created by an act of the Confederate Congress meeting in Montgomery on February 26, 1861. The organizational plan was patterned after that of the United States Army.[10] There were three grades of medical officers: surgeon general, surgeon, and assistant surgeon. The surgeon general had the rank and privileges of colonel with an annual salary of $3,000. Surgeons had the rank of major with a pay range from $1,944 to $2,400 per year, and assistant surgeons ranked as captain and were paid $1,320 to $1,800 per year.

Assistant surgeons supervised the administration of first aid and directed litter bearers in the removal of casualties to field hospitals. Regimental surgeons stayed with their brigades at the field infirmaries to care for the wounded brought in from the battle arenas. The most urgent cases were handled immediately by the surgeons; the other wounded were taken by ambulances (canvas-covered wagons) to interior receiving hospitals or to general hospitals located in most cities.

The permanent and semipermanent hospitals in the interior were better equipped and staffed than the field infirmaries. The best general hospitals were usually located in the larger towns, and Richmond had more hospitals than any city of the Confederacy.

An effort was made to house all the patients from a given state together in a separate hospital. Most of the hospitals derived their names from the state from which their patients originated.[11] The famous Chimborazo Hospital in Richmond, where Juliet Opie Hopkins served, had a section that housed mostly soldiers from Alabama.

Dr. David C. DeLeon of Mobile, one of a group of twenty-four medical officers who had resigned from the United States Army early in the war, was appointed acting surgeon general on May 6, 1861.[12] His successor, Dr. Samuel Preston Moore of South Carolina was appointed surgeon general on July 30, 1861, and served with distinction in this capacity for the duration of the war.[13]

Medical officers were assigned to administrative, field, hospital, or supply positions. Field physicians in Alabama regiments were usually residents from the areas of Alabama in which their regiments were organized. The proportion of state physicians to other Southern physicians serving in the Alabama Confederate hospitals was not as great as was those serving in the army field hospitals. Medical supply positions within the state were usually occupied by Alabama residents. The capital of the Confederacy was moved from Montgomery, Alabama, to Richmond, Virginia, in 1861, and the carefully prepared and completed records of the Confederate Medical Department were destroyed when Richmond burned on April 2, 1865. The record of where each Alabama physician served was lost.

Alabama Physicians Who Served in the Confederate States Army

Several Alabama physicians occupied high positions in the Medical Department of the Confederate States Army. Dr. LaFayette Guild (1825–1870), the personal choice of General Robert E. Lee, was medical director of the Army of Northern Virginia. He occupied a position probably next in importance to that of surgeon general.[14] Dr. Guild, a native of Tuscaloosa, graduated from the University of Alabama in 1845 and from Jefferson Medical College in 1848. He entered the United States Army as an assistant surgeon and remained until the outbreak of the Civil War, at which time he resigned his commission and joined the Confederate Army.

Dr. James Fountain Heustis (1829–1891), Professor of Anatomy at the Medical College in Mobile, graduated from the Medical Department of the University of Louisiana in 1848 and from 1850 to 1857 was an assistant surgeon in the United States Army. With the outbreak of the Civil War, he entered the Confederate Army Medical Department and served as medical director of hospitals in the Department of the Gulf with headquarters in Mobile.[15]

Dr. Elias Davis (1833–1864), a native of Jefferson County, was a physician who chose to fight with the army rather than minister to the sick and wounded.[16] After graduating from the University of Georgia Medical Department in 1853, he practiced in Jefferson County until

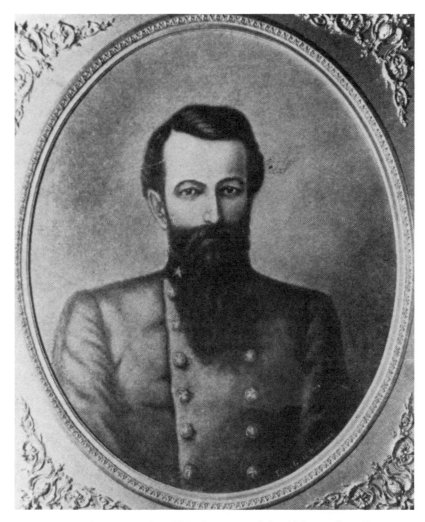

LaFayette Guild, M.D., 1825–1870 (Courtesy of the Alabama State Department of Archives and History)

1861, when he enlisted as a private in Company B, 10th Alabama Regiment. He rose to the rank of major and was killed in battle at Petersburg, Virginia.

Dr. William H. Anderson of Mobile served as medical purveyor of the military district that included Alabama.[17] He entered the Confederate Army with the rank of surgeon of the 21st Alabama Regiment, which was mustered into service at Mobile on October 13, 1861. He was appointed medical purveyor (purchaser or provider of drugs) in January, 1862. He was cofounder of the Medical College of Alabama, Professor of Physiology and Pathology, and dean of the college at the time he entered the Confederate Army.

Dr. Josiah Clark Nott, principal founder and Professor of Surgery at the Medical College, joined the Confederate Army as a medical inspector in General Braxton Bragg's Second Corps of the Army of Mississippi and served throughout the war.

Charles Theodor Mohr (1824–1901) of Mobile, born and educated in Germany, was one of the best trained chemists in the South.[18] At the beginning of the Civil War, the Confederacy established several pharmaceutical laboratories to manufacture drugs for the Medical Department of the Army. Dr. Mohr operated the laboratory at Mobile and described his role as follows:

> the government requested me to meet the challenge by taking an active part in the direction of a laboratory for the preparation of pharmaceuticals and indigenous products. I agreed to do so. There was no lack of materials for the construction of apparatus; a drug grinding mill, a steam distillation apparatus and a contrivance for the production of high-grade alcohol from corn whiskey; only glass vessels for the laboratory were largely absent. The task of examining the medical supplies smuggled in through the blockade from Europe, like opium, morphine, quinine, and others, were also assigned to me.[19]

Dr. Mohr found that French quinine was "highly adulterated." Medical personnel frequently confused the drugs quinine sulfate and morphine sulfate, which resulted in harm to the patients.[20] He is best known for his extensive studies of the flora of Alabama, published in *Plant Life of Alabama*. He began this work in 1860 and continued it throughout his lifetime.

Dr. George Augustus Ketchum, Professor of Principles and Practice of Medicine at the Medical College in Mobile, volunteered as a surgeon with the First Company of State Artillery in Pensacola and was commissioned surgeon of the Fifth Alabama Infantry. On his way through Mobile to Virginia, Dr. Nott offered him the position of surgeon of an organization formed for the defense of Mobile. Dr. Ketchum held this position until the end of the war.[21]

Dr. John William Mallet (1832–1912) joined the Medical College faculty in 1861 as Professor of Chemistry. He entered the Confederate States Army as a private, was promoted to first lieutenant, and made aide-de-camp to General R. E. Rodes of the Fifth Alabama Infantry on November 16, 1861. He saw action at Williamsburg and at Seven Pines, Virginia. At the request of Josiah Gorgas, he became superintendent of the Confederate States Ordnance Laboratories on May 21, 1862. His duties included reorganizing Southern arsenals and depots and planning the ordnance laboratory at Macon, Georgia. He formulated standard procedures for the different laboratories and arsenals and supervised the manufacture of powder and percussion caps. Mallet designed a new type of shell with a polyhedral cavity, which was introduced in the army in September, 1862. He developed explosive caps using potassium chlorate and sulfur as a substitute for mercury fulminate. Dr. Mallet was promoted to major in 1862 and to lieutenant-colonel in 1864. He was wounded while inspecting a fort at Charleston in 1863.[22] After the Civil War, Dr. Mallet made a survey for petroleum in Louisiana and Texas. He served on the faculty at several southern universities including the University of Virginia. In 1882, he was president of the American Chemical Society.

Very little is known as to what part Alabama medicine played in the medical care in the Confederate States Navy. There is, however, a poignant story of Dr. David Herbert Llewellyn, a courageous physician from Westshire, England, who gave his life caring for the injured crew aboard the famous Confederate raider, the C.S.S. *Alabama* at the time of its fatal engagement with the U.S.S. *Kearsarge* off Cherbourg, France, June 19, 1864. Disregarding his own safety, Llewellyn continued to give aid and assistance to the ship's wounded. Llewellyn, who was twenty-six years old at the time, had joined the predominately English crew on the ship's maiden voyage. He lost his life for a dying cause in the service of a country he had never seen.[23]

Nursing Care in the Confederate Army

In the Confederate Army, women provided an increasing amount of nursing care. The role of the female as nurse to the family was a familiar one, but authorities only reluctantly accepted the service of women in hospitals. Many women in Alabama, as well as in other states, made great personal sacrifices in order to minister to sick and dying soldiers.

Originally, women other than those in the holy orders of the Catholic church were reluctant to serve as nurses in hospitals due to public criticism. However, women did serve as matrons since such positions were considered respectable. In 1862, the Confederate Congress authorized the employment of female nurses in the Medical Corps. Men served as apothecaries, stewards, ward masters and attendants. Slaves were employed as cooks and laundresses, and sometimes captured black soldiers were assigned to hospitals as aides.

Although the Confederate Government was slow in organizing its medical service for the care of the sick and wounded, Alabama authorized hospitals to be organized near the field of battle action early in the war. Governor John Gill Shorter (governor of Alabama, 1861–1863) appointed Arthur F. Hopkins of Mobile as superintendent of the Alabama hospitals.[24] His wife, Juliet Opie Hopkins, was his able assistant.[25]

Juliet Opie Hopkins (1818–1890) and Kate Cumming (1835–1909), both natives of Mobile, are women never to be forgotten for their courage and dedication to the care of sick and wounded Confederate soldiers.

The example of Mrs. Hopkins, who gave her time, money, and service to Alabama soldiers of the Confederacy, was unique.[26] From early 1861 to the end of the war, she devoted most of her time to sick and wounded soldiers in the Alabama section of the famous Chimborazo Hospital in Richmond. From her own fortune, from private contributions, and from Alabama state appropriations, a hospital supply depot was maintained in Richmond under her supervision. She gave her entire fortune, estimated at $200,000–$500,000, to provide for the needs of Alabama soldiers. Mrs. Hopkins was wounded at the Battle of Seven Pines while assisting a wounded officer and remained partially crippled for the rest of her life. When Mrs. Hopkins died on March 9, 1890, in Washington, D.C., the entire congressional delegation from Alabama attended her funeral.[27]

Miss Kate Cumming is Alabama's most prominent representative of the small group of women who braved public criticism to supply nursing care for sick and wounded Confederate soldiers.[28] Miss Cumming, born in Leith, Scotland, in 1835, was brought to America as an infant and reared in Mobile. She served with the Army of Tennessee from early 1862, soon after the Battle of Shiloh, until the end of the war. She wrote extensively of her experiences.*

Drugs and Medical Supplies

One of the most controversial military measures instituted against the seceded Southern States during the Civil War was the inclusion of

---

*She wrote *A Journal of Hospital Life in the Confederate Army of Tennessee* which was published by J. P. Morton Co. in Louisville, 1866, and was considered to be one of the best intimate views of the Civil War as seen in the Medical Corps. Later, she revised her *Journal,* and entitled it *Gleanings from the Southland,* which was published by Roberts & Son in Birmingham, 1895.

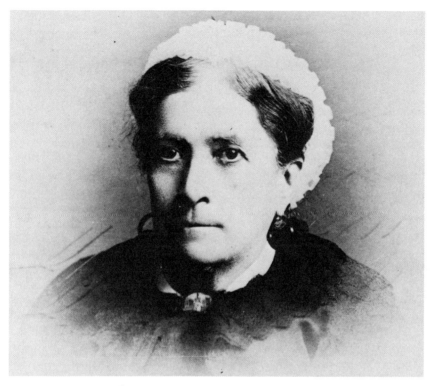

Juliet Opie Hopkins, 1818–1890 (Courtesy of the Alabama State Department of Archives and History)

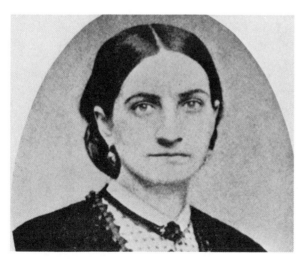

Kate Cumming, 1835–1909

medical supplies as contraband of war in the naval blockade of southern ports. This action had its origin in the famous proclamation signed by President Abraham Lincoln on August 16, 1861. In addition to arms of war, this decree forbade traffic in medical and surgical supplies to the Confederacy.[29]

This naval blockade of southern ports gradually strangled foreign commerce in the South and doomed the Confederacy to defeat. The embargo of drugs and medical supplies imposed severe hardships on the Medical Department of the Confederacy in caring for both the sick and wounded Confederate soldiers and the Union prisoners. The civilian population also suffered greatly from the loss of the necessities of life and most seriously from the lack of medicines. Indeed, survival at home was no less difficult than survival in the army.

Supplies were obtained, however, through the blockade from northern states and from Mexico. They were also manufactured by the Confederacy and secured by capture from the enemy. But some supplies obtained through the blockade or through trading with the enemy were held by speculators seeking exorbitant profits. After 1862, this latter situation became so prevalent that General Robert E. Lee ordered that medical supplies found in the possession of speculators be confiscated and turned over to the purveyors for redistribution.

The Medical Purveyor Department was responsible for securing, storing, and distributing medical supplies; and medical officers attached to this service were under the authority of and reported directly to the Surgeon General's Office.[30] Large sums of money were needed for procuring and distributing supplies, which ranged from cots, bedding, pots and pans to surgical instruments, drugs, bandages, and crutches.

Early in the war, Surgeon General Samuel Preston Moore placed Richard Potts, a medical purveyor in Montgomery, in charge of all internal trade of medical supplies and drugs on the Mississippi River. This project appears to have been poorly managed, and Potts encountered competition from other purveyors as well as from the Confederate Army Medical Department in Richmond. Despite his pleas for more cooperation and freedom in the conduct of traffic with the enemy, his efforts remained ineffective, and he was relieved of his duties, February, 1865.[31]

The scarcity of drugs and medicines also seems to have come, in large part, from poor distribution. Deficiencies in drugs and medical supplies were inevitable with the breakdown of transportation, communication, and record keeping. Surgical instruments, probably because they were furnished by their owners, did not seem to be in short supply.

The three most important drugs and those in greatest demand were morphine, quinine, and chloroform. There were numerous incidences of maldistribution. For example, quinine was overabundant in South Carolina in 1864 while in Georgia it was scarce. In October of that same year, Surgeon E. H. C. Bailey, who was in charge of the supply depot at Demopolis, Alabama, reported that he had adequate supplies, including 1,966 ounces of quinine sulfate, 245 drams of morphine sulfate, and 34 pounds of chloroform.[32]

Surgeon W. H. Anderson, who served as medical purveyor for the district that included Alabama, had established pharmaceutical laboratories at Montgomery and Mobile with supply depots at Montgomery and Demopolis.[33] Some of the chemicals and drugs produced under the direction of C. T. Mohr at the Mobile and Montgomery laboratories were alcohol, silver chloride, sulfuric ether, nitric ether, podophyllin resin, silver nitrate, sweet spirits of nitre, iodide of potassium, and blue mass.[34] Some of the plants from which medicine substitutes were made were:

Jamestown, commonly known as Jimson weed, used for pain
Maypop root, for relief of pain
Boneset, for reducing fever
Yellow Jasmine, for nervousness
Queen's root, as a tonic
Alder vine bark and pith, for making salve
Slippery elm bark, for making poultices
Prickly pear, despined and macerated, for poultices

Other plants used were Georgia bark, white willow, Indian physic, skunk cabbage, wild cherry bark, and cranesbill.[35]

A pill containing equal amounts of red pepper and crude resin, called the "Diseremus Pill," was concocted by an Alabama medical officer. It was handed to the weakened men with the instructions to "take two after each loose operation."[36] The result of such treatment was not reported.

A medicine made from a combination of dogwood, poplar, and willow bark was found unsatisfactory as a substitute for quinine. Families were urged to plant beds of red garden poppy and to collect medicinal plants for sale to the government. (A good grade of raw opium resin could be obtained from the seed pods of the poppy plants and was then made into laudanum.) Thousands of pounds of indigenous plants were bought by agents of the Medical Department and made into remedies. Medical purveyors were requested to include drug substitutes in all drug orders.

Gross shortages did occur late in the war when breakdown of communication and transportation made it impossible to supply the needs of the rapidly retreating armies. Also, the massive number of Union sick and wounded, in prison hospitals already inadequately staffed and supplied, further complicated the local shortages.[37] When supplies were available and transportation by railway and wagon could be obtained, drugs and medical supplies often arrived in poor condition or deteriorated in therapeutic value because of lack of packing boxes and bottles.[38]

Alabama suffered greatly from the blockade due to the inadequacy of its transportation system and its geographical position. Its railroad connections with the other states were poor and were generally appropriated by the Confederate Government for military use. Some relief from the blockade might have been obtained by contraband trade with the Federals on the northern border of the state; however, there were no railroads connecting North Alabama with central and southern sections. The result was that the people had to survive as best they could with the meager resources at hand.[39]

Hospital Care of the Confederate Soldier
in Alabama

The first hospitals were converted homes, hotels, stores, churches and barns, usually organized and administered by women's aid societies.[40] Newspaper advertisements appeared for the purchase of clean rags at six cents per pound. Women prepared food for the hospitals, knitted socks and other garments, and children went to work rolling bandages and making dressings for soldiers.[41]

Many military hospitals in the state were closed in March, 1863, when the Confederate Medical Department assumed authority over all hospitals. After this, Alabama ranked third in the number of hospitals within its borders, Virginia being first and Georgia second. The types of hospitals were field, general, and wayside hospitals. Field hospitals located in North Alabama were closed early in the war as the area was occupied by enemy soldiers. General hospitals were located throughout the state, far removed from the fighting area. Wayside or way hospitals were established to serve the sick, traveling soldiers, and civilian refugees fleeing from enemy occupied territory. Alabama hospitals were small in size in comparison to those in Virginia and Georgia.

Alabama Confederate Hospitals

CITY	LOCATION	HOSPITAL	BED CAPACITY	MEDICAL OFFICERS
Auburn	Auburn University Campus	Texas Hospital[42] (occupied main college building)	unknown	Surgeon Dudley D. Sanders Assistant Surgeon L. A. Bryan
Cahaba	unknown	Prison Hospital[43] (part of a prisoner of war camp—established in 1864)	unknown	Isaiah H. White
Calera-Columbiana	Shelby Springs	Shelby Springs General Hospital[44] (formerly a popular health resort)	350	Surgeons B. H. Thomas, D. Warren Brickell Assistant Surgeons Bradbury, Jones, and John P. Furniss
Courtland	unknown	Hospitals[45] (established in Simpson and Barclay homes)	unknown	unknown
Demopolis	Franklin Street, opposite railroad depot	Demopolis Wayside Hospital[46] (converted hotel)	unknown	Surgeon H. Hinckley Assistants Perrin, Randal, and Rew
Eufaula (The city was originally called Irwinton.)	old Bailey House	Eufaula Wayside Hospital[47] (established 1863)	34	Surgeons H. M. Weedon and Paul De Lacey Baker

CITY	LOCATION	HOSPITAL	BED CAPACITY	MEDICAL OFFICERS
Florence[48]	Court Street	(factory building)	unknown	unknown
Florence	corner of Seminary Street and Old Jackson Highway, now Military Avenue	(home of a Miss Dyas)	unknown	unknown
Gainesville[+]	unknown	Buckner Hospital[49] (opened spring, 1862—Gainesville Academy and the American Hotel were jointly occupied by this hospital—closed December 5, 1863)	unknown	Surgeons Francis Thornton, W. T. McAllister; Drs. S. W. Lee, Fla., R. D. Jackson of Selma, Drs. Reese of Alabama, and Yates of Texas were on the staff.
Greenville	¼ mile west of present Louisville and Nashville Railway Station, southwest side of Highway 10	Greenville General Hospital[50] (built during fall and winter of 1863)	150	Surgeon John T. Broughton Assistants Caldwell and Murphy (two local physicians)
Huntsville[+]	Jefferson and Holmes streets	Tennessee Valley Hospitals[51] (several houses converted for hospital use; also the Easley Hotel which closed early due to enemy occupation)	unknown	unknown

CITY	LOCATION	HOSPITAL	BED CAPACITY	MEDICAL OFFICERS
Marion	Washington Street	Marion General*[52] (established August, 1863, in 2 dormitories of Howard College; then located in Marion, now Marion Institute)	unknown	Dr. James M. Green Dr. Albert Russell Erskine
Mobile[53]	unknown	Nidelet Hospital (formerly the U.S. Naval Hospital)	250	Surgeon L. L. Nidelet Assistant Surgeons D. E. Smith, E. Young
Mobile	St. Anthony and Broad streets	County Hospital (until late 1960s Mobile City Hospital)	160	Surgeon William Henderson Assistant Surgeon C. O. Helwig Acting Assistant Surgeon E. D. Fenner
Mobile	southeast corner of Lipscomb and Conception streets	Levert Hospital[54] (originally used as a private infirmary by Dr. Henry S. Levert)	40	Surgeon R. H. Redwood
Mobile[53]	Conti Street	Conti Hospital (formerly a hotel)	140	Surgeon I. F. G. Payne Assistant Surgeon E. M. Erwin

*Ann D. England, A Compilation of Documented Information About The Confederate Hospital in Marion, Alabama, May 20, 1863–May 20, 1865 ([Marion]: n.p., circa 1950).

CITY	LOCATION	HOSPITAL	BED CAPACITY	MEDICAL OFFICERS
Mobile	Royal Street	Nott Hospital (formerly Dr. J. C. Nott private infirmary)	63	Surgeon G. W. Nott
Mobile	Royal Street	Moore (formerly a hotel)	123	Surgeon W. C. Cavenegh
Mobile	unknown	Heustis Hospital (converted hotel)	100	Surgeon J. M. Heard; Assistant Surgeon I. B. Hinkle
Mobile	unknown	Hospital built by Confederate Government for blacks who worked on the fortification of Mobile	156	Surgeon G. A. Moss; Assistant Surgeon L. L. Newsom
Montgomery[+]	unknown	Montgomery Wayside Hospital[55] (known as Soldiers' Home—established June 14, 1861, by Ladies Aid Society of Montgomery)	unknown	unknown
Montgomery[53]	opposite corners of Perry Street and Dexter Avenue (then Main Street)	Madison Hospital (2 buildings—hotel and Masonic building)	292	Surgeons C. I. Clarke, G. W. McDade, O. B. Knod
Montgomery	corner of Perry Street and Monroe (then Market) Street	Concert Hall Hospital (3-story building)	250	Surgeons W. I. Hobb, A. P. Hall; Acting Assistant Surgeons

CITY	LOCATION	HOSPITAL	BED CAPACITY	MEDICAL OFFICERS
Montgomery	corner of Bibb and Commerce streets	St. Mary's Hospital (3-story building)	325	Surgeons John H. Walters, John H. Britts, John W. Keys Acting Assistant Surgeon A. A. Homer
Montgomery	corner of Bibb and Commerce streets, opposite St. Mary's Hospital	Ladies Hospital (3-story building—established April 1, 1862)	265	Surgeons T. F. Duncan, T. A. Healey, B. F. Blount
Montgomery	near depot of Alabama & Florida Railroad at corner of Coosa and Tallapoosa streets	Watts Hospital (tent hospital)	250	Surgeon F. M. Hereford Assistant Surgeon I. B. Kelly Acting Assistant Surgeons I. A. Thomas, A. P. Ryall
Montgomery	unknown	Stonewall Hospital (adjoined Watts Hospital)	300	Surgeons R. J. Taliaferro, T. F. Fromm Assistant Surgeons H. T. Winn, I. C. Sneed
Notasulga	2 miles from Notasulga and ¼ mile to the right of the Notasulga-Tuskegee Highway	Conscript Hospital[56] (established fall of 1863 on the grounds of Camp Watts; torn down in 1955)	unknown	Surgeon U. R. Jones

CITY	LOCATION	HOSPITAL	BED CAPACITY	MEDICAL OFFICERS
Point Clear	Point Clear Hotel	Point Clear General Hospital[57] (established in portion of old Point Clear Hotel in 1864)	unknown	unknown
Selma	southwest corner of Broad and Water streets, adjacent to Alabama River	Selma Wayside Hospital[58] (established by Selma Ladies Military Aid Society, Sept., 1863)	100	Surgeon J. C. Curry Assistant Surgeons E. B. Freeman, Rogers, Kilpatrick, Leonard
Selma	Alabama Avenue	Selma General Hospital[59] (converted boys' school—after the war became Selma Military Institute)	200	Surgeon W. Hurt
Springhill (suburb of Mobile)	Springhill	Miller General Hospital[60]	170	Surgeon Goronwy Owen
Talladega	northwest corner of Court and North streets	Talladega Wayside Hospital[61] (formerly Exchange Hotel—converted to hospital April 1, 1862)	unknown	Surgeon G. S. Bryant Assistant Surgeon Reuben H. Dugger

CITY	LOCATION	HOSPITAL	BED CAPACITY	MEDICAL OFFICERS
Town Creek[+]	unknown	Town Creek Hospital[45] (home of Colonel Pruitt and Town Creek Methodist Church)	unknown	unknown
Tuscaloosa	Bryce Hospital	Tuscaloosa General Hospital[62] (established spring of 1864 in 2 wings of the Alabama Hospital for the Insane)	unknown	Surgeon R. N. Anderson Dr. William A. Leland, a local physician
Tuscumbia[+48]	west of city near Memphis Highway	Old James Throckmorton house	unknown	Drs. B. S. Newsum, William H. Newsum, William C. Cross, William Desprez
Tuscumbia[+]	502 East 5th Street	Stonecraft—John D. Inman home	unknown	(These physicians served the Tuscumbia Hospitals)
Tuscumbia[+]	Ivy Green	Ivy Green—Helen Keller home	unknown	
Uniontown	unknown	Uniontown Officers' Hospital[63]	unknown	Surgeon G. C. Gray

[+]Confederate hospitals discontinued by December 31, 1864. A partial list of Confederate hospitals in Alabama is given in H. H. Cunningham, *Doctors in Gray: The Confederate Medical Service* (Baton Rouge: Louisiana State University Press, 1958), p. 289.

Georgia Confederate Hospitals Relocated in Alabama in 1864

The retreat of General Joseph E. Johnston's and later General John Bell Hood's Confederate Army from Chattanooga to Atlanta resulted in many field hospitals being moved to Alabama.[64] It was the mobility of the Confederate hospitals that kept them in existence at all, but the necessity of repeated moves was detrimental to the health and comfort of the patients and added greatly to the trials of the medical staff. The whole situation was trying in the extreme.[65] It was in the field hospitals of this retreating army that the indefatigable Miss Kate Cumming served with distinction.

HOSPITAL	GEORGIA LOCATION	ALABAMA LOCATION
Kingston	Kingston	Opelika
Erwin	Barnesville	Opelika
Empire	near Macon	Opelika
Fairground	near Macon	Opelika
Institute	near Macon	Opelika
Flewellen	unknown	Opelika
Bemiss	unknown	Opelika
St. Mary's	LaGrange	Union Springs
Cannon	LaGrange	Union Springs
Oliver	LaGrange	Union Springs
Law	LaGrange	Union Springs
Bell	Greensboro	Eufaula
Shorter	unknown	Eufaula
Milton	unknown	Eufaula

Medical Care of War Prisoners

For the most part, medical treatment of wounded captives, both Union and Confederate, was considered humane. Dr. Jonathan Letterman, the Union Army's medical director, expressed the sentiment of most army medical officers in the following statement: "Humanity teaches us that a wounded and prostrate foe is not then our enemy."[66]

It appears reasonable to conclude that the Confederacy cared for its disabled prisoners about as well as it did for its own sick and wounded— Andersonville notwithstanding. Both were victims of severe privation from inadequate food and medical care in the latter part of the conflict. As the Union Army dealt blow after blow at the Confederacy, the transportation and supply systems broke down almost completely. The shortage of manpower, which had been so apparent on the battlefield, also extended to hospital personnel.[67] However, the Medical Department of the Confederacy was so well organized that it continued to function until the end of the war even though most of the other departments disintegrated as defeat approached.

Summary

Alabama contributed a great deal to the Confederacy in the operation of hospitals within her borders and in the service rendered by Alabama physicians in all areas of the Confederacy.

It is not possible, now, to compute with exactness the cost of the Civil War. Deaths from all causes took a grisly toll of over 600,000 in the Federal and Confederate Armies. Disease, neglect, malnutrition, and exposure are known to have produced far more casualties than did firearms. Of Alabamians who fought in the Confederate Army, approximately one out of four did not return. The State of Alabama Department of Archives and History has a record of 122,000 men from Alabama who served in active duty in the Confederacy, of which 35,000 died. This, of course, does not take into account loss of life in the "back home" population due to lack of medical care and scarcity of drugs. The intangible costs cannot be calculated.

We lost not only these men, but their children, and their children's children. . . . We have lost the books they might have written, the scientific discoveries they might have made; the inventions they might have perfected. Such a loss defies measurement.[68]

Notes

1. James O. Breeden, *Joseph Jones, M.D.: Scientist of the Old South* (Lexington: University Press of Kentucky, 1975), pp. 228–29.

2. Cunningham quoted the figures at three-fourths. H. H. Cunningham, *Doctors in Gray: The Confederate Medical Service* (Baton Rouge: Louisiana State University Press, 1958), p. 5.

3. Bell Irvin Wiley, *The Life of Johnny Reb, The Common Soldier of the Confederacy* (Baton Rouge: Louisiana State University Press, 1978), p. 244.

4. Ibid., p. 245. Seventeen-year-olds and those who were between the ages of forty-six and fifty years were drafted, although they were to serve only as a reserve force.

5. Wiley, p. 254.

6. Ibid., p. 252.

7. Ibid., p. 253.

8. Ibid., p. 400.

9. Cunningham, p. 20.

10. Ibid., pp. 21–44.

11. Wiley, p. 266.

12. Cunningham, p. 27.

13. Ibid., pp. 27–28.

14. Thomas McAdory Owen, *History of Alabama and Dictionary of Alabama Biography* (Chicago: S. J. Clarke Pub. Co., 1921), 3: 711–12.

15. Ibid., pp. 804–05.

16. Ibid., p. 461.

17. "William H. Anderson," *Representative Men of the South* (Philadelphia: Charles Robson Co., 1880), pp. 136–43.

18. Richard C. Sheridan, "Alabama Chemists in the Civil War," *Ala. Hist. Quart.* 37 (Winter 1975): 270.

19. Ibid., pp. 270–71.

20. Ibid., p. 271.

21. Owen, pp. 968, 971.

22. Sheridan, pp. 269–70.

23. Howard L. Holley, "A Study in Courage," *New Physician* 14 (June 1965): 161.

24. Arthur F. Hopkins was a chief justice of the Alabama Supreme Court from 1837 to 1838. He was also elected a United States Senator but was not listed on the official roll of the Senate.

25. Lucille Griffith, *Alabama: A Documentary History to 1900* (University, Ala.: The University of Alabama Press, 1972), p. 433.

26. Lucille Griffith, "Mrs. Juliet Opie Hopkins and Alabama Military Hospitals," *Ala. Rev.* 6 (1953): 99–120.

27. W. J. Donald, "Alabama Confederate Hospitals, Part 2," *Ala. Rev.* 16 (1963): 75.

28. Ibid., pp. 75–76.

29. Howard L. Holley, "Narration: The Civil War: The AMA and Embargo on Medicine for the Confederacy," *JAMA* 182 (Dec. 1962): 204, 208.

30. Cunningham, p. 146.

31. Ibid., pp. 136–37.

32. Ibid., p. 159.

33. Ibid., pp. 146–47.

34. Ibid., pp. 147–48.

35. Ibid., pp. 148–49.

36. Ibid., p. 187.

37. Ibid., pp. 159–60.

38. Ibid.

39. Albert Burton Moore, *History of Alabama* (Tuscaloosa: Alabama Book Store, 1951), p. 446.

40. W. J. Donald, "Alabama Confederate Hospitals," *Ala. Rev.* 15 (1962): 271–81; Part 2, 16 (1963): 64–78; and Cunningham, p. 45.

41. E. Grace Jemison, *Historic Tales of Talladega* (Montgomery, Ala.: Paragon Press, 1959), p. 139.

42. Donald, Part 2, 16 (1963): 67.

43. Donald, 15 (1962): 271; and F. T. Miller, ed., *The Photographic History of the Civil War* (New York: Review of Reviews Co., 1912), 7: 86.

44. James F. Sulzby, Jr., *Historic Alabama Hotels and Resorts* (University, Alabama: University of Alabama Press, 1960), pp. 209–12.

45. Donald, Part 2, 16 (1963): 69.

46. Ibid., pp. 65–66; and Mrs. W. G. Winn, letter to Dr. T. M. Owen, 25 February 1911, Alabama Department of Archives and History, Montgomery.

47. Donald, Part 2, 16 (1963): 64; M. T. Thompson, *History of Barbour County, Alabama* (Eufaula, Ala.: n.p., 1939), p. 140; and Sulzby, pp. 238–39.

48. N. Leftwich, Tuscumbia, Ala., interview with Dr. William J. Donald, 1962, and Donald, Part 2, 16 (1963): 64–78.

49. Donald, Part 2, 16 (1963): 71; and Sulzby, p. 15.

50. Donald, 15 (1962): 278.

51. Ibid., Part 2, 16 (1963): 68.

52. G. V. Irons, "Howard College as a Confederate Military Hospital," *Ala. Rev.* 9 (1956): 22–32.

53. Mobile and Montgomery military hospitals are described in an inspection report by Surgeon R. L. Brodie, medical director, Division of the West, 26 December 1864, Alabama Department of Archives and History, Montgomery.

54. *Directory For the City of Mobile, For 1861* (Mobile: Farrow and Dennett, 1861), p. 21.

55. Donald, Part 2, 16 (1963): 69–70.

56. Ibid., p. 64; and W. P. Hodnette, Notasulga, Ala., interview with Dr. William J. Donald, 1962, cited in Donald, Part 2, 16 (1963): 64–78.

57. Donald, Part 2, 16 (1963): 67; C. G. Godard, Fairhope, Ala., interview with Dr. William J. Donald, 1962, cited in Donald, Part 2, 16 (1963): 64–78; and Sulzby, pp. 136–37.

58. Donald, 15 (1962): 279; and G. M. Callen, Selma, Ala., interview with Dr. William J. Donald, 1962, cited in Donald, Part 2, 16 (1963): 64–78.

59. Donald, 15 (1962): 280; and Lela Legare, Montgomery, Ala., interview with Dr. William J. Donald, 1962, cited in Donald, 15 (1962): 251.

60. Donald, 15 (1962): 279.

61. Ibid., Part 2, 16 (1963): 65.

62. Ibid., 15 (1962): 280.

63. Donald, Part 2, 16 (1963): 65.

64. Ibid., 15 (1962): 272.

65. K. Cumming, *Kate: The Journal of a Confederate Nurse* (Baton Rouge: Louisiana State University Press, 1959), p. xvi.

66. Cunningham, p. 129.

67. Ibid., pp.104–05.

68. Allan Nevins, "The Glorious and the Terrible," *Saturday Review* 44 (2 Sept. 1961): 46–47.

Chapter 5

Medical Practice after the Civil War

Advances in Surgery

Demoralization resulting from the Civil War and reconstruction had delayed the steady scientific advances in medicine and surgery in Alabama. Surgical experiences in the Civil War did, however, give newer insights into the problems of shock and infection.

After the Civil War, the boundaries of surgery were gradually expanded. The introduction of anesthesia (1846) immeasurably simplified the surgeon's operative problems and made possible more complicated procedures while removing from patients the pain and anxiety associated with surgical procedures. Unfortunately, the enthusiasm that originally greeted the introduction of anesthesia lasted only a few years. By the 1860s, it was readily apparent that infection and shock still were the major roadblocks to successful surgery. These dangers remained so great that when a major operation was attempted, it was often considered tantamount to signing the patient's death certificate.

In the immediate post–Civil War years, American physicians made relatively few contributions to the advancement in surgery. The United States was still largely rural, and most surgery was performed in private homes—either the surgeon's or the patient's. As in many medical developments, surgery required hospitals and a large patient population in order to become a specialty. Hence, urban areas were the first to support physicians who wanted to specialize in surgery and later other specialties. Although a few large hospitals and urban centers provided an opportunity for surgery, America had nothing comparable to the great European hospitals. The large crowded European hospitals, however, were plagued with repeated infections. This was undoubtedly a factor in the European's early acceptance of the antiseptic principle. The fact that this danger was not so acute in America may help to explain the reluctance of American surgeons to adopt measures to prevent surgical infection—the Listerian method.

Aseptic techniques, a fundamental modern surgical introduction, were originally met with scorn and ridicule. It was not until the last decades of the nineteenth century that the seeds sown by Pasteur and Lister began to bear fruit. The surgical profession's grudging acceptance of the most basic postulate of the Listerian method was due in large part to its continuing delay in acceptance of the germ theory of disease. The highly complicated nature of Lister's methods may have also deterred many surgeons who, although still dubious of the germ theory, might have given the Listerian technique an empirical trial. Most surgery was performed in private homes; therefore, it was exceedingly difficult to guarantee aseptic conditions for an operation even where the technique was used. Certainly, a few unsuccessful operations added a further note of discouragement. The indifference or outright hostility of the leading British surgeons toward the Lister techniques undoubtedly adversely influenced American surgeons.

It should be pointed out, however, that much of the Listerian ritual gradually found general acceptance. Cleanliness became the order in surgical procedures, a step that eventually paved the way for asepsis. Diluted carbolic acid solution became the preferred antiseptic.

In the years following 1865, even before Lord Joseph Lister's (1827–1912) work, cleanliness in dealing with open wounds and the value of carbolic acid as an antiseptic had gradually become recognized. It was not until the latter decades of the nineteenth century, however, that Lister's principles of aseptic surgery were fully accepted by physicians in Alabama.

The methods used sought to create a sterile operating field in order to prevent the entrance of pathogenic organisms. They involved sterilizing all instruments, dressings, sponges, gowns, and other items in the operating room. These were cleaned and soaked most commonly in diluted carbolic acid, a solution of bichloride of mercury or alcohol. The value of steam sterilization was also recognized. A major item that did not lend itself to sterilization was the surgeon's hands. In 1889, Dr. William Stewart Halsted (1852–1922) of Johns Hopkins suggested the use of rubber gloves to protect his nurse's hands from the antiseptic solution to which she was allergic. Later, Dr. Joseph C. Bloodgood, one of Halsted's assistants, began using sterile rubber gloves routinely for surgery. The use of facial masks in the operating room was a later development. An extant photograph of an operating room team at the Hillman Hospital around the turn of the century shows the surgeon and nurses without masks.

Anesthesia

In 1884, Sigmund Freud (1856–1939) made the first detailed study of the physiological effects of cocaine. Dr. Carl Koller (1857–1944), also from Vienna, reported his pioneering work on the value of cocaine as a local anesthetic in the same year. Dr. William S. Halsted introduced the field of local and conduction anesthesia by demonstrating the use of a cocaine solution with which he injected himself and his associates.

Dr. James Leonard Corning (1855–1923) of New York began experimenting with spinal anesthesia in 1885. In 1899, Dr. Rudolph Matas (1860–1957) of New Orleans first employed this technique for surgical purposes. However, he found that cocaine was too toxic for intraspinal use. Dr. Matas also devised an improved method for local nerve block and massive infiltration anesthesia.

Dr. Frank Dubose of Selma wrote in the *Transactions of the Medical Association of the State of Alabama* in 1914 that the difficulties and harmful consequences of spinal anesthesia had placed an extreme limit on its use.[1] It was only after the introduction of new anesthetic agents for spinal anesthesia that this procedure became safe and its use became widespread.

Surgery

While it is true that to single out a few physicians is to do an injustice to many, it would likewise be unjust not to identify individuals who originally reported their findings in medicine. Therefore, we have used the *Transactions of the Medical Association of the State of Alabama (Transactions), New Orleans Medical and Surgical Journal, American Surgeon,* and *The Journal of the Medical Association of the State of Alabama* to identify the original reports of advancements in medicine and surgery that took place in Alabama.

Successful practitioners are often more occupied with diagnosing and treating disease than with reporting their experiences. Unfortunately, it is the lot of such men who are invaluable when alive to be soon forgotten after they are dead. Certainly this may explain in some instances the absence of reports about recent advances in the practice of medicine.

One of the early reports on Alabama surgery was made in 1869 by Dr. J. Paul Jones, Sr. (1837–1903), of Camden, who reviewed the surgery performed in still largely rural Wilcox County.[2] As to be expected, amputations were common and were usually of the leg, thigh, and hand. No mention was made of the use of aseptic techniques. Dr. Jones successfully repaired two acutely strangulated hernias. He also removed a breast for carcinoma. However, the patient expired about six months later with what he considered to be metastases. In a remarkable surgical procedure, he successfully removed an osteosarcoma of the jaw in a young black female without using anesthesia. He considered that the tumor was so large that the expected excessive loss of blood could result in tracheal aspiration. As there was then no means of suction available, he hoped the patient, without anesthesia, could clear her respiratory tract.

One of the most outstanding early surgeons in Alabama and a colorful adventurer in the pre–Civil War years was William Joseph Holt (1829–1881) of Montgomery.[3] Dr. Holt was highly respected not only by the members of the medical profession but also by the young men in Montgomery who aspired to study medicine. Of the young men who read medicine under his direction, no doubt Luther Leonidas Hill became the most renowned. Dr. Holt, a native of Georgia, originally read medicine with Dr. L. A. Dugas, one of the founders of the Medical College of Georgia. He received the M.D. degree from the Georgia school on February 28, 1852. After graduation, Dr. Holt went to Europe and studied in the schools and hospitals in Berlin and Vienna. He also studied in Paris in the first half of the nineteenth century. Paris was the undisputed center of medical training where such giants of the medical world as Pierre Louis, Jean Civiale, Claude Bernard, and Alfred Velpeau practiced.

While in Paris, Dr. Holt attended Emperor Napoleon III's coronation in Notre-Dame de Paris; and on January 30, 1853, he witnessed the emperor's marriage to Eugénie de Montijo, a Spanish countess. Dr. Holt tendered his services to Nicholas I, tsar of Russia, while the tsar was in Paris. During the Crimean War, he entered the medical department of the Russian Army. Little seems to be recorded of his services as a surgeon in the Russian Army; however, he was decorated by the tsar. Dr. Holt was admitted into four of the seven orders of Russian knighthood: the orders of St. Anne, St. Stanislaus, St. Andrew, and St. George.

Dr. Holt offered his services to the Confederate States Army in 1861 and was with the first state troops that reached Pensacola. After the war, he and his family moved to Montgomery where he entered the practice of medicine.

Dr. James Fountain Heustis (son of Dr. Jabez Wiggins Heustis) was one of Mobile's outstanding surgeons and Professor of Anatomy and Surgery at the Medical College of Alabama during the latter half of the nineteenth century. Writing in the *Transactions* in 1881, he commented on the use of Lister's antiseptic method in surgical operations, stating that "while recognizing its great value in [successful] operations, I cannot say that I see its special need in [oophorectomy], though statistics show that the mortality from [this] operation is reduced to minimum [when it is used]."[4] He further observed that if all precautions for preventing shock were taken—including exclusion of cold air from the peritoneal cavity, careful removal of blood and cystic contents, and suturing the peritoneal surface of the incision with silver wire or catgut—the necessity of antiseptics could scarcely be required. On another occasion he was more emphatic in his praise of the Lister technique as he wrote that

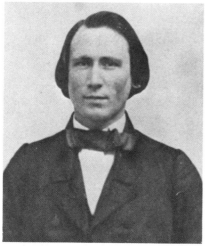

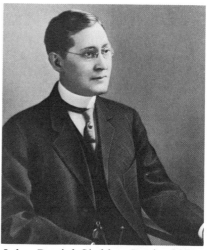

William Joseph Holt, M.D., 1829–1881 (Courtesy of the Alabama Museum of the Health Sciences, Lister Hill Library, Medical Center, The University of Alabama in Birmingham)

John Daniel Sinkler Davis, M.D., 1859–1931 (Courtesy of the Alabama State Department of Archives and History)

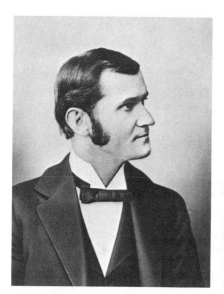

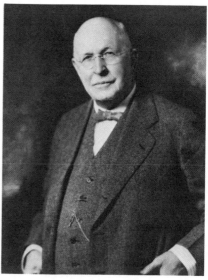

William Elias Brownlee Davis, M.D., 1863–1903 (Courtesy of the Alabama State Department of Archives and History)

Luther Leonidas Hill, M.D., 1862–1946 (Courtesy of Mrs. Amelie Hill Laslie (Mrs. C. G.), Daughter, Montgomery, Alabama)

Of all the recent advances in surgery, Lister's antiseptic system maintains the first place, and the wonderful reputation made for it by him has spread to every part of the world, and has been added to by such brilliant results everywhere, there can be no doubt of its complete success, and of its deserving all its claims.[5]

In a review of surgery that he had performed (1881), Dr. Heustis described the successful removal of a large ovarian tumor from a young female using aseptic precautions.[6] In the same report, he described a cesarean section on a fourteen-year-old female with an infantile pelvis. The mother and infant succumbed, which he thought was due, at least in part, to the fact that the surgery had been too long delayed in order to allow for an attempted normal delivery. Likewise, he reported successful surgical repair of a congenitally absent vagina in a sixteen-year-old female. Dr. Heustis apparently rebuilt a vaginal canal and maintained its patency with repeated dilations. He used diluted carbolic acid solution to irrigate the vagina routinely. Dr. Heustis also reported on the closure of urethrovaginal, vesicovaginal, and vesicouterovaginal fistulas using a modification of the Sims and Bozeman surgical techniques.

Probably two of the most remarkable surgeons of this period were Dr. John Daniel Sinkler Davis (1859–1931) and his brother, Dr. William Elias Brownlee Davis (1863–1903), both natives of Jefferson County. Dr. J. D. S. Davis had graduated in 1879 from the Medical College of Georgia. He was a member of the surgical faculty of the Birmingham Medical College where he was an active surgical investigator. Dr. W. E. B. Davis attended the Medical Department of Vanderbilt University in 1882, and the following year he attended the Kentucky School of Medicine at Louisville. In 1884, he entered Bellevue Hospital Medical College, New York City, and was awarded an M.D. degree the following spring. In 1887, he attended surgical clinics in London, Berlin, and Vienna. He served as Professor of Gynecology and Abdominal Surgery at the Birmingham Medical College. He and Dr. J. D. S. Davis were the founders of the *Southern Surgical and Gynecological Association* (1887), and he served as its president in 1901.[7] It is now known as the *Southern Surgical Association*. The brothers founded the *Alabama Medical and Surgical Journal* (1886). Dr. W. E. B. Davis served as editor of the *Transactions of the Southern Surgical and Gynecological Society* from 1887 until his death in 1903 (see Chapter 9, "Medical Journals in Alabama").

As early as 1889, the Davis brothers experimented in intestinal surgery using dogs. In a remarkably erudite study, they reported successful intestinal anastomoses of ileoileostomy, jejunoileostomy, ileocolostomy and gastroenterostomy.[8] The results were obtained using a catgut plate or ring to approximate and stabilize the anastomosis. In this study, Dr. J. D. S. Davis also reported some of his and his brother's experiences in intestinal closure in humans after penetrating gunshot and knife wounds. They advocated immediate closure of perforated wounds of the abdominal viscera.

In 1892, Dr. W. E. B. Davis performed experiments upon dogs for the purpose of determining the safest treatment of common bile duct obstruction.[9] The principles established by these experiments were that sterile bile is inoffensive to the peritoneum and that after removal of calculi from the common duct, suture of the duct is not necessary and indeed may be harmful. The observations of Dr. Davis lessened the dangers and simplified the technique of choledochostomy. Dr. William J. Mayo said of Dr. Davis's work, "his original experimental and clinical investigations on the infection of the common duct were of international import." The Davis brothers also emphasized that intestinal sounds were a good indication of abdominal disease: a silent abdomen is found in generalized peritonitis, whereas high-pitched sounds may be heard in intestinal obstruction.

Unquestionably, the Davis brothers' remarkable experiments helped to advance surgery of the abdominal cavity and its contents. After Dr. W. E. B. Davis's death in 1903, Dr. J. D. S. Davis continued to perform excellent and innovative surgery well into the twentieth century.

Dr. Luther Leonidas Hill (1862–1946), a native of Montgomery, Alabama, was one of the giants of surgery in Alabama in the latter part of the nineteenth century and the early decades of the twentieth century.[10] Prior to entering medical school, he served an apprenticeship with Dr. William Joseph Holt of Montgomery. He was educated at the Medical Department of the University of the City of New York, receiving his M.D. degree in 1881. Dr. Hill was not satisfied with his training and acquired a second M.D. degree from the Jefferson Medical College of Philadelphia. In 1883, Dr. Hill studied at King's College Hospital in London under the famous surgeon, Lord Joseph Lister, known for his antiseptic surgical techniques. Returning to Montgomery, he practiced medicine for more than fifty years until a short time before his death in 1946. In 1897, he became the surgeon-in-chief at the Laura Croom Hill Hospital, a private hospital, which he and his brother, the gynecologist, Dr. Robert S. Hill, operated for more than 35 years.

When Dr. Hill entered practice in 1881, surgical operations consisted chiefly of amputations, tracheotomy, trephining, lithotomy, lithotrity, hernia repairs, ligating aneurisms, removing foreign bodies, dressing fractures, and reducing dislocations.

Dr. Hill was apparently the first surgeon to use aseptic techniques in Montgomery and to promote their use over the entire state. The first operation he performed after returning to Mongomery in 1883 was a laparotomy, in which he no doubt used the technique he had learned from Lister. He said of Lister's work "mankind owes to Sir Joseph Lister an everlasting debt of gratitude which it can never repay."

In 1893, in an address before the State Medical Association, Dr. Hill reviewed the status of the field of surgery and its recent developments.[11] He also reported on some of his own work. This report demonstrates both how young the field of surgery was and how remarkable was Dr. Hill's surgical versatility. Some examples of procedures he had performed included section of the fifth cranial nerve for trigeminal neuralgia and various operations for hernia for which he emphasized the value of a radical cure technique. He also reported on the use of homologous tissue transplants.

The reluctance to enter the abdominal cavity and its viscera is readily evident in reading the files of the antebellum surgical journals. Even where the abdominal viscus had been penetrated, most surgeons would only close the wound and hope for the best. Obviously, most of these patients died of peritonitis. Dr. Hill reviewed the use of laparotomy for gunshot wounds and perforations of the intestines, pointing out that the conservative therapy still widely used in these patients resulted in an 88 percent mortality. He recognized that resection of the perforated area or simple closure of the intestine was the best course of treatment, and his results were encouraging. He reviewed the use of surgery for appendicitis but concluded that conservative care was still the best course to adopt. Surgery for this disease was still considered hazardous.

Dr. Hill was especially interested in wounds of the human heart. In 1900, he published a review of the subject in the *Medical Record*, detailing an account of seventeen known cases of suture of heart wounds, two of which he had witnessed.[12] As early as 1881, one Dr. John B. Roberts conceived the idea of suturing the human heart but was scoffed at by the great Viennese surgeon, Christian Albert Theodor Billroth (1829–1894): "No surgeon who wishes to preserve the respect of his colleagues would ever attempt to suture a wound of the heart." Several attempts were made by Europeans, but it was not until 1896 that Dr. Ludwig Rehn of Frankfurt, Germany, performed the first closure of a human heart wound in which the patient recovered.

On the night of September 15, 1902, Dr. Hill sutured a wound in the human heart for the first time in America, and the patient lived.[13] Dr. Hill had been called to attend a young black boy, Henry Myrick, who had been "stobbed in his heart." The patient was bleeding excessively, and there was no available hospital. Dr. Hill knew that his only hope to save the boy's life was to close the lacerated heart. With the consent of the parents, Dr. Hill placed the boy on the kitchen table about one o'clock in the morning. In the meantime, several physicians, one of whom was his brother, had arrived to assist. By the light of a kerosene

HENRY MYRICK, 13 YEAR-OLD B— OF MONTGOMERY, STAB—
THE HEART SEPTEMB—. 14, AND NOW WELL.

MONTGOMERY, October 25.—(Special.)—No branch of the medical profession is just now attracting so much attention as surgery of the heart and the very rare cases are given in detail by the great news organizations. An account of an opperation of this sort sent out from New York only this week suggests that a detailed description of a re-ient successful operation here may be of value to the profession and of interest o everybody. The subject is a thirteen-ear-old negro boy, who was stabbed in the heart at the city cemetery on September 14 last, by a little boy named John Conners. He is now, so far as any one can tell, as well and healthy a little negro as goes about Montgomery.

The Southern Alabama Medical League met in annual session at Dothan last Tuesday, and Dr. L. L. Hill, the operating surgeon, was present with the boy and read a paper describing the operation, the boy, himself, stripped to the waist in order to illustrate the lecture. From this public and authentic account the following facts are gathered:

The boy, whose name is Henry Myrick, was stabbed at 5 p. m. He walked off a few steps and fell. He was carried to his home, a common negro cabin a short distance from the cemetery. At 1 a. m., just eight hours afterward, he was taken from the bed and placed on an improvised operating table. The operation was performed by the light of two oil lamps borrowed from neighboring cabins. At the time the extremities were cold, the pulse imperceptible, the respiration sighing and the boy partially unconscious. A small quantity of chloroform was given. Examination showed that the knife had entered a little to the right of the left nipple and had penerrated the cavity.

An incision was first made one-half inch from the breast bone and carried out four inches along the third rib. A similar incision was made along the sixth rib, and the outer ends of these joined by a verticle incision. The third, fourth and fifth ribs were then cut in two and the door thus made was turned back and gave access to the cavity. The lines of these incisions are brought out in the accompanying photograph taken just before the stays were removed.

The pericardium or sac surrounding the heart was found to be filled with blood from the wound in the heart. The wound in the sac was enlarged two and a half inches and eight ounces of blood removed. The condition of the boy at once improved. The surgeon then passed his hand into the sac and pulled the heart up, when a hole one-half inch long was discovered in the left ventricle. From this hole there came a stream of blood at every contraction. The hole was closed with a cat gut suture and this stopped the bleeding. The pericardium was then closed and the door or flap brought down and stitched in position.

The boy was delirious for three days and his pulse averaged 145. On the fifteenth day he sat up for the first time, and on October 21 went to Dothan, more than a hundred miles away, in perfectly good physical condition to enjoy his nevel experience with the doctors.

The operating surgeon has been president of the Alabama State Medical Society, Dr. R. F. Michel, one of the oldest and most eminent practitioners in the state, was present to assist, and Dr. E. C. Parker and several other local physicians were also there.

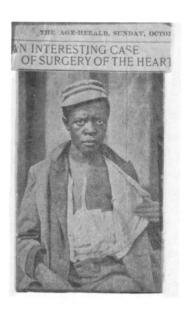

THE AGE-HERALD, SUNDAY, OCTO—

AN INTERESTING CASE
OF SURGERY OF THE HEART

The first successful heart surgery in the United States was performed by L. L. Hill on September 15, 1902. (Newspaper clipping from *The Birmingham Age-Herald,* October 26, 1902)

lamp, the surgery was performed. Chloroform was used as the anesthetic. Dr. R. S. Hill held the beating heart, "to steady it sufficiently . . . to allow the passage of a cat-gut suture through the center of the wound."[14] In 45 minutes, the operation was over. The boy recovered only to succumb to a similar wound acquired in a fray years later in Chicago. Dr. Hill thus became the first American physician to suture successfully a wound of the human heart that involved one of the heart chambers.

In 1898, Dr. Hill proposed the establishment of the Jerome Cochran Memorial Lecture to be given annually at the State Medical Association meeting to honor the first State Health Officer. Dr. Hill gave the lecture in 1913.

On June 7, 1959, the Society for Vascular Surgery honored Dr. Hill in Atlantic City when the Luther Leonidas Hill Memorial plaque was presented to his son, Senator Lister Hill of Alabama, commemorating the pioneering contributions of his father in cardiovascular surgery.[15] A cardiovascular surgical research unit at The University of Alabama in Birmingham was dedicated to his memory in October, 1959.

Hillman Hospital Surgical Training Program

During the first three decades of the twentieth century, the excellent quality of the Hillman Hospital house staff training was widely recognized. One of those responsible for this training was Dr. James Monroe

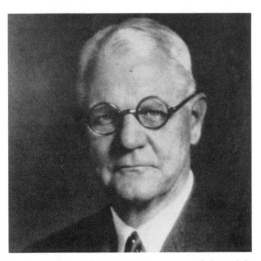

James Monroe Mason, M.D., 1871–1952 (Courtesy of the Alabama Museum of the Health Sciences, Lister Hill Library, Medical Center, The University of Alabama in Birmingham)

Mason (1871–1952), a native of Alabama.[16] He originally matriculated at the Medical College of Alabama at Mobile but transferred to the School of Medicine of Tulane University. In 1899, he received his M.D. degree from Tulane. He served as a resident in surgery at Charity Hospital in New Orleans (1897–1899) and entered the practice of medicine in Birmingham in 1899. In 1902, he entered Johns Hopkins University for a period of postgraduate study. Dr. Mason visited the foremost clinics of Europe in 1910, 1911, and 1928.

The standards of surgery not only in Birmingham but in the entire state were elevated because of Dr. Mason. He served as attending surgeon, surgeon-in-chief, and a member of the Medical Advisory Board of Hillman Hospital. He also made major contributions in the surgical interns' and residents' training at Hillman Hospital.

Dr. Mason served in World War I as a major of the United States Army Medical Corps. He was chief of Surgical Services at the United States Army General Hospital at Des Moines, Iowa. While he was stationed there, this hospital was designated an Empyema Center.

Dr. Mason was a member of the Founder's Group of the American College of Surgeons in 1913. He was a member of the Board of Governors for nine years and also served for twelve years as a member of the Board of Regents. He became president of the Southern Surgical Association in 1930. In 1935, at the 100th anniversary of the School of Medicine of Tulane University, the honorary degree of Doctor of Science was conferred upon Dr. Mason.

In 1945, when the Medical College of Alabama became a four-year institution in Birmingham, Dr. Mason became Professor of Surgery and chairman of the Department of Surgery there. He served in this capacity until 1949, when Dr. Champ Lyons was appointed the first full-time Professor of Surgery.

Dr. H. Earl Conwell (1893–1973) and his colleague Dr. John D. Sherrill (1892–1968), both prominent orthopedic surgeons, were active in the Hillman Hospital orthopedic training program. Dr. Conwell was also active in the program at Lloyd Noland Hospital. He is best known for his work, "Injuries to the Elbow," published in an internationally known textbook, Key and Conwell's *The Management of Fractures, Dislocations, and Sprains.* The book went through seven editions.

Dr. Cecil Gaston (1887–1940), a Birmingham surgeon who graduated from Vanderbilt and Jefferson Medical College, Philadelphia, became interested in proctology training at the Hargis Clinic in Detroit.[17] He was

---

* *The Management of Fractures, Dislocations, and Sprains* was originally published in 1934 by C. V. Mosby Co., St. Louis. The seventh edition was also published by C. V. Mosby Co. in 1961.

allegedly the first Birmingham physician to use the proctoscope routine-ly, and he established the Hillman Proctology Clinic. These surgeons were only three of many prominent physicians who gave of their time and knowledge to make Hillman Hospital justly well known.

Appendectomy

The diagnosis and treatment of appendicitis is one area of abdominal surgery in which American surgeons deserve the most credit. During the nineteenth century, the disorder was referred to as typhlitis or inflam-mation of the cecum, based on the assumption that the problem lay in the cecum, the blind pouch in which the large intestine begins.

Beginning in the last decade of the nineteenth century, appendicitis became recognized as a hazardous disease. The diagnosis of "cramp colic," as the disease was referred to, was frequently viewed with alarm by most laymen. Appendiceal abscesses were occasionally recognized and drained, but it was not until the 1890s that appendectomies were performed in Alabama.

In 1887, Dr. E. P. Earle of Birmingham published a definitive article on typhlitis.[18] He obviously was aware of the pathology and the symp-tomatology of appendicitis. He described the rupture of the appendix and the resulting general peritonitis and death. Dr. Earle recognized the necessity of surgical intervention in acute disease, but commented that surgical operations were hazardous and that the surgeon should make sure that he was dealing with an acutely involved or necrosed appendix before he would be justified in intervening surgically. Dr. Earle no doubt reflected the prevailing opinion in as much as he recommended surgical intervention only where it was the last possible recourse.

By early 1900, physicians realized that early appendectomies rarely proved fatal, but that when the treatment was medical rather than surgical, mortality ran from fifteen to twenty percent. Newer methods of diagnosis were gradually coming into use, and the value of the white blood count was recognized.

Although individual American physicians had diagnosed perforation of the appendix in cases of so-called typhlitis, it remained for Reginald Herber Fitz (1843–1913) of Boston to pinpoint the source of the prob-lem. In 1886, he analyzed 466 cases involving this type of abdominal distress and showed that in the vast majority of them inflammation of the appendix was the primary cause. So convincing was his study that by the 1890s the term typhlitis was being replaced by appendicitis. The next development was the work of Charles McBurney (1845–1913) of New York. In 1889, he identified McBurney's point, the area of the abdomi-nal wall in which tenderness indicated inflammation of the appendix. In

1894, he described an operative method for removing the appendix that is still called McBurney's incision. This procedure was first cited in an article in the *Transactions* by Dr. L. L. McArthur of Chicago.

Dr. J. D. S. Davis in 1890 had discussed the surgical technique of appendectomy. He stated: "It (the appendix) should be amputated closely, just as you would a diverticulum in any other portion of the bowel, pushed in, and then closed with Lembert sutures—serosa to serosa. The best results will attend this procedure."[19] Dr. W. E. B. Davis observed: "In these cases (appendicitis cases) the surgeon has a fertile field, and one in which many lives can be saved by timely operation."[20]

In 1899, Dr. George Summers Brown (1860–1913) of Birmingham addressed the State Medical Association on the subject of appendicitis.[21] He stated that appendicitis should be considered a surgical disease, and that the attitude of the general practitioners that medical treatment would suffice was the cause of the high mortality. Dr. Brown further observed that those operated on early usually lived. He reviewed his experience with this disease and pointed out that rupture of the appendix is the most common cause of death; whereas early operations were usually followed by cure and uneventful recovery. He described sixteen cases in which he operated early after onset of symptoms. Only one had died. The next year, 1900, he again addressed the association on the importance of bolder measures in the treatment of appendicitis.[22] He stated that he had had a total experience in appendicitis of eighty cases of which he had operated on thirty-one with five deaths. He postulated that all of these most certainly would have lived if they had had early surgical removal of the appendix. The early operation in all instances reduced the death rate. Dr. Brown also described a case of retrocecal appendix with rupture.

All of these early practitioners used drastic purges to empty the colon in treatment of patients suffering with appendicitis. It was only recognized after long observation that this frequently precipitated rupture of the involved appendix. The routine use of purges was then discontinued.

Physicians were beginning to realize the seriousness of a ruptured appendix. Dr. W. P. Jackson, a prominent surgeon from Mobile, discussed the complications of ruptured appendix in 1922.[23] Dr. William Wade Harper (1868–1941) of Selma stated in a discussion of Dr. Jackson's paper that more deaths were caused from the results of appendicitis than any other disease in Alabama other than, of course, tuberculosis.

In 1929, Dr. L. J. Johns of Birmingham addressed the State Medical Association on the occurrence of appendicitis in children.[24] He pointed out the difficulty in diagnosis and the high rate of mortality resulting from ruptured appendix. Again Dr. Harper of Selma stated that the high mortality rate in children caused by appendicitis was the result of the failure to recognize that the clinical manifestations of this disease in children could be entirely different from that in adults.

Blood Transfusions

Blood transfusions had been attempted as early as the nineteenth century. However, it was not until 1900 that Karl Landsteiner (1868–1943) of Vienna—and later of the Rockefeller Institute—found that there are different types of human blood.[25] Because of Dr. Landsteiner's discovery, blood transfusions became relatively safe when only like blood types were used. The footnotes in the 1900 Landsteiner report contained information on one of his most important discoveries, namely, that the agglutination occurring between serum and blood cells of different humans was a physiological phenomenon which he explained by individual differences. In an article the following year, Landsteiner described a simple technique of agglutination, whereby he divided human blood into three groups: A, B, and C (later O). Two of his co-workers, the clinicians Descastello and Sturli, examined additional persons and found the fourth blood group, later named AB.

As transfusion techniques improved, storing blood became possible. Indirect transfusions became commonplace. In 1937, the first blood bank was established at Chicago's Cook County Hospital, where blood was stored at a temperature of 4° to 6° centigrade.

Another major step was made when heparin was discovered. In 1916, Jay McLean, a sophomore medical student at Johns Hopkins, discovered a substance with anticoagulant properties that Dr. Howell, in whose laboratory he worked, named heparin in 1918. Heparin's anticoagulant qualities have made it invaluable in both surgery and medicine. This discovery along with the emergence of hematology as a specialty and improvements in blood transfusion techniques, have made open heart surgery and other complicated operative procedures feasible.

As early as 1909, Dr. J. D. S. Davis in a report published in the *Transactions* discussed the use and technique of direct blood transfusions.[26] One of the difficulties encountered then in direct blood transfusions was the cumbersome technique of uniting an artery of the donor to a vein of the recipient. The force of the blood flow of the artery then filled the venous system of the recipient. Clotting of the blood at the site of the junction of the artery and vein was a common occurrence. Dr. Davis used a cannula, similar to the one originally described by Dr. George Crile of Cleveland, to effect a vascular union. It was inserted in the radial artery of the donor and in the basilic vein of the recipient.

No attempt was made to cross-match the blood of the recipient and donor. Dr. Davis observed that there was no accurate means to estimate the amount of blood given by the direct method. However, he used indirect measurements to monitor the procedure in the donor including the estimation of the hemoglobin, cell count, and pulse rate. He felt that measuring the blood pressure of both donor and donee frequently was the most reliable guide available to determine the amount administered. If the blood pressure fell to 80 mm of mercury in the donor, the transfusion was promptly terminated.

The agglutination of either donor or donee's blood cells was an important index to danger. If the transfused blood hemolyzed or agglutinated the blood of the patient, harm could result; and the transfusion was stopped immediately. The use of close relatives of the patients as donors in these transfusions possibly resulted in fewer reactions. Dr. Davis cited newer developments indicating that certain interesting phenomena of agglutination and lysis sometimes occurred on mixing the red cells from the blood of one individual with the serum from another. This finding eventually resulted in using blood types to make blood transfusions relatively safe. Dr. Davis had further observed that, in infants with hemorrhagic diathesis and hemophilia, the transfusion of fresh blood would frequently check the hemorrhage.

Writing in the *Transactions* of 1917, Dr. Philip Ball Moss (1883–1936) of Selma pointed out that one of the most important procedures in blood transfusions was choice of donor.[27] He warned of the presence of agglutinins and hemolysins that caused reactions in blood transfusion. Dr. Moss, in quoting recent work that described the four distinct groups of blood (I, II, III, and IV) and how they could be identified, pointed out that even after typing and before using the blood in transfusions, one should always retype it to make doubly sure the blood was compatible.

Dr. Earle Drennen (1882–1957) of Birmingham wrote in the *Transactions* in 1920 that the citrate technique was the best procedure for preserving the blood for transfusions.[28] This had the advantage that blood did not have to be given immediately and thus could be collected at one site and transported to another. The citrate technique made possible the blood banks after the 1930s.[29] He also noted that direct transfusions between patients and donors were no longer used.

The Development of Neurology and Neurosurgery

Dr. Eugene DuBose Bondurant and Dr. William Henry Hudson were pioneers in the fields of neurology and neurosurgery; Dr. Bondurant was a neurologist and Dr. Hudson was a neurosurgeon.[30] Both men brought a level of neurological eminence and innovation to Alabama that was unknown to most of the country at that time. Dr. Bondurant, born in Gallion, Alabama, attended Southern University of Greensboro, Alabama, and graduated from the University of Virginia School of Medicine in 1882. In 1884, he entered graduate training at the New York Insane Hospital. Later he studied in England and on the continent under some of the leading clinicians of that day.

In 1885, Dr. Bondurant was appointed to the staff of the Alabama Hospital for the Insane in Tuscaloosa where, in 1892, he became assistant superintendent. In 1895, while still at Bryce, he observed endemic beriberi in the patient population. This was the "first time a nutritional disease was recognized in the United States."[31] Sir William Osler cited this observation in the third edition of his textbook of medicine published in 1898. Dr. Bondurant also held academic positions at the Medical College of Alabama in Mobile and the University of Alabama School of Medicine in Tuscaloosa. (See Chapter 3, "Efforts in Medical Education" and Chapter 13, "The History of the Mental Health Movement in Alabama.")

Dr. William Henry Hudson (1862–1917), a contemporary of Dr. Bondurant, was dubbed by a biographer as the "Itinerant Neurosurgeon."[32] He was born in Chipley, Georgia. In 1886, he received his M.D. degree from the Atlanta Medical College and undertook two years of postgraduate training in Baltimore, Philadelphia and New York. In 1888, he began his practice in Lafayette, Alabama; however, in 1892, he went to London for further training. While in London, he probably met Sir William Richard Gowers and possibly came under Sir Victor Horsley's influence.

In 1893 and 1894, Dr. Hudson studied in Berlin where he gained some expertise in the microscopical examination of surgical specimens. Upon returning to Lafayette in 1894, his welcome was far from friendly in that before he left, he had neglected to pay some of his outstanding debts. After the turn of the century, he moved to Montgomery.

By 1913, Dr. Hudson had performed 152 craniotomies and craniectomies with no mortality. Also he devised techniques for the following: decompression of the skull, closure of the dura, and fixation of bone flaps using scrupulous antiseptic procedures. Also a number of "ingenious skull instruments" were developed by Dr. Hudson such as a perforator, burr, drill and osteotome. Some of these instruments are still widely used.[33]

Surgical neurology came into its own through various individuals who followed in the wake of Dr. Hudson. Most neurosurgeons came from the ranks of the general surgeons of the early twentieth century. One of these was Dr. Charles Edward Dowman (1882–1931). Dr. Dowman was born in Quincy, Florida. He was educated at Emory University and in 1905, he received his M.D. from Johns Hopkins. Between 1905 and

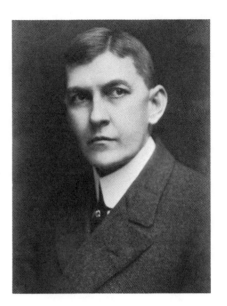

Eugene DuBose Bondurant, M.D., 1862–1950, Dean 1912–1916 (Courtesy of the Heustis Medical Museum, Mobile, Alabama)

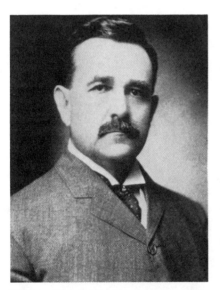

William Henry Hudson, M.D., 1862–1917 (Reproduced with permission from Fincher, E. F.: "William Henry Hudson, M.D., Itinerant Neurosurgeon, 1862–1917," *J. Neurosurg.* 16: 123–34, 1959)

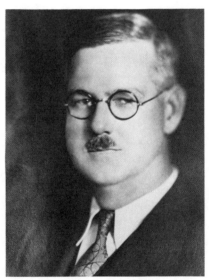

Charles Edward Dowman, M.D., 1882–1931 (Courtesy of Dr. Charles E. Dowman III, Atlanta, Georgia)

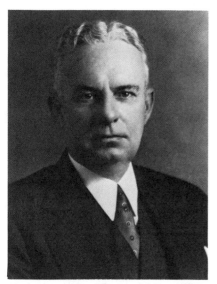

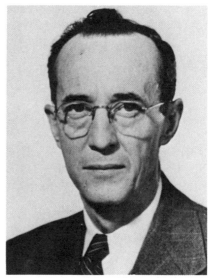

Chalmers Hale Moore, M.D., 1889–1945 (Courtesy of Mrs. Chalmers Hale Moore, Sr., Carlsbad, California)

James Owen Foley, Ph.D., 1897–1961 (Courtesy of Mary Foley Holland, Daughter)

1907, Dr. Dowman took pathological and surgical training in Berlin and Breslau. A portion of 1907 was spent at the National Hospital at Queen Square, London. During this time, he did experimental work in Sir Victor Horsley's laboratory.

From 1909 through 1913, Dr. Dowman was visiting surgeon and pathologist at Hillman Hospital, and neurosurgeon from 1913 to 1915. He was also professor of pathology at the Birmingham Medical College from 1911 to 1913. In 1913, Dr. Dowman was a member of the faculty at Emory University School of Medicine in the department of surgery and later in neurosurgery. In October 1917, he entered the army and was part of the Emory unit which was stationed in France. Upon discharge, he rejoined the faculty of Emory University School of Medicine.[34]

Dr. Chalmers Hale Moore (1889–1945) succeeded Dr. Dowman as chief of neurosurgery at Hillman Hospital. Dr. Moore was born in Jefferson County, Alabama. He attended Washington and Lee University, and in 1913 he received his M.D. degree from Johns Hopkins. By 1935, he had changed his practice from general surgery to neurosurgery due principally to the influence of former classmates, Drs. Gilbert Horrax and Walter Edward Dandy. Dr. Moore also served as consultant to several other hospitals in Birmingham.

Any discussion of the neurological sciences should include neuroanatomy and neurophysiology. Three anatomists, James Owen Foley, Ph.D., Dr. Elizabeth Caroline Crosby and Dr. Tryphena Humphrey made major contributions to this field. Dr. Foley (1897–1961) was a Rockefeller Research fellow at Cornell in 1938. During his career, he came in contact with such eminent scientific researchers as Drs. S. W. Ranson, H. W. Magoun, W. R. Ingram, and C. J. Herrick. Most of Dr. Foley's research publications dealt with aspects of the peripheral and autonomic nervous systems.

Dr. Foley was professor of anatomy both at the Tuscaloosa and Birmingham medical schools. He is best remembered by the medical students for his outstanding teaching ability. In 1960, the University of Alabama conferred on Dr. Foley the honorary degree of Doctor of Science in recognition of his many outstanding contributions to science. Dr. Foley was responsible in large part for Dr. Elizabeth C. Crosby (1888–) coming to the Medical Center in Birmingham. She received her master's degree in 1912 from the University of Chicago and a doctorate in 1915. Dr. Crosby has held appointments at several colleges and universities. She received awards for her outstanding research in comparative anatomy and neurology from various medical and scientific organizations. In 1960, The University of Alabama appointed her Professor Emeritus of Anatomy at the Medical Center. Until ill health forced her retirement, she was an active participant at the clinical conferences on neurology and neurosurgery. She has continued to write, however, and had an article published as late as 1979.

Dr. Tryphena Humphrey (1902–1971), a former student and close friend of Dr. Crosby, also came to the Medical Center. She attended the University of Michigan and received her M.D. in 1931 and her Ph.D. degree in 1936. Dr. Humphrey went to Europe for further study, and while there she became interested in research pertaining to neuroanatomy and neuroembryology. Dr. Humphrey became a full professor at the University of Pittsburgh. In 1962, Dr. Humphrey and Dr. Crosby collaborated on a remarkable book, *Correlative Anatomy of the Nervous System*.* This book is still in use today. Dr. Humphrey was appointed Career Professor of Anatomy at The University of Alabama in Birmingham Medical Center where she continued her research work.

Obstetrics and Gynecology

Gynecological surgery ranged from simple exploratory incisions to cesarean section. The removal of cystic ovarian tumors, some of which weighed over 100 pounds, was frequently performed. After the antebel-

---

Correlative Anatomy of the Nervous System was published in 1962 by Macmillan in New York.

lum years, cesarean sections were still performed but apparently not on the scale that had been previously reported.

As it had been in the pre–Civil War years, the practice of midwifery after the Civil War remained largely in the hands of relatively untrained midwives. Probably due to their low fees and availability, midwives continued to hold sway in the vast majority of maternity cases; physicians were called in only when complications occurred.

Physicians gradually became involved in childbirth. The advent of anesthesia undoubtedly contributed to this fortunate state of affairs. Anesthesia had been used for obstetrical cases in Alabama as early as the 1850s, and its use steadily increased with the passing years.

In a general discussion at the 1886 annual meeting of the State Medical Association, it was observed that aggressive use of antiseptics in obstetrics before and during labor was of little value and might actually be harmful.[35] Irrigation of the vagina and uterus with an antiseptic solution in a routine delivery was condemned. It was pointed out that the hands of the accoucheur and his assistant should be thoroughly cleaned and rinsed with antiseptics. Dr. Jerome Cochran advised against aggressive antiseptic techniques being used routinely in normal labor. He noted that the immense majority of women will pass through childbirth without becoming septic. Dr. Richard Fraser Michel (1827–1907) of Montgomery observed that irrigation of the vagina and uterus with disinfectants after routine normal childbirth could introduce infection and should be abandoned.

The Alabama medical profession made real progress in the area of women's disorders during the post–Civil War period. In Alabama as elsewhere, the nature and cure of puerperal fever continued to be a major problem. Physicians and surgeons of the South who read medical journals were kept abreast of the work of Ignaz Semmelweis and other leaders who had demonstrated the contagious nature of puerperal fever. Sadly, they remained mostly unconvinced.

The prevailing schools of thought on the nature of puerperal fever included those who believed it to be a local inflammation arising from the process of parturition. Another school of thought considered it analogous to a traumatic fever, with the more severe forms caused by pyemia and septicemia. A third group considered it primarily a blood disease like other zymotic diseases occurring as epidemics, with contributing endemic and contagious factors. All were convinced of the serious nature of this disease.

The reluctance with which physicians surrender traditional ideas and methods was again demonstrated in the latter part of the nineteenth century. The therapeutic value of drastic bloodletting and purging in the treatment of puerperal fever was still being stressed.

By the turn of the century, it was evident that no well-informed Alabama physician questioned the infectious etiology of puerperal fever. The State Medical Association had sharply criticized the lack of aseptic techniques and surgical cleanliness among physicians in the private practice of obstetrics. It was agreed that in maternity hospitals where antiseptic techniques were rigorously followed, deaths of parturient mothers from puerperal fever were remarkably low. Fortunately, in the ensuing years the rising level of medical education and improving socio-economic status of the populace brought a sharp reduction in maternal and infant mortality. Unfortunately, it was only after the introduction of antibiotics that this dread complication of childbirth lost most of its frightening aspects.

Improved treatment of newborn infants was not immediately forthcoming. For years, the routine usually followed at the time of delivery of a baby was that the midwife bathed the infant in frequently soapy water in front of an open fire. After bathing the baby, the midwife would place some saliva on the navel to "help it heal." Then she would apply tight navel bandages and layer after layer of clothing. Newborn babies were tightly wrapped with an abdominal binder and dressed with close-fitting clothes so that the infant might not "move its hands or feet too freely and thereby distort the bones which [were] very flexible . . ."[36]

Near the turn of the century, a new breed of physicans was gradually beginning to supervise infant care, yet swaddling clothes and tight navel bandages remained customary until well into the twentieth century. Intelligent physicans advised against tight navel bandages and suggested that cleanliness was the best means of healing the navel. This sound advice gradually gained acceptance, but it was not until the advent of trained nurses and midwives that any concrete progress was made.

Radiology

Wilhelm Conrad Röntgen (1845–1923), a German physicist, first announced his discovery of the X ray on December 28, 1895. In January, 1896, Professor M. I. Pupin of the Columbia University Physics Department made the first diagnostic radiograph in the United States. The X ray as a diagnostic and therapeutic modality was immediately seized upon by the American medical and dental professions, and Americans played a significant role in its development and technology. Suffice it to say, the evolution of the X ray into a major diagnostic instrument and therapeutic device was an important contribution to medical knowledge in the twentieth century.

William Herbert Rollins (1852–1929), a New England physician and dentist, was among the first to recognize the danger involved in the use of X rays. In 1901, he reported that in his laboratory work with guinea pigs, X rays were capable of causing death. These experiments led him to warn about the danger of overexposure and made him one of the leading advocates of protective X-ray housing devices.

In 1902, Dr. E. D. Bondurant of Mobile gave a paper at the annual meeting of the Alabama Medical Association entitled "Some of the Therapeutic Uses of the X-Ray."[37] He stated that he used a motor-driven static X-ray machine with a low vacuum German X-ray tube. In another part of his paper, he mentioned the use of the Crookes tube. Likewise, he stressed methods of protecting the healthy parts of the treatment area to prevent X-ray burns. Dr. Bondurant recommended this modality for treatment of squamous epithelioma, as well as lupus of the face. He used the X ray to relieve the pain of malignant diseases of internal organs and reported good results in the treatment of facial neuralgia and intercostal neuralgic pain. Dr. Bondurant referred also to favorable reports of the use of X ray in curing chronic headaches!

In 1906, Dr. William Allen Pusey (1865–1940), Professor of Dermatology at the University of Illinois, addressed the Alabama Medical Association on the status of X ray as a therapeutic modality.[38] He reported on the results of X-ray therapy for superficial lesions such as acne, lupus vulgaris, and tuberculous adenitis. In malignancies of the skin, he stressed that X ray was not the treatment of choice. Surgical excision was still the preferred treatment. Dr. Pusey observed that the results of X-ray therapy of carcinoma of the deep body structures was often difficult to evaluate. He had treated carcinoma of the breast with metastasis with good results although he considered surgery the treatment of choice for early disease. He also felt that X rays were of value in treatment of pseudoleukemia, leukemia, and pruritus of the vagina and rectum.

Dr. Eugene Garland Northington (1880–1933), a native of Prattville, Alabama, practiced in Birmingham from 1904 until 1908. He joined the United States Army Medical Corps and retired as lieutenant-colonel in 1930. Dr. Northington was an officer in the Army Medical Corps for 22 years. He was one of the early users of roentgen rays in Alabama and apparently suffered extensive X-ray burns while experimenting with this modality. He eventually lost both hands and arms as surgeons attempted to stop the spread of X-ray-induced malignancies. Northington General Hospital in Tuscaloosa, named for him, was built in 1943 and was operated by the United States Army. The hospital closed after World War II.[39]

In the 1910 *Transactions*, Dr. William H. Oates (1871–1936) of Mobile reviewed the use of X rays as a diagnostic tool.[40] He pointed out that foreign bodies and bone fractures were easily identified. Dr. Oates also suggested the use of the fluoroscope to determine the exact position of a bone fracture. He emphasized the importance of X rays in medico-legal medicine. Dr. Oates discussed calculi in the kidneys, ureters, and urinary bladder and stated that gallstones were frequently invisible in the skiagraph (early term for a roentgenogram). He also commented on the value of X ray in the diagnosis of disease of the abdominal viscera using a bismuth paste as a contrast medium. In the discussion of Dr. Oates's paper, Dr. J. Sellers (1872–1955) of Jefferson County mentioned that he had been using diagnostic X ray since 1903. It is possible that he was one of the earliest physicians to use diagnostic X rays in Jefferson County. Dr. J. D. Gibson (1863–1929) of Birmingham was listed as a member of the American Roentgen Ray Society in 1903. Nothing further is known concerning this physician.

In the 1912 issue of the *Transactions*, Dr. John H. Edmondson (1880–1956) of Birmingham described his experiences with X ray in the diagnosis of disease of the colon.[41] He had used bismuth orally and by enema as a contrast media.

At the annual State Medical Association meeting in 1916, Dr. Walter A. Weed (1883–1947) of Birmingham discussed X ray in the diagnosis of early tuberculosis of the lung and concluded that this method would play a very important future role in the diagnosis of pulmonary tuberculosis.[42] Dr. Weed stated in 1917 that he had used radium since 1913.[43]

Dr. John H. Edmondson, in 1922, again reviewed his experiences on the use of X ray as a diagnostic procedure.[44] He also considered that X rays were particularly valuable in identifying diseases of the chest. In 1923, Dr. Irwin P. Levi (1888–1960) of Anniston addressed the annual meeting of the State Medical Association on the value of roentgen rays as an aid in diagnosis of cardiac lesions.[45] He pointed out that fluoroscopy of the chest was valuable in diagnosing heart lesions. Dr. Levi repeatedly emphasized that this modality should be only an adjunct to the proper clinical evaluation of the patient.

Dr. Virgil Dark (1887–1940) and Dr. Fred Boswell (1888–1942) of Montgomery, in 1923, reported their therapeutic results in patients suffering from deep-seated malignancies and treated with X ray.[46] They observed that the treatment of lung cancer by X ray in other than inoperable disease was usually not recommended. In their experiences, primary malignancies of the uterus responded better with combined radium and deep X-ray therapy. They observed that when this combined treatment was used, inflammation of the bladder and rectum was a common occurrence. In treatment of early cancer of the cervix, the results were uniformly good. They commented that treatment of cancer of the prostate had been unsatisfactory, whereas results in primary malignancies of the neck such as Hodgkin's disease were only fair.

Metastatic lesions in this area also did not respond well. Cancer of the bladder responded poorly, but good results had been obtained in treatment of sarcoma of the neck.

In 1924, Evarts Ambrose Graham (1883–1957) and Lewis Gregory Cole (1874–1954) opened up a promising field in roentgenology of the gallbladder.[47] They injected tetraiodophenolphthalein intravenously. The dye was then excreted into the biliary tract—including the gallbladder. A failure to obtain pictures usually indicated a diseased gallbladder. Gallstones could be visualized as a contrast with this procedure.

During the next decade, there was an increasing number of reports in the *Transactions* of experiences with the use of X rays in diagnosis and treatment of disease.

Advances in Medicine

During the last half of the nineteenth century, there were very few contributions to the advancements of scientific knowledge in America. Little or no research was under way in the medical schools in this country. Therefore, study abroad was a necessity for medical graduates who wished to keep abreast of the latest developments in medicine. From 1820 to 1860, American students went to France to study in the great medical centers in Paris. After the Civil War, however, Germany and Austria became the great centers for learning that attracted American physicians.

American medicine was late in reaping the results from major scientific developments in Europe. However, near the end of the nineteenth century a gradual revolution in medicine and surgery occurred. The grudging acceptance of Pasteur's work paved the way for identification of microscopic organisms as a causative factor in disease.

It was not until the 1890s that William Henry Welch (1850–1934), who was at the newly opened Johns Hopkins University, introduced the principle that laboratory training and research were fundamental to effective medical education. Soon after this, American medicine began to move into the mainstream of world medicine. Welch was joined by Drs. T. Mitchell Prudden (1849–1924), George M. Sternberg (1838–1915), and Theobald Smith (1859–1934). Dr. Prudden introduced experimental pathology and bacteriology to America. Dr. Sternberg was appointed United States Army Surgeon General in 1893. He was vitally involved in the work on yellow fever and malaria control during the Spanish-American War and later in Cuba. Theobald Smith was the first director of the United States Department of Agriculture's pathological laboratory and the organizer of the Departments of Bacteriology at

George Washington and Cornell Universities. Obviously, there were other intelligent and progressive individuals who also contributed to this development.

The average American physician knew little of these developments and was even less concerned with what was happening in the laboratories. Newer developments in medical science were rarely reported even though there were a few medical journals available.

Medical practice in the second half of the nineteenth century did not differ too greatly from that of earlier days. The average physician had only a vague notion of etiology and treated empirically all symptoms of disease. The rapid march of scientific medicine abroad during the latter years of the nineteenth century widened the gap between medical discoveries and most medical practice, especially in rural areas where physicians still adhered to the old ways. The rural doctor continued to compound and sell his medicines and on occasion served as veterinarian as well as dentist.

Long after Pasteur disproved the theory of spontaneous generation, Alabama and other American physicians grudgingly accepted the germ theory of disease origin. A paper appeared in the *Transactions* (1882) that used flawed reasoning to systematically disprove the germ theory of disease.[48] It would be fair to say, however, that this opinion was not shared by the leaders of medicine in the state.

The management of the major infectious diseases demonstrates the extent of the revolution that had occurred in medical practice during the latter part of the nineteenth century. It became apparent that diseases were separate entities and that specifics rather than cure-alls were needed. Caution and moderation gradually became the preferable method of treatment. The comfort and support of the patient became paramount. In the last quarter of the century, it remained for the bacteriologist to identify the specific pathogenic organisms and pave the way for effective therapy and preventive medicine.

Drugs such as quinine, aconite, opium, alcohol, mercury, strychnine, arsenic, and other potentially dangerous drugs still formed the basis of *materia medica*. Opium, frequently used for bowel complaints, came to rival calomel as a cure-all. It was administered in one form or another for most all diseases. Opium was sold wholesale as raw gum opium, laudanum, paregoric, and morphine. Also it was an ingredient in Dover's Powder as well as in dozens of prescriptions and readily available patent medicines. Medical texts seldom warned medical students about the danger of addiction. John Duffy states that opium was so popular in this country that "the annual importation of [this drug] increased from 24,000 pounds in 1840 to 416,864 pounds in 1872. By the 1890's, Americans were using half a million pounds of crude opium per year."[49]

It is not surprising that there was a growing number of opium addicts. Some physicians blamed these addictions on quacks and irregulars, but many physicians were likewise to blame because of indiscriminate prescribing of opium derivatives. Dr. Peter Bryce and later Dr. J. T. Searcy, superintendents of Bryce Hospital in Tuscaloosa, spoke out about drug addiction and its relationship to the indiscriminate dispensing of opium by physicians.

There was a wide gap between the top physicians and those conducting an ordinary practice, and this division steadily increased as the century approached its close. Most physicians eked out a bare living. Many supplemented their income by operating a pharmacy, farm, or some other business. Far too many of these physicians were poorly trained and knew little of the scientific advances in medicine. On the other hand, affluent physicians came from well-to-do families and had studied abroad. They generally held professorships in the medical schools and had the additional advantage of an entrée into a middle- or upper-class practice. These later became the specialists in the profession. However, it was not uncommon for even the specialists to maintain a concurrent general practice.

American medicine, which had lagged behind that of Western Europe, suddenly began to forge ahead in the early 1900s. This was brought about by discoveries in bacteriology and pathology, by vast developments in basic science, by major reforms in medical education, and by a combination of improved transportation and economics in the United States.

Meanwhile, many states and municipalities, following the example of New York City, which had established a diagnostic laboratory in 1893, began making practical use of new laboratory techniques. In 1907, the Alabama State Public Health Department established such a laboratory in Montgomery. It became operational in 1908, and Dr. E. M. Mason was employed as the first bacteriologist.

Of the diagnostic devices coming into use after the Civil War, the thermometer was one of the first. Interestingly enough, there is very little comment about its use in the *Transactions* of that period. Dr. J. S. Wilkinson of Flomaton declared in 1890 that "since the clinical thermometer had come into general use, accurate temperature records have been kept on [severely ill patients] throughout the civilized world."[50]

Infectious Diseases

Respiratory Diseases

Respiratory diseases such as influenza, pneumonias, pleurisies, and common colds were a perennial health problem, but it is doubtful that they were any more serious in the late nineteenth century than they had been earlier. Influenza, generally in a mild form, appeared almost annually. In Alabama, tuberculosis was the chief cause of death at the turn of the century and remained so until 1918. Pneumonia was the second leading cause of death.

Of all the endemic respiratory diseases, none proved as fatal in the late nineteenth and early twentieth centuries as tuberculosis, "the white plague." The pattern of its incidence in the state followed that of the United States as a whole. The end of slavery, combined with urbanization, caused a radical increase in the spread of this disease. The susceptibility of the blacks to lung complaints undoubtedly accounted for the high tuberculosis death rate. Improvements in medical care, public health, and the general standard of living gradually brought a radical change in tuberculosis among both whites and blacks (see Chapter 12, "The Development of Public Health in Alabama").

The last epidemic in the state to result in mobilization of all state and local resources was the brief onslaught of "Spanish Influenza" in 1918–1919. It apparently appeared in three separate waves. A mild form occurred in the spring of 1918. The second, and most deadly, occurred in the fall of 1918. At that time, the combined causes of influenza and pneumonia accounted for 11,328 deaths in Alabama. Of these deaths, influenza was the cause of death in 5,446 of the cases. A third wave of a milder nature occurred again in the spring of 1919. The disease apparently began in areas of overcrowding such as at the troop cantonments at Fort McClellan. The building of a nitrate plant at Muscle Shoals and Florence was under way, and many individuals had come from all over the country to obtain jobs. As in any boom town, there were inadequate accommodations for this vast influx of people. The disease struck a devastating blow to this area.

The death rate was highest in the age group fifteen to forty years. The young adults from rural areas were apparently more susceptible to the disease. In late summer and autumn of 1918, during the most severe onslaught, the mortality was excessively high in the twenty- to forty-year-old population, which included the military age group. It has been estimated that fifty percent of those who contracted Spanish influenza succumbed.

The great pandemic swept throughout the state and temporarily disrupted all social and economic activities. All public schools, theatres, churches, and colleges were closed. Just as suddenly the disease subsided. The improved transportation of the twentieth century probably explains the exceptionally rapid dissemination of the disease throughout the state.[51]

Yellow Fever

By 1900, yellow fever as an epidemic disease had disappeared from Alabama. The last yellow fever epidemic occurred in Mobile in 1897. A few cases were reported in Alabama in 1905, but there were none in Mobile. The effective quarantine measures and the aggressive anti-mosquito campaign undertaken by Dr. Jerome Cochran had finally paid off. Yellow fever was no longer a problem in Alabama (see Chapter 1, "Early Medical Practice in Alabama").

Malaria

In 1870, the State Medical Association decided to issue a plea through the newspapers addressed to the planters and landowners of the state pointing out the need for a thorough system of land drainage for the purpose of diminishing the prevalence of malaria. An article in several local newspapers stated in part:

> All doctors agree, notwithstanding their different theories as to what the poison is, that you must have three conditions acting in conjunction to produce malarial fevers, viz: heat, moisture, and decaying vegetable matter. Now it is evident that we cannot get rid of heat; but it is equally evident that we can control in a great measure, the other two elements necessary to the production of malarial poison. By a proper system of drainage we can get rid, . . . of the superabundant moisture, and with a little labor judiciously directed, the superabundant vegetable matter can be destroyed previous to its natural death.

This notice was signed by Drs. J. S. Weatherly, chairman; R. F. Michel; and J. B. Gaston.

Job Sobieski Weatherly (1828–1891), a native of South Carolina, was one of the early leaders in preventive medicine in Alabama.[52] He was a private pupil of Dr. P. A. Aylett in South Carolina and was later a student in the Medical Department of the University of New York, from which he graduated in 1849. He began to practice medicine in Adairsville, Georgia, in 1851. From there, he moved to Palmetto, Georgia, and in 1857 to Montgomery, Alabama. In 1875, Dr. Weatherly contended that malarial fever was a disease that could be prevented by drainage and cultivation of swampy areas and ponds. Unfortunately, little implementation of this public health measure was begun in Alabama until after 1900.

The control of the vector (*Anopheles* mosquito) was probably the most important factor in the elimination of malaria in Alabama. This was accomplished by several means, including: education of the population on the use of screen doors and windows, the elimination of reservoirs for

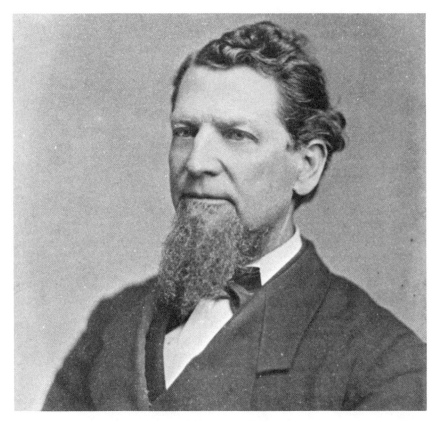

Job Sobieski Weatherly, M.D., 1828–1891 (Courtesy of the Alabama State Department of Archives and History)

the breeding of mosquitoes, and later by the use of insecticide during and after World War II. By the 1940s, malaria had all but disappeared from the region.

It should not be overlooked, however, that several other factors contributed to the decline and finally the elimination of malaria in Alabama. There was a large reservoir of immunity in the black population in that there existed a natural resistance to some types of malaria. The best understood of these is a genetically inherited hemoglobinopathy, sickle cell anemia trait, which provides a partial barrier to proliferation of parasites in the red blood cells. Ten percent of the black population in Alabama is thought to have the sickle cell anemia trait.

An equally impressive, though poorly understood, variety of natural immunity is an innate resistance in most of the black population to the *Plasmodium vivax* strain of malaria. This is probably a genetically controlled phenomenon but not one related to the hemoglobinopathies. There is also evidence of an acquired immunity to the parasites in all infected individuals. This unquestionably deterred the spread of malaria in the inhabitants of Alabama.

One of the factors that should not be overlooked is the frequency of inaccurate diagnoses. Certainly many fevers of undetermined origin were originally thought to be malaria. Thus, increasing availability of capable laboratories that could identify the malarial parasite in the blood resulted in a decreased number of patients reported as suffering with malaria. Likewise, prompt and adequate treatment eliminated the source of the causative organism.

Diphtheria

The story of diphtheria demonstrates the difficulty in recording historical incidence of a disease due to inadequacy of diagnosis. The terminology used in the medical literature of "true croup" and "false croup" had no real significance. The basic difference was between diphtheria, the so-called true croup, and the many other laryngeal disorders. Due to this fact, it is difficult to determine the incidence of this disease prior to 1900. Treatment with diphtheria antitoxin was introduced during Dr. William Henry Sanders's term as State Public Health Officer (1896–1917). It was made available free of charge to those unable to purchase it. Since this time, diphtheria has not been a widespread problem in the state.

Typhoid Fever

The early attempts to eliminate typhoid fever illustrate some of the difficulties in translating scientific discoveries into medical practice. A British medical report in the latter part of the nineteenth century pointed out that typhoid was spread almost entirely from discharges of the bowels. Chloride of lime and other disinfecting agents were recommended for bowel discharge, and the necessity for providing pure drinking water and milk was recommended. This discovery should have opened the way for prevention of typhoid fever, but some medical essayists continued to ignore the relationship between sewage and typhoid.

As typhoid fever spread slowly throughout the South in the latter years of the nineteenth century, its presence was often obscured by the high incidence of malaria. The differentiation of these two diseases was difficult and often perplexed the physician. In the Black Belt area where malaria was widespread, quinine proved effective in most cases of malaria, but it had no value in "continued fevers" (that is, typhoid fever).

Beginning in 1914, the diagnosis of typhoid fever was one of the services offered by the new State Department of Health Laboratory in Montgomery. It was in that year that the State Board of Health made a contract with a manufacturer, Alexander & Company of Marietta, Pennsylvania, to "keep a supply of [typhoid vaccine] on hand at several drug stores in the various counties of the state." The cost of sufficient vaccine at that time to immunize one person was between forty cents and sixty cents. In 1922, the State Laboratory in Montgomery began to manufacture typhoid vaccine for free distribution.[53]

Smallpox

The Mobile Board of Health successfully fought the threat of smallpox epidemics during the years preceding and immediately following the Civil War. But the carpetbagger regime in Mobile in 1871 had "dispensed almost contemptuously with the services of the Board of Health," and even went to the extreme of repealing the Mobile health ordinances. In the winter of 1873–1874, smallpox in Mobile became a grave menace, probably as a result of the large influx of nonimmune individuals—particularly the recently freed plantation slaves. Dr. Cochran, when asked to serve as city health officer, accepted the offer and promptly set to work to stem the epidemic. His efforts succeeded, and he was widely acclaimed for his direction of the program, his plan of control, and the detailed analysis that he published on this major health project.[54]

A smallpox epidemic devastated Jefferson County in 1897 and 1898. Beginning in May, 1897, approximately 745 people contracted the disease, and sixteen died. The epidemic was of such ferocity that in November, 1896, the United States Marine Hospital Service took charge of its control. The disease seemed to die out but reappeared spontaneously, due no doubt to the lack of vaccination in the surrounding counties and mining communities; approximately fifty-four new cases were reported between January 1, 1899, and April 15, 1899.[55]

Syphilis

One of the most significant medical achievements of the present century is in the field of chemotherapy.[56] The chemotherapeutic field grew primarily out of the work of one man, Paul Ehrlich (1854–1915).

Ehrlich very early attempted to synthesize a chemical compound that would specifically bind and destroy the spirochete *Treponema pallida*, the causative organism of syphilis, while remaining sufficiently innocuous to the unhappy carrier of the spirochete. Mercury had been used in the treatment of syphilis, but this drug frequently did not eliminate the disease and often there were disastrous side effects. Work on the spirochete *Treponema pallida* grew out of earlier, partly accidental observations that certain other spirochetes were particularly sensitive to dyes and their derivatives. After trying hundreds of chemical combinations, Ehrlich finally obtained an effective drug in 1910. This drug, first called "606" because it was the 606th combination tried, was later named Salvarsan (arsphenamine). Dr. Courtney William Shropshire was apparently one of the earliest physicians in Birmingham to introduce Salvarsan for the treatment of syphilis.[57]

Writing in the *Transactions* of 1924, Dr. Barney Burns Rogan (1875–1933) of Selma reported on his experiences with Salvarsan.[58] His article, entitled "The Responsibility of the General Practitioner in Reference to Syphilis," detailed the prescribed dosage of arsphenamine in the treatment of syphilis.

In 1906, August Paul von Wasserman (1866–1925), Albert Ludwig Siegmund Niesser (1855–1916), and Carl Bruck (1879–1944), all from Germany, developed the first serologic test for syphilis, originally known as the Wasserman. The test was soon made available by public health laboratories, and in 1911, it was made available in Alabama by the State Laboratory in Montgomery.[59]

Infectious Diseases in Birmingham

Early Birmingham and Jefferson County (1870–1900) were apparently subjected to abnormal numbers of infectious diseases—probably because of their boom town conditions. Poor nutrition, exposure, polluted water, inadequate sewage disposal, and overcrowding contributed to this condition.

In the summer of 1873, Asiatic cholera devastated the city of Birmingham.[60] Contamination of the drinking water was considered the source of infection. There are no surviving records showing the number of individuals who developed the disease, but the death rate was extremely high. It is estimated that between 128 and 175 died during this epidemic. People fled the city, leaving the sick and dying in the care of clergymen, nurses, and physicians.

An epidemic of jaundice occurred in Birmingham in 1882. This was described by Dr. John William Sears (1830–1896) in the *Transactions* of that year.[61] He made a significant observation that pregnant women who were usually in their third trimester were more seriously affected. Of the seventeen pregnant women who contracted the disease, twelve recovered and five died. Dr. Sears commented on the mild character of the disease, with the exception of that occurring in the pregnant women. In regard to the cause of death of the pregnant women, he commented that the patients died not from the disease but from delirium, convulsions, and coma. He apparently was describing liver coma and ammonium intoxication. Although he had no autopsy findings to confirm his suspicion, he felt that these patients died of acute yellow atrophy of the liver.

In an interesting observation, Dr. Sears noted that the jaundice epidemic was prevalent at the same time and under the same circumstances as that of an outbreak of typhoid fever. He erroneously postulated that the jaundice was caused by the same "germ" that caused the typhoid fever but presented with different clinical manifestations. Obviously, he was commenting on two different diseases that occurred simultaneously. Contamination of water, milk, and food with raw sewage was the probable cause of both diseases.

Sulfanilamide

A short article in the November, 1937, issue of the *Journal of the Medical Association of the State of Alabama* was of momentous portent.[62] The subject was a new drug imported from Germany called sulfanilamide. Dr. J. N. Baker, the State Health Officer and author, called attention to the remarkable therapeutic results that had been obtained in treating infections with the new drug. He also called attention to the fact that a number of deaths had been attributed to sulfanilamide both in the state and throughout the nation. However, these deaths occurred after the sulfanilamide was mixed with diethylene glycol. Apparently, glycol was the agent that caused renal failure and death.

Both the American Medical Association and the American College of Surgeons meetings in the summer of 1937 had already called attention to the remarkable curative effects of sulfanilamide in the treatment of infectious diseases such as meningitis, gonorrhea, scarlet fever, pyelitis, erysipelas, puerperal fever, and type III pneumonia.

The introduction of sulfanilamide marked the beginning of a new era of chemotherapy for infectious diseases, and a number of related agents appeared on the market in rapid succession. The advent of penicillin and its remarkably wide spectrum of effectiveness was still almost a decade away, but the era of the long sought "magic bullet" had begun, in which specific drugs were used for a specific causative organism.

The advent of blood transfusions, sulfa drugs, antibiotics, the artificial heart-lung machine, and a host of other innovations have dramatically altered surgery in the past fifty years. Aside from a tremendous increase in the spectrum of surgical procedures and an equally great reduction in mortality, there has been remarkable growth in the number of patients either cured or given some measure of relief.

Health Problems

Mental Diseases

One of the early Alabama physicians interested in mental diseases was Benjamin Leon Wyman (1856–1930), who was born in Tuscaloosa, Alabama, and received his M.D. degree from the University of Virginia in 1878.[63] He also graduated in medicine from the University of New York and became assistant physician in the New York Lunatic Asylum and later resident physician at Randall's Island Hospital in New York. Afterwards, he was associated with Bryce Hospital in Tuscaloosa. Dr. Wyman moved to Birmingham in 1886 and had a large practice, chiefly in nervous and mental diseases.

He was one of the founders and original stockholders of the Birmingham Medical College and was named dean of this institution in 1898, succeeding Dr. William H. Johnston, who had served as the first dean. Dr. Wyman resigned as dean in 1912. Dr. Wyman was elected second president of the Southern Medical Association at the first official meeting in Birmingham in 1907 and presided over the second meeting in Atlanta the following year. He was one of the organizers of the Section on Neurology and Psychiatry of the Southern Medical Association, which held its first meeting in 1921. He served as section chairman in 1927.

His chairman's address, entitled "Crime and Delinquency in Relation to Mental Disorders," was a plea for a much-needed reform of the system of introducing expert testimony, particularly psychiatric testimony, in criminal cases. He wished to eliminate the abuse of the expert witness, such as that employed in the famous Leopold and Loeb murder trial in Chicago, in which distinguished alienists called by the defense rose to testify before a jury that the defendants were insane, and equally distinguished alienists called by the prosecution testifed that they were sane and wholly responsible for their acts. Dr. Wyman believed that

> under no circumstances should the psychiatrist be a partisan or accept employment by the defense in a criminal trial where the plea of insanity is the defense. . . . [But that legal] provision should be made for the examination of all offenders by a competent psychiatrist before the defendant is arraigned for trial.[64]

Psychiatry

A number of physicians practiced both neurology and psychiatry at the beginning of the twentieth century.[65] The combining of the two fields was not uncommon at that time. Dr. Henry Silas Ward was one such physician. Dr. Ward, one of the founders of the Norwood Clinic in

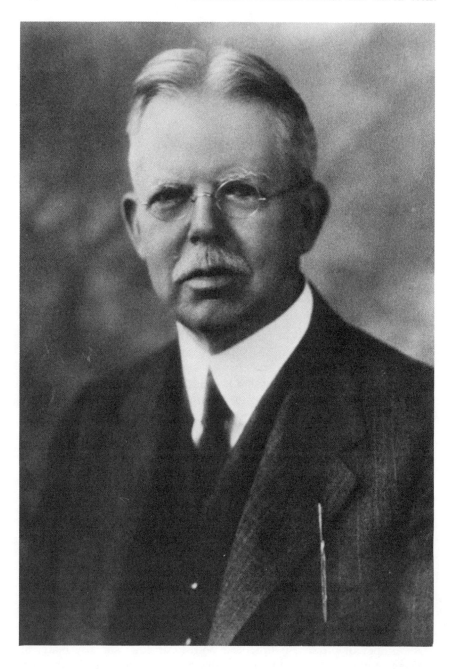

Benjamin Leon Wyman, M.D., 1856–1930 (Courtesy of the Birmingham Public Library)

1925, was born in Smith County, Tennessee. In 1887, he received his B.S. from Southern Normal School, and in 1888, his M.D. degree from the University of Nashville Medical College. He took his postgraduate training at Johns Hopkins from 1902 to 1903. Several years later he went to London and took postgraduate training at the National Hospital at Queen Square. From 1912 to 1916, Dr. Ward was professor of clinical medicine and neurology at the Birmingham Medical College. After 1916, he served as professor of medicine and neurology at the University of Alabama School of Medicine in Tuscaloosa. Dr. Ward was also chief-of-staff at Hillman Hospital where he practiced neuropsychiatry and medicine.

Dr. Frank Alfred Kay (1899–1968) was a psychiatrist but was also interested in all diseases of the nervous system. Dr. Kay was born in Birmingham and was educated at Birmingham-Southern College. He received his M.D. degree from Emory University in 1922. In 1923, he became affiliated with Bryce Hospital in Tuscaloosa. Dr. Kay also held academic appointments at the University of Alabama School of Medicine in Birmingham where he was chairman of the Department of Psychiatry. Even though his primary interest was psychiatry, he continued to show considerable interest in neurology.

Dr. Wilmot Shipp Littlejohn (1897–1979) practiced both psychiatry and neurology. His major interest lay in neurology, however. Dr. Littlejohn was born in Cordele, Georgia, and was educated at Emory University where he received his M.D. He began his postgraduate training in Georgia. However, in 1929, he continued his training at the Neurological Institute in New York under Dr. Foster Kennedy. In 1930, Dr. Littlejohn moved to Birmingham where he was in charge of the neurological service at the Jefferson-Hillman Hospital. In 1942, he entered the United States Navy where he received special training at the United States Naval Hospital at Bethesda. He returned to Birmingham in 1945 and became a member of the faculty at the University of Alabama School of Medicine. Dr. Littlejohn became chairman of the joint Department of Neurology and Psychiatry. Later the department was divided with psychiatry becoming an independent department. Neurology became a division of the Department of Medicine with Dr. Littlejohn as head of this section. Until ill health forced Dr. Littlejohn to retire, he was active in the Medical School and was also a consultant to several hospitals in Birmingham.

Nutrition

One of the nation's outstanding nutritionists was James Sommerville McLester (1877–1954) of Birmingham, Alabama.[66] He graduated in 1899 from the school of medicine at the University of Virginia, after

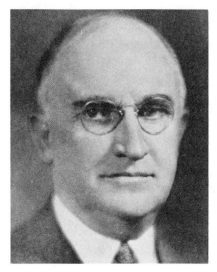

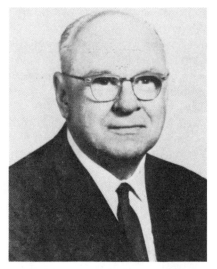

James Sommerville McLester, M.D., 1877–1954 (Courtesy of the Alabama Museum of the Health Sciences, Lister Hill Library, Medical Center, The University of Alabama in Birmingham)

Frank Alfred Kay, M.D., 1899–1968 (Courtesy of the Alabama Museum of the Health Sciences, Lister Hill Library, Medical Center, The University of Alabama in Birmingham)

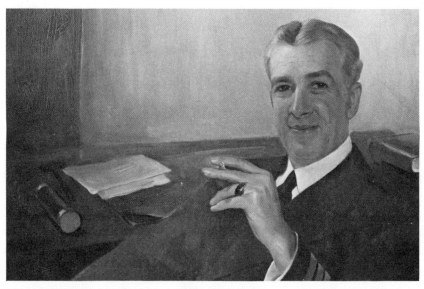

Wilmot Shipp Littlejohn, M.D., 1897–1979 (Courtesy of the Alabama Museum of the Health Sciences, Lister Hill Library, Medical Center, The University of Alabama in Birmingham)

which he did postgraduate studies at the universities of Göttingen and Freiburg, Germany. He returned to become Professor of Pathology on the faculty of the Birmingham Medical College in 1902 and later became Professor of Medicine there. He was also active in the Hillman house staff training program. In 1907 and 1908, he returned to Europe for further postgraduate work in Berlin and Munich, at which time he studied under Dr. Emil Fischer (1852–1919), whose work on sugars, nucleoproteins, amino acids, and polypeptides is regarded as representative of major advancements in biochemistry. Dr. Fischer synthesized Veronal (phenobarbital). However, most of the investigations by Fischer and his contemporaries centered around the problem of nutrition. His work in this field made possible the discovery of vitamins.

After the Birmingham Medical College closed in 1915, Dr. McLester was appointed Professor of Medicine at the two-year medical school at Tuscaloosa in 1920, a position he held until 1945. After the school was moved to Birmingham in 1945, he was appointed Professor of Medicine and chairman of the department and became Professor Emeritus in 1949. He was author of *Nutrition and Diet in Health and Disease* and *The Diagnosis and Treatment of Disorders of the Metabolism.**

In 1929, Dr. McLester was a member of the Council on Medical Education and Hospitals of the American Medical Association (AMA), serving until his election to the presidency of that association in 1934. He served as chairman of the Council on Foods and Nutrition of the AMA from 1940 to 1952. On November 28, 1953, he was awarded the Joseph Goldberger Award for outstanding contributions in the field of clinical nutrition. Dr. McLester was further cited for his outstanding role in translating the results of nutrition research into human values, the integration of nutrition into the teaching of all phases of medicine, and his contribution to nutrition during World War II.

Dr. McLester was probably the first physician in Birmingham to use raw liver in the treatment of pernicious anemia. He had been present when Dr. George Richard Minot had presented a paper on this subject in 1923.

The Hillman Hospital Nutrition Clinic

In 1937, Dr. Conrad Elvehjem (1901–1962) and his colleagues in the Agricultural Chemistry Department of the University of Wisconsin reported the discovery of nicotinic acid. The first use of nicotinic acid was for "black tongue" in dogs, but its discovery was to have a wide

---

Nutrition and Diet in Health and Disease was published by W. B. Saunders Company, Philadelphia, 6th edition, 1952. *The Diagnosis and Treatment of Disorders of the Metabolism* was published by Oxford Press, New York, 1935.

impact in the treatment of pellagra. Although the immediate result was a sharp reduction in the death rate from pellagra, the disease remained a problem until the economic status of the population of the South improved.

By the late 1930s, the way was open to eliminate nearly all the nutritional diseases. Dr. Harry Steenbock (1886–1967) of the University of Wisconsin had found a way to create vitamin D artificially in 1924. Within a few years, irradiated milk and other foods were widely available. As World War II approached, interest was expressed in fortifying bread and flour with vitamins. The war itself accelerated the movement, and by 1945, pellagra and beriberi were no longer serious problems in the United States.

The Nutrition Clinic in Birmingham was established at the invitation of the staff of the Hillman Hospital and on the recommendation of Dr. Tom D. Spies. In 1937, the Department of Internal Medicine of the University of Cincinnati sponsored the clinic in Birmingham. The clinic operated in the new clinic and laboratory building at the hospital each summer, the season when pellagra was prevalent in Alabama, and was funded with grants and private donations. It served as a widely recognized postgraduate training facility in nutrition.

Tom Douglas Spies (1902–1960) was born in Ravena, Texas, but his name will always be associated with medicine in Alabama because of his clinical research work on nutrition at the Hillman Hospital.[67] Dr. Spies graduated from Harvard Medical School in 1927 and did an internship at Lakeside Hospital in Cleveland, Ohio. During this time, he became interested in nutritional diseases, especially pellagra. From 1936 to 1947, Dr. Spies, who developed the Hillman Nutrition Clinic, held the position of Assistant Professor under Dr. Marion Blankenhorn, who was Chairman of the Department of Medicine at the University of Cincinnati. In 1947, Dr. Spies moved to Chicago where he was Professor and Chairman of the Department of Nutrition and Metabolism at Northwestern University Medical School. At the same time, he served as director of the Nutrition Clinic at Hillman Hospital, and from 1945 to 1960, he was Visiting Professor of Medicine at the new medical college in Birmingham, Alabama.

Dr. Spies began visiting the Hillman Hospital Clinic as early as 1934, when he became interested in nutrition deficiency diseases in Jefferson County. He came to Birmingham at the invitation of Dr. James S. McLester, then president of the AMA. Dr. Spies spent much of his career after 1935 working at Hillman Hospital. The clinic closed soon after his death in 1960. Early in his career at Hillman Clinic, he successfully treated patients critically ill with endemic pellagra using an intensive diet of meat, eggs, milk, and fresh vegetables.

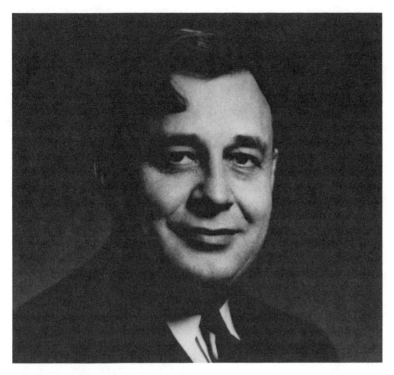

Tom Douglas Spies, M.D., 1902–1960
(Courtesy of Dr. William Niedermeier)

Dr. Spies pioneered the use of nicotinic acid in the treatment and prevention of pellagra. He also recognized the potential value of folic acid in the treatment of tropical sprue in 1945. For his work in tropical sprue, Dr. Spies received official recognition by the governments of Cuba in 1950 and the Commonwealth of Puerto Rico in 1951. The Modern Medicine Award was given to him in 1957 "in recognition of outstanding contributions to the progress of Medicine." In the same year, he also received the Distinguished Service Award of both the AMA and the Southern Medical Association. In March, 1939, he was awarded the John Phillips Memorial Medal by the American College of Physicians.

Later, while using nicotinic acid as a possible remedy for pellagra, Dr. Spies became aware of the existence of multiple vitamin deficiencies in individuals previously thought to be suffering from single vitamin deficiencies. Over a period of time, evidence mounted supporting the validity of this idea. Elimination of multiple vitamin deficiency as a national problem was accomplished in part due to Dr. Spies's continuing efforts to require cereal and dairy product manufacturers to enrich their products.

Dr. Spies was elected to the presidency of the Southern Medical Association, but he died before he assumed office. Dr. Spies was a maverick and rugged individualist in medicine, and he continually waged a war against parochial medical dogma. Paul deKruif, the science writer, described him as "a mentally tough man who was exceedingly gentle; a famine fighter of the first order."

Preventive Medicine

One of the first major American medical accomplishments of the twentieth century was the demonstration in 1900 that yellow fever was carried by a particular mosquito.

The Spanish-American War, which required the occupation of Cuba by our troops, raised the specter of serious losses due to yellow fever. United States Army Surgeon General George M. Sternberg, an American bacteriologist, had been involved in research on yellow fever—as had Dr. Aristides Agramonte, a Cuban bacteriologist and a United States Army contract surgeon. In 1900, Sternberg created a full-time medical team to study this problem; the team was headed by Major Walter Reed (1851–1902) and included James Carroll (1854–1907) and Jesse W. Lazear (1866–1900). Dr. Agramonte also joined Major Reed and his medical team. Dr. Reed had studied under Dr. William H. Welch at Johns Hopkins and had worked closely with Sternberg. In 1881, Carlos Finlay (1833–1915), a Cuban physician, discovered strong evidence to prove that a particular mosquito, the *Aedes aegypti* was responsible for transmitting yellow fever. In spite of his impressive evidence, little immediate attention was accorded Finlay's theory. After reviewing the various possibilities, Reed and his associates centered their efforts on the mosquito thesis and with the help of Finlay were able to demonstrate the validity of his hypothesis. Few medical breakthroughs have had so great an impact as the work of the Reed Commission.

The Spanish-American War rendered the elimination of yellow fever imperative. Major William Crawford Gorgas (1854–1920), a native of Mobile and the Chief Sanitary Officer in Havana, soon rid that city of yellow fever, a disease that had been endemic since the eighteenth century.[68]

Likewise, it is questionable whether the Panama Canal could have been completed without the elimination of yellow fever. Malaria and yellow fever were the major reasons for the failure of the French to build an interoceanic canal in Panama in the 1880s and the major obstacles

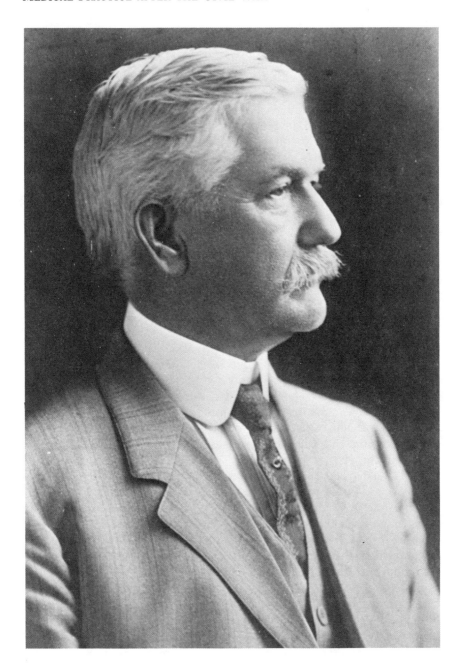

William Crawford Gorgas, M.D., 1854–1920 (Courtesy of the Alabama State Department of Archives and History)

facing the American effort in 1904. The dramatic conquest of these diseases was of inestimable value in terms of its economic, social, and psychological impact on the southern United States, the Caribbean area, South America and other tropical and semitropical regions.

Admiral John G. Walker, chairman of the Isthmian Canal Commission, and General George W. Davis, first governor of the Canal Zone, were not proponents of the mosquito theory of malaria and yellow fever but were advocates of the more traditional "filth and miasma" origin of the disease. The early American attempt at digging the canal was disastrous, as disease, mostly malaria and yellow fever, devastated the workers. Colonel Gorgas was originally named chief sanitary officer of the Canal Zone by President Theodore Roosevelt but was not made a member of the commission. Neither Walker nor Davis would cooperate with Gorgas's goals and his sanitation efforts. Gorgas was finally appointed to the Isthmian Canal Commission in 1907 and implemented his policies on prevention of disease. These were successful in controlling yellow fever as well as malaria in the Canal Zone and ultimately allowed construction of the canal. It is estimated that during the ten years of construction Dr. Gorgas's work saved seventy thousand lives and eighty million dollars.

In 1908, Dr. Gorgas was chosen president of the AMA. The AMA, in commenting on this election, stated that "in thus honoring Colonel Gorgas, the Association has also honored not only itself, but the Medical Corps of the U. S. Army, the profession of medicine, and the government that was wise enough to recognize that . . . it is to the voice of the sanitarian that industrial and engineering enterprise must look."[69] Dr. Gorgas received many honors before his death in 1920. In 1951, he was elected to the Hall of Fame at New York University.

In 1914, Colonel Gorgas was appointed surgeon general of the United States Army. While serving in this capacity, he reshaped the Medical Corps to meet the challenge of World War I. "Foremost among these achievements was that in an era when deaths from illness in the military often equaled or exceeded deaths from battle, Gorgas and the Medical Corps reduced mortality resulting from illness to the lowest in history."[70]

In 1904, Dr. Lloyd Noland (1880–1949) joined the American Medical Mission to the Panama Canal Zone on the staff of General William Crawford Gorgas.[71] A native of Virginia, he had graduated from the Baltimore Medical College with an M.D. degree in 1903. Dr. Noland first served at the Ancon Hospital, but was later appointed executive officer to General Gorgas's health and sanitation program in the Canal Zone. In 1905, he was made chief surgeon of the Colon (Panama) Hospital.

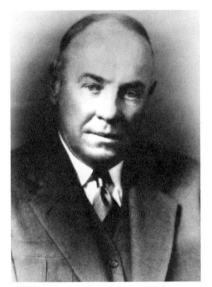 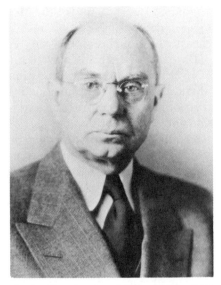

Lloyd Noland, M.D., 1880–1949
(Courtesy of the Alabama Museum of
the Health Sciences, Lister Hill Library, Medical Center, The University
of Alabama in Birmingham)

Seale Harris, Sr., M.D., 1870–1957
(Courtesy of the Alabama Museum of
the Health Sciences, Lister Hill Library, Medical Center, The University
of Alabama in Birmingham)

In 1912, Dr. Noland accepted the post of superintendent of Tennessee Coal and Iron's Health Department in Fairfield. Here he led the first
extensive experiment in industrial medicine in the South. He was a
familiar figure in medical and political circles in Alabama and on the
national scene until his death (see Chapter 2, "Development of Hospitals").

Seale Harris (1870–1957) was born in Cedartown, Georgia, and
graduated with an M.D. degree from the University of Virginia in
1894.[72] Dr. Harris originally practiced medicine in Union Springs,
Alabama, where he was elected health officer of Bullock County in 1898
and served for eight years. In 1906, he matriculated at Johns Hopkins
University for a postgraduate course in medicine and later studied in
Europe. The following year he returned to Mobile where he was

appointed to the faculty of the Medical College of Alabama as Professor of the Practice of Medicine and Clinical Medicine. He served as physician-in-chief of the Mobile City Hospital for the same year.

Dr. Harris began his private practice of medicine in Birmingham in 1915. In 1917, he was commissioned major in the United States Army Medical Corps. He was assigned to the staff of General William Crawford Gorgas in the Surgeon General's Office in Washington. During this time, he edited a publication known as *War Medicine*. He served overseas from 1918 to 1919, during which time he accompanied President Woodrow Wilson's party on its tour of Italy. After his return, Dr. Harris served again in the Surgeon General's Office in Washington, where he wrote the chapters on gastrointestinal diseases in the *Medical History of World War I*. He returned to his private practice in Birmingham in 1919. Dr. Harris was active in the early medical publications of Alabama (see Chapter 9, "Medical Journals in Alabama").

Dr. Harris served as president of the Southern Medical Association in 1922. He also was cited by the Medical Association of the State of Alabama for his work in describing the new disease syndrome, "hyperinsulinism." In 1939, while visiting in Sir Alfred Bantings's laboratory, Dr. Harris observed symptoms in patients who had received too much insulin. The symptoms and signs were similar to a syndrome he had commonly observed in his private practice; he designated the syndrome "hyperinsulinism" and correctly identified it as having been caused by low blood sugar.

In 1949, Dr. Harris was awarded the American Medical Association's Distinguished Service Medal for his research work. The Southern Medical Association awarded him its Research Medal in 1949. The University of Alabama conferred the LL.D. degree on Dr. Harris in 1950. Being a prolific author, he was a frequent contributor to medical literature. He probably is best known for his books *Bantings Miracle* published in 1946 and *Woman's Surgeon, The Life Story of J. Marion Sims* in 1950.*

Conclusion

Medical progress during the first half of the twentieth century has been stupendous. The elimination of many infections, with the consequent prolongation of the average life, has led to an unprecedented prevalence of cancer and degenerative cardiovascular diseases, against which medicine's ability to fight successfully is still limited. Heart disease became the leading cause of deaths in the state in 1926 and since has remained the first ranked cause.

Bantings Miracle was published by J. B. Lippincott Company, Philadelphia, and *Woman's Surgeon, The Life Story of J. Marion Sims* was published by the Macmillian Company, New York.

We should recognize, however, that in spite of the unprecedented achievements of this century, some of the most prominent and "modern" accomplishments of present-day medicine actually were already well in evidence in the nineteenth century.

Notes

1. F. G. Dubose, "Local Anaesthesia in Major Surgery with Report of Cases," *Trans.* (1914), p. 445. Dr. Dubose was chief surgeon at the Vaughan Memorial Hospital in Selma.

2. J. Paul Jones, "Report on Surgery in Wilcox County," *Trans.* (1869), pp. 111–18.

3. Emmett B. Carmichael, "William Joseph Holt," *Ala. J. Med. Sci.* 1 (1964): 451–54.

4. James Fountain Heustis, "Surgical Cases," *Trans.* (1881), pp. 498–508 (hereafter cited as Heustis, "Surgical Cases").

5. James Fountain Heustis, "Recent Progress in Surgery," *Trans.* (1882), p. 329.

6. Heustis, "Surgical Cases," pp. 499–500.

7. Robert M. Moore, "The Davis Brothers of Birmingham and the Southern Surgical and Gynecological Association," *Trans. South. Surg. Assoc.* 74 (1962): 4, 7.

8. John D. S. Davis, "An Experimental Study of Intestinal Anastomosis," *Trans. South. Surg. & Gyn. Assoc.* 2 (1889): 142–73.

9. Moore, p. 10.

10. Emmett B. Carmichael, "Luther Leonidas Hill," *South. Surg.* 14 (1948): 659–69.

11. Luther Leonidas Hill, "Progress in Surgery," *Trans.* (1893), pp. 327–41.

12. L. L. Hill, "Wounds of the Heart with a Report on Seventeen Cases of Heart Suture," *Med. Record* 58 (15 Dec. 1900): 921–24.

13. L. L. Hill, "A Report of a Case of Successful Suturing of the Heart, and Table of Thirty-Seven Other Cases of Suturing by Different Operators with Various Terminations and the Conclusions Drawn," *Med. Record* 62 (29 Nov. 1902): 846–48.

14. Ibid., p. 846.

15. Dr. Hill's son, Senator Lister Hill, named for Lord Lister, became one of the most famous men in the United States Senate during the post–World War II years; he was noted for sponsoring legislation on health affairs. Senator Hill is known as the Father of the National Institutes of Health and the National Library of Medicine.

16. J. M. Donald, "James Monroe Mason, 1871–1952," *Trans. South. Surg. Assoc.* 64 (1952): 406–9.

17. Dr. Julius E. Linn, Sr., personal communication, 1980.

18. E. P. Earle, "Typhlitis, Peri-Typhlitis, and Appendicitis," *Trans.* (1887), pp. 351–58.

19. E. P. Hogan, "The Appendix Problem," *Trans.* (1928), p. 495.

20. Ibid.

21. George Summers Brown, "Appendicitis," *Trans.* (1899), pp. 415–33.

22. G. S. Brown, "Appendicitis," *Trans.* (1900), pp. 449–59.

23. W. R. Jackson, "Complications of Acute Appendicitis Due to Delayed Operation," *Trans.* (1922), pp. 236–43.

24. L. J. Johns, "Appendicitis in Children," *Trans.* (1929), pp. 222–30.

25. "Karl Landsteiner," *Dictionary of Scientific Biography* (New York: Charles Scribner's Sons, 1973), 7: 622–25.

26. J. D. S. Davis, "Blood Transfusion," *Trans.* (1909), pp. 499–510.

27. P. B. Moss, "Some Practical Points on Blood Transfusion," *Trans.* (1917), pp. 480–83.

28. Earle Drennen, "Blood Transfusion," *Trans.* (1920), pp. 143–49.

29. The Blood Bank opened at the Hillman Hospital in 1942 and was directed by Dr. Albert Casey.

30. Samuel C. Little, "A History of Neurology in Alabama," *Ala. J. Med. Sci.* 11 (1974): 360–62.

31. Emmett B. Carmichael, "Eugene DuBose Bondurant," *Ala. J. Med. Sci.* 1 (1964): 326.

32. Edgar F. Fincher, "William Henry Hudson, M.D., Itinerant Neurosurgeon, 1862–1917," *J. Neurosurg.* 16 (1959): 123–34.

33. Ibid.

34. Miriam H. Libbey, librarian, A. W. Calhoun Medical Library, Emory University School of Medicine, Atlanta, personal communication, April 1981.

35. "The Omnibus Discussion, Antiseptic Surgery," *Trans.* (1886), pp. 96–100.

36. John Duffy, ed., *The Rudolph Matas History of Medicine in Louisiana* (Baton Rouge: Louisiana State University Press, 1962), 2: 351.

37. E. D. Bondurant, "Some of the Therapeutic Uses of the X-Ray," *Trans.* (1902), pp. 283–87. The *Transactions* of 1899 states that a paper entitled "The X-Rays in Diagnosis" was presented by Dr. J. Grey Thomas of Mobile and was discussed by Drs. Jackson and Inge. Unfortunately the paper is not available.

38. William Allen Pusey, "The Present Status of Roentgentherapy," *Trans.* (1906), pp. 418–31.

39. Marie Bankhead Owen, *The Story of Alabama: A History of the State* (New York: Lewis Hist. Pub. Co., Inc., 1949), 1: 517; and "Deaths," *JAMA* 101 (1933): 154.

40. William H. Oates, "The Value of the X-Rays in Diagnosis," *Trans.* (1910), pp. 455–66.

41. J. H. Edmondson, "X-Ray Diagnosis in Colon," *Trans.* (1912), p. 514.

42. Walter A. Weed, "The Value of the X-Ray in the Diagnosis of Incipient Tuberculosis," *Trans.* (1916), p. 420.

43. Walter A. Weed, "The Present Status of the Local Application of Radium and X-Rays," *Trans.* (1917), p. 434.

44. John H. Edmondson, "The Present Status of the X-Ray in Diagnosis," *Trans.* (1922), pp. 214–17.

45. Irwin P. Levi, "The Roentgen Ray as an Aid to Diagnosis in Cardiac Lesions," *Trans.* (1923), pp. 341–53.

46. Virgil Dark and Fred Boswell, "Results Observed in 125 Cases of Deep Seated Malignancies Treated with High Voltage X-Rays," *Trans.* (1923), pp. 330–36.

47. John P. Long, "The X-Ray Diagnosis, Its Uses and Limitations," *Trans.* (1925), p. 332.

48. John W. Blow, "Micro-Organisms and Their Relation to Disease," *Trans.* (1882), pp. 429–47.

49. John Duffy, *The Healers, A History of American Medicine* (Chicago: University of Illinois Press, Illini Books, 1979), p. 233.

50. James Anthony Wilkinson, "Some Thoughts on Our Modern Therapeutics," *Trans.* (1890), p. 311.

51. Geraldine Emerson, "A Spanish Lady in Alabama, 1918–1919," MS., n.d.

52. Thomas McAdory Owen, *History of Alabama and Dictionary of Alabama Biography* (Chicago: S. J. Clarke Pub. Co., 1921), 4: 1735.

53. Ira Myers, state health officer, letter 20 September 1979.

54. Carey V. Stabler, "The History of the Alabama Public Health System" (Ph.D. diss., Duke University, 1944), p. 35.

55. Howard L. Holley, "A Century and a Half of the History of the Life Sciences in Alabama; Smallpox Epidemic in Jefferson County," *Ala. J. Med. Sci.* 16 (1979): 140–42.

56. Ira Myers, state health officer, letter 23 May 1980.

57. Dr. Shropshire founded the Civitan International and was the first president of the Civitan International (*Birmingham Post-Herald*, 13 February 1953).

58. B. B. Rogan, "The Responsibility of the General Practitioner in Reference to Syphilis," *Trans.* (1924), p. 212.

59. See Note No. 56.

60. Howard L. Holley, "A Century and a Half of the History of the Life Sciences in Alabama; Cholera in Birmingham," *Ala. J. Med. Sci.* 15 (1978): 288–89.

61. John William Sears, "The Birmingham Epidemic of Jaundice," *Trans.* (1882), pp. 472–80.

62. J. N. Baker, "Sulfanilamide," *J.M.A. Ala.* 7 (Nov. 1937): 192–93.

63. T. M. Owen, pp. 1817–18.

64. "Dr. Benjamin L. Wyman, In Memoriam," *South. Med. J.* 23 (1930): 175.

65. Little, pp. 360–62.

66. Emmett B. Carmichael, "James Sommerville McLester: Nutritionist-Physician," *Bull. Hist. Med.* 36 (March-April 1962): 141–47.

67. William Niedermeier, "Tom D. Spies: Physician, Scientist, Humanitarian, A Biographical Note," *Ala. J. Med. Sci.* 1 (1964): 329–31; and "Symposium to Honor Dr. Tom Spies," *U. Ala. Med. Center Bull.* 10 (March 1966): 5.

68. Michael H. Ellman, "William Crawford Gorgas and the American Medical Association," *JAMA* 243 (15 Feb. 1980): 659–60. Major Gorgas was a famous sanitarian. He attended Bellevue Medical College, New York City, and received his M.D. degree in 1879. After a year of postgraduate study, he entered the Medical Department of the United States Army.

69. Ellman, p. 660.

70. Ibid.

71. Emmett B. Carmichael, "Lloyd Noland—Sanitarian, Surgeon and Hospital Administrator," *Ala. J. Med. Sci.* 7 (1970): 114–17. Dr. George Searcy accompanied the Gorgas expedition to Panama, but after contracting malaria, he was forced to return home. Emmett B. Carmichael, "Pellagra Story in the United States of America," *J.M.A. Ala.* 49 (March 1980): 23, 26, 31, 33.

72. T. M. Owen, 3: 759.

Part II
Organizational Efforts

Chapter 6

Local Medical Societies

Highly skilled members of the medical profession emigrated to the settlements in the fertile areas of the Gulf Coast, the Tennessee River Valley, and the Black Belt region of the state. The difficulties of communication and transportation between these areas and the Mobile area and early regional isolation favored the development of local medical societies rather than a centralized state organization.

No doubt, from the early era, physicians in the state had been in the habit of meeting informally to discuss the common problems that they had encountered in their daily practices. The desire to make these meetings more formal was voiced in a letter addressed "To The Medical Men in Huntsville," printed in the *Huntsville Republican* on June 15, 1821:

> Would it not be a good thing for you and the physicians in your vicinity, to form a *Medical Society* for the purpose of uniting in procuring an extensive library, with chemical and all other apparatus necessary for the mutual instruction of each? Let the Society meet at stated times, and each member deliver a medical lecture.[1]

Six years later, the **Medical Society of North Alabama** came into being. At a convention of physicians held in the town of Huntsville on December 3, 1827, this society was organized, a constitution adopted, and the following officers elected:

Thomas Fearn, M.D., president
John R. Lucas, M.D., 1st vice-president
Young A. Gray, M.D., 2nd vice-president
E. Picket, M.D., corresponding secretary
M. S. Watkins, M.D., recording secretary
Alex Erskine, M.D., treasurer
George R. Wharton, M.D., librarian[2]

The object of this society was

> to give its best efforts toward the improvement of the Science of Medicine,
> by concentrating the amount of medical experience and observation that
> may be diffused throughout our section of the country, and to increase
> our common knowledge by such means as may appear to us, most
> conducive to such an end . . . the establishment of a medical library
> consisting of such rare and valuable writings as are not usually found in
> the private libraries of physicians and the collection of such facts and
> observations, as may be thought worthy of preservation by its members.[3]

From time to time, an examining committee would select such papers
as were deemed pertinent. These were then placed in the care of the
corresponding secretary for publication in some medical journal.

The society felt it was important to establish a permanent medical
library in the town of Huntsville. All the members of the society were to
have free access to this library, and it was confidently believed that such a
selection of works would render it a source of valuable and important
information. The constitution determined that every member of the
society, upon his admission to membership, should pay to the Treasurer
ten dollars, which, along with an annual contribution of a smaller sum
fixed by the society, would be used to purchase books for a library.

The regular meetings of the society were held in Huntsville on the
first Monday in May and December. The physicians of Alabama and of
the adjoining counties of Tennessee who wished to become members of
this organization were invited to attend.

Nothing is known about the later history of this society, but it seems
that similar forces were at work in other sections of the state. It is
probable that the medical boards created by the "1823 Law" helped to
further this movement by bringing together physicians in an official
capacity. (See Chapter 11, "Regulation of Medical Practice.")

The **Mobile Medical Society** was organized in 1839 and incorporated
on December 21, 1841. The incorporators were Drs. Henry S. Levert,
Josiah C. Nott, Solomon Mordecai, and John H. Woodcock. It was
organized at the instigation of the city of Mobile in an effort to amelio-
rate and, indeed, if possible to prevent a repeat of the disastrous yellow
fever epidemic of 1839.[4]

The organization of the Mobile society was to have a profound and
lasting influence on organized medicine in all of Alabama. The General
Assembly granted the society the powers of a board of health in Mobile.
The Assembly stipulated also that the society would be required to carry
out such ordinances as the city of Mobile might adopt in regard to health
measures. Here, then, was the first attempt in Alabama to organize a
board of health. Indeed, it was this organization that Dr. Jerome

Cochran used thirty years later as a prototype for a unique board of health system in the state of Alabama. It is believed that this was the first instance in the United States that a partnership between the medical profession and a state government was formed to protect the public's health.

The society was incorporated a second time on February 23, 1866, with Drs. George A. Ketchum and Josiah C. Nott named among the members.

The **Medical Society of South Alabama** was declared on January 30, 1839, to be "a body corporate" and constituted the medical board of Selma. In an act that was approved by the General Assembly on April 28, 1841, the powers and privileges of this board were "transferred to and vested in" the **Alabama Medical Society**. The act set forth, in part, that the Alabama Medical Society is

> . . . body corporate and politic, by the name and style of the Alabama Medical Society; and under this name shall have perpetual succession of officers, sue and be sued, plead and be impleaded, and have a common seal with power to change or alter the same at pleasure . . . to adopt a constitution and pass such by-laws, as may be deemed necessary for its good government; . . . to hold by purchase, gift, grant, or otherwise, property, real, personal and mixed, not exceeding in value sixty thousand dollars, . . . the members of this society shall be known and styled, Fellows of the Alabama Medical Society.[5]

It is thought that the Alabama Medical Society was intended to be a statewide organization; however, it was in reality a local Selma society. After January 28, 1867, it became the **Selma Medical Society** with state legislation that stated:

> To revive the charter of the Alabama Medical Society, and to change its name. [Said the Legislature:] . . . the charter of the Alabama Medical Society shall not be deemed and held as forfeited, on account of any failure on the part of said society to do and perform such acts as may have been required of them by the charter under which they are made a body corporate, but all the powers and privileges heretofore granted to said society are hereby revived and affirmed and its name changed to that of 'The Alabama Medical Society' to 'The Selma Medical Society.'[6]

The **Sydenham Medical Society** of Montgomery was organized February 1, 1850. Its bylaws allowed any licensed physician to be elected to its membership upon complying with the rules and regulations of the society.

The duties and powers of the society were:

> . . . the said corporation shall be required to carry into effect such ordinances as the corporation of the city of Montgomery may adopt in regard

to it, to organise a board of health and procure necessary information and advice upon the subject of the health of the city and the precautionary measures necessary to procure the same.[7]

The incorporators were Drs. William M. Boling, R. Rush Jones, Henry M. Jackson, William O. Baldwin, Mathew Bozeman, and J. Marion Sims.

The society was incorporated again on February 8, 1866, as the **Medical and Surgical Society** of the city of Montgomery.[8] Drs. W. O. Baldwin, J. F. Johnson, T. R. Hill, R. F. Michel, Samuel E. Norton, A. A. Wilson, J. G. Scott, E. A. Semple, W. J. Holt, and P. C. Lee were among the organizers of the society. The society was authorized to organize a board of health and to examine annually applicants seeking certificates of qualification to practice medicine. In 1878, it became the **Montgomery County Medical Society**.

The **Montgomery Social Medical Club** was organized in 1872 and had ten members.[9] The club was in existence for twenty years, during which time it promoted and maintained the harmony and high ethical tone that characterized the medical profession of Montgomery. During the cooler months of the year, the club held meetings every two weeks— usually at the home of one of the members. These meetings were unique in that they were purely social, with all medical discussions being strictly forbidden. There was a meal and much conversation at each meeting. The members attended in formal attire.

The first medical society in Jefferson County was organized in 1865, with Dr. Joseph R. Smith, president, and Dr. G. T. Deason, secretary.[10] In the years between 1865 and 1869, the society appeared to be inactive. There are no extant records. In 1869, the **Jefferson County Medical Society** was reorganized with Dr. F. M. Prince, of Jonesboro, president, and Dr. R. N. Hawkins, secretary. The organization apparently did little until the year 1873, when it was reactivated to aid in the cholera epidemic.

In the year 1873, Dr. J. W. Sears was elected president of the Jefferson County Medical Society, and Dr. M. H. Jordan, secretary. Dr. Sears held the office of president until 1879, and Dr. Jordan remained secretary until 1878 when S. M. Gillespie, Ph.D., was elected to serve until 1879.

In 1879, Dr. M. P. Taylor was elected president and Dr. W. H. Cook, secretary. This election was under the new constitution of the Medical Association of the State of Alabama. Dr. Taylor remained president until 1881. Dr. S. L. Ledbetter was elected secretary for the year 1880.

Dr. M. H. Jordan was made president in 1881, and Dr. Ledbetter was reelected secretary. Dr. Jordan remained president until 1883, when Dr. Henry N. Rosser was elected to the presidency and Dr. Ledbetter was reelected secretary.

Officers of the
Jefferson County Medical Society
(1884–1887):

1884—Dr. H. P. Cochran, president; Dr. A. J. Douglass, secretary.
1885—Dr. J. C. Dozier, president; Dr. B. G. Copeland, secretary.
1886—Dr. Charles Whelan, president; Dr. E. P. Earle, secretary.
1887—Dr. John D. S. Davis, president; Dr. B. L. Wyman, secretary.

The **John A. Andrew Clinical Society** was founded in 1912 in Tuskegee under the direction of Dr. John A. Kenney and conducted annual clinics for evaluation of patients with difficult diagnoses.[11] It was primarily for black physicians in the city of Tuskegee and in Macon County, but white physicians were welcomed.

The society was organized by a committee consisting of Drs. John A. Kenney, chairman; H. C. Bryant; L. B. Palmer; U. G. Daitey; and J. A. McMillian.

In 1918, the John A. Andrew Clinical Society was reorganized and its scope enlarged. Its first officers were Drs. C. V. Roman, president; C. W. Powell, vice-president, and John A. Kenney, secretary and treasurer. Other members included Drs. C. Wayman Reeves, Atlanta, Georgia; Rupert O. Roett, Houston, Texas; G. N. Woodward, Fort Valley, Georgia; Louis T. Wright, New York City; Charles E. Thomas, Anniston, Alabama; John Hall, Nashville, Tennessee; and Morgan Norris, Kilmarnock, Virginia.

The aims of the society were the advancement of the science and art of medicine and surgery and dedication to the study of diseases. Since 1921, the society has sponsored an annual postgraduate course in medicine and surgery for black physicians in the South. Its annual professional symposium continues to be one of the most prestigious scientific events in Alabama.

Notes

1. "To The Medical Men in Huntsville," *Huntsville Republican*, 15 June 1821.
2. "Medical," *Southern Advocate of Huntsville*, 7 December 1827.
3. Ibid.
4. William H. Brantley, Jr., "Alabama Doctor," *Ala. Lawyer* 6 (1945): 253.
5. Acts of Alabama, 28 April 1841, p. 14.
6. Acts of Alabama, 28 January 1867, p. 247.
7. Acts of Alabama, 1 February 1850, p. 314.
8. Acts of Alabama, 8 February 1866, pp. 263–64.

9. Jerome Cochran, "The Medical Profession," *Memorial Record of Alabama: Historical and Biographical* (Madison, Wisconsin: Brant and Fuller, 1893), 2: 139.

10. John D. S. Davis, "The Medical Profession," *Jefferson County and Birmingham* (n.p.: Southern Historical Press, 1877), pp. 97–111. Jefferson County was organized in 1820. Birmingham was not chartered until 1871.

11. H. W. Kenney, M.D., medical director, Tuskegee Institute, Tuskegee, Ala., letter, 28 August 1969.

Chapter 7

Organization of the Medical Association of the State of Alabama

Early Days of the State Medical Association

The Medical Association of the State of Alabama was founded December 1, 1847. It had become increasingly apparent that the state needed a collective body of physicians that could speak with knowledge and authority on health matters. Efforts to regulate the practice of medicine had been far from successful. Lack of effectiveness of the 1823 licensure law convinced many Alabama physicians that only a strong and united medical profession could insure improvement in the standards of medical practice.

A Selma physician, Dr. Albert Gallatin Mabry (1810–1874), acting at the behest of the Alabama Medical Society—a local society founded in Selma, was directly responsible for initiating a meeting of physicians from many parts of the state. The Medical Association of the State of Alabama was organized at this meeting.

On December 7, 1846, the Alabama Medical Society of Selma met in the office of Drs. Drewry Fair and Mabry (in Selma) and adopted the following resolution:

> Resolved, that the society recommend a State Medical Convention to be held in the town of Selma, on the fourth monday in March next, and the secretary of the society be instructed to correspond with other medical societies of the State on the subject, and the result of his correspondence be made known to this society at its next meeting.[1]

The following letter was sent to the Mobile Medical Society:

Selma, April 8th, 1847

To the President of the Mobile Medical Society:
Sir:—

> At the annual meeting of the [Alabama] Medical Society held in Selma on the 7th December last, the question of the advantage which might result

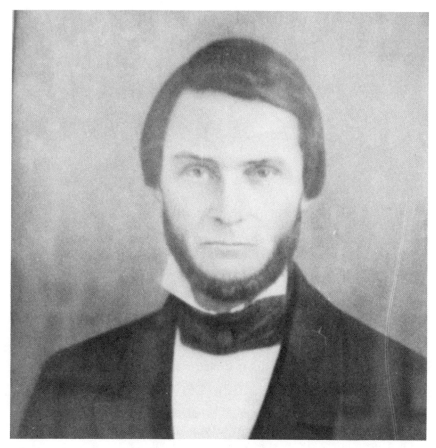

Albert Gallatin Mabry, M.D., 1810–1874 (Courtesy of Bryce Hospital, Tusca-loosa, Alabama)

from a State Medical Convention, where the members of the Profession, being assembled from all parts of the State, and freely interchanging their sentiments and opinions upon its present condition, its wants and future prospects, was raised and considered, and a resolution finally adopted, instructing the secretary of the society to correspond with the medical societies of the State, and ascertain their views upon the subject.

The time and place of holding the Convention, are, by this society, held as subjects of comparatively little importance. If, however, their views meet a general concurrence, they respectfully suggest Selma as the place, and the second Monday in December as the time. But they will cheerfully yield to the general wish and meet their brethren of the Profession in Mobile, Montgomery or any other place of easy access, that may be desired.

We have the example of our professional brethren of Mississippi, Virginia and some other States not only for holding such a Convention, but for the establishment of a State Medical Society. This latter is considered a measure of much importance to the future interests of the Medical Profession. If properly organized and conducted, such a society it is confidently believed would not fail to increase its usefulness, elevate its dignity, and aid much in the restoration of it to its former high place in the estimation of the public.

A Code of Medical Ethics for the guidance and government of the members of the profession in their intercourse with each other and their patients is supposed to be much needed and very generally desired. The adoption and recommendation of such a code by a State Convention, would give it authority and insure its reception.

Medical Education and the means by which it may be improved, are deemed worthy of the most serious attention, and might very properly be brought before a State Convention—such as we propose to hold. The [burden] of the medical treatment of the poor of the country rests upon the shoulders of the members of our profession, and while we are allowed no privilege adequate to compensate us for this burthen [sic], we are by the laws of the state required to pay a tax upon the amount received as a reward for the arduous duties performed by us, and Quackery, in all its hideous deformity suffered to stalk over the country, untramelled and unrestrained. This is wrong—and while we would deprecate every thing like a complaining spirit, we believe it a duty we owe to ourselves to impress [express] our sentiments freely upon this subject.

The fact that a Lunatic Asylum is needed in Alabama as much as it is in the other States of this Union cannot be denied,—and although we would not presume to dictate to the Legislature in regard to the establishment of such an institution, yet we deem it our duty to place this subject in its proper light before the people—that its importance may be understood.

A report upon this subject by a State Convention would unquestionably procure for it that attention from the public which its importance deserves.

You will please lay this communication before your society and report the result of their action to

Your Obt. Servt.

A. G. Mabry Sect.
Ala. Med. Society.

P.S. I avail myself of this opportunity to call your attention and that of the members of your Society to the offer of the Alabama Medical Society of "A copy of Pancosts' Surgery, or other book of equal value," as a Premium for the best Essay on the Convulsions of Children. The Essay and the name of the writer to be deposited with the Secretary of this Society on or before the first Monday in December next.[2]

At a meeting of the Alabama Medical Society held in Selma on June 23, 1847, Dr. Mabry submitted the following report:

The secretary having been instructed at the last annual meeting of the society, to correspond with the different medical societies of the state, for the purpose of ascertaining their views upon the subject of the propriety of holding a State Medical Convention, reports that so far as he had been able to learn there was but one medical society in the state except our own, and that one was the Mobile Medical Society. He read a copy of a communication which he had, in obedience to instructions, addressed to that society, containing a proposition for the holding of a State Medical Convention, and the reply thereto, agreeing to the suggestion of this society for the holding of such a convention on the second [Monday] in December next, and proposing Mobile as the place.[3]

The secretary presented to the society the letters from Dr. James Guild (1799–1884) of Tuscaloosa and Dr. Hardy Vickers Wooten (1813–1856) of Lowndesboro, who expressed their approval of the suggestion. Then the following motion was made:

Resolved, 1st. That a State Medical Convention be called to be held in Mobile on the second Monday in December next, 2nd. That all gentlemen of the medical profession in this state, and particularly the members of the different examining boards, be invited to attend the convention, and that we earnestly request the cooperation of the Mobile Medical Society in extending this invitation.[4]

The following notice appeared in the *Alabama Tribune*, Mobile, December 1, 1847:

Alabama State Medical Convention.

The Delegates, accredited from Medical Societies or Association of this State to the Medical Convention to be [held] in the city of Mobile, are requested to meet at the Waverly House on WEDNESDAY, December 1st, at 11 o'clock, A.M., for organization, election of officers, and other preliminary business.

Delegates and gentlemen of the REGULAR FACULTY visiting the city for this purpose, are requested to leave their names and addresses with any one of the Committee of Reception to wit:

[William] B. Crawford, M.D., Conti [St.], Josiah C. Nott, M.D., corner St. Francis and St. Joseph Sts., George A. Ketchum, M.D., Conception [St.], opposite the Public Square.

By order

JOHN F. INNERARITY, M.D.
Secretary Mobile Medical Society[5]

A group of twenty-one physicians met Wednesday morning, December 1, 1847, at the Waverly House in Mobile. Dr. Aaron Lopez (1800–1873) of Mobile was selected as temporary chairman. A convention was organized, which, after adopting a constitution and electing officers, declared itself "The Medical Association of the State of Alabama."[6] Elected officers were:

> President, W. B. Johnson, M.D., of Perry County.
> First Vice-President, R. L. Fearn, M.D., of Mobile.
> Second Vice-President, A. G. Mabry, M.D., of Selma.
> Secretaries, George F. Pollard, M.D., of Montgomery
> and W. B. Crawford, M.D., of Mobile.
> Treasurer, George A. Ketchum, M.D., of Mobile.[7]

Proceedings of the convention for December 2nd and 3rd appeared in the *Alabama Tribune* of Mobile, and the following quotations from that paper are of interest:

> Medical Convention—This body met yesterday morning pursuant to adjournment on the previous day. . . .
> After the convention was thus organized, on motion of Dr. Lopez, of Mobile, a committee was appointed to prepare a code of ethics, taking for its basis the code adopted at the general medical convention held [in] Philadelphia last May.*
> During the sitting of the convention several very able speeches were delivered by Dr. Johnson, the President, Dr. Lopez, Dr. Mabry and Dr. Fearn.
> There were twenty-four delegates present yesterday.[8]

Dr. Lopez, along with nine other members of the Medical Association of the State of Alabama, was selected to represent the new organization at the next annual meeting of the American Medical Association in May, 1848, in Baltimore, Maryland.[9]

The first regular meeting of the newly organized society was in 1848, in Selma, with Dr. William B. Johnson of Marion, Perry County, presiding.[10] In 1849, two sessions were held, the first on March 6–7, 1849, in Wetumpka and the other in Montgomery on December 13, 1849. At the Wetumpka meeting, Dr. A. G. Mabry of Selma, the president, was absent, and Dr. S. D. Holt, who was second vice-president, was elected president and presiding officer. Dr. Holt also presided at the Montgomery session. Some of the papers read at these two sessions were published in the *New Orleans Medical Journal*.[11]

The Association was incorporated by the General Assembly on February 13, 1850.[12] The incorporators were Drs. N. L. Meredith, Thomas W. Mason, J. A. English, T. A. Bates, W. B. Johnson, and H. M. Jackson.

---

*This was the organizational meeting of the American Medical Association.

Regular meetings were held yearly until 1856. At these meetings members presented papers and representatives were chosen to the American Medical Association. The organization continued to pursue such causes as the improvement of the quality of medical practice, the establishment of a hospital for the insane and a medical school. In order to stimulate interest in the work of the Association, the *Transactions of the Medical Association of the State of Alabama* were published beginning in 1850. The 1850 session was held in Mobile, December 10–13, with Dr. Aaron Lopez as the presiding officer. Proceedings of this session, together with the papers presented, were published in the first edition of the *Transactions*, a pamphlet of 150 pages.[13]

It was at the 1850 session that a renewed effort was made to interest the General Assembly in establishing a hospital for the insane. Drs. A. Lopez, S. Holt, W. H. Anderson, H. V. Wooten, W. O. Baldwin, and William Boling were appointed as a committee to "memorialize" the General Assembly, urging the importance of such an institution and to aid Miss Dorothea Lynde Dix, who was then making earnest efforts to accomplish the same goal.[14] (See Chapter 13, "The History of the Mental Health Movement in Alabama.")

On December 8, 1851, the State Association met in Montgomery. Dr. W. O. Baldwin presided, due to the death of Dr. Charles E. Lavender, the elected president. On December 10, 1852, the State Association met in Selma. Dr. William McFarland Boling who had been elected president of the Association for that year, was absent and Dr. A. G. Mabry presided.[15]

At the 1852 session, the committee for establishment of a hospital for the insane, of which Dr. Aaron Lopez was chairman, reported that the General Assembly had passed an act providing for this facility and had approved plans for construction of the hospital at Tuscaloosa.[16] Dr. Lopez had been appointed by the governor to visit various hospitals for the insane in the United States. He had complied with this commission and reported to the governor. At this time, five members of the State Medical Association were appointed to the first Board of Trustees of the new institution. The hospital opened its doors in 1861 under the superintendency of Dr. Peter Bryce.[17]

The Association was to meet in Montgomery in 1853, but probably due to a yellow fever epidemic in the autumn of the year, no meeting was held. No mention is made of who had been elected president for 1853. The Association met in Montgomery on January 10–12, 1854, with Dr. A. Denney presiding.[18]

At the 1852 session, the treasurer had reported that the Association was $800 to $900 in debt. At the 1854 session, at least $1,000 was due from delinquent members.[19]

When the 1855 session was held in Mobile, February 5–7, with Dr. L. H. Anderson presiding, the treasurer reported that more than half of the members were delinquent in dues. At this session it was resolved to make Mobile the permanent home for the meetings and to establish a pathological museum and medical library there. Each year the State Association selected a prominent member to give an oration on an important medical topic. Dr. William Taylor (1824–1907) of Talladega was the annual orator for this session. The theme of his address was "an able and exhaustive plea to demonstrate the value and necessity for the South to have her own Medical College, and to bring to bear the many advantages which Mobile offered as a site for the Medical College."[20] In 1859, the support of the Association members was essential for the passage of a bill that chartered the Medical College of Alabama in Mobile and granted it a subsidy of $50,000.[21]

The session of 1856 was presumably held again in Mobile, and Dr. T. W. Mason of Wetumpka was president. No transactions were printed for this session.[22]

The fledgling Association was short-lived. Its membership was never large—at the most 150—and the organization faced many problems. Physicians were elected to membership whether they were present at the meetings or not and were apparently kept on the membership rolls indefinitely. Moreover, members were drawn almost exclusively from the southern and central parts of the state, largely from the cities of Mobile, Selma, and Montgomery. There were no railroads; and travel, except on the rivers, was slow, inconvenient, and expensive. This was especially true for practitioners in northern Alabama. Most of the meetings were held in the winter or the early spring months, which added to the difficulties of travel. The summer months were avoided most probably due to the danger of yellow fever. No doubt the burdens placed on already overworked physicians by the duties of the Association were difficult to bear. Only about two-thirds of the members ever paid their dues regularly. The rest, claiming that they had not authorized their names to be entered for membership, refused to pay dues at all.

In spite of voluntary contributions, the treasury had a deficit as early as 1851. The major expenditures were for printing the *Transactions* and for expenses of delegates sent to the annual American Medical Association meetings. In 1855, the Association, in a major effort to increase its membership, ordered 1,500 copies of the *Transactions* printed. It was this ambitious project that brought about the bankruptcy of the Association. The Association never recovered from its financial crisis.[23]

The overwhelming financial indebtedness prevented any further publication of the *Transactions*, and it is not known whether the Association met after 1856.[24] Certainly, the outbreak of the Civil War spelled the doom of the struggling organization. Many of its members joined the armed forces of the Confederacy. All men were caught up in the strife, and it was not until 1868 that the Medical Association of the State of Alabama met again.

The State Medical Association After 1868

Representatives of Mobile, Montgomery, Greensboro, and Selma medical societies, together with other physicians from surrounding areas, met in Selma on March 3–4, 1868, to reorganize the Medical Association of the State of Alabama. The ranks of Alabama physicians had been sadly depleted by the war, and only six prewar members were present. These were Drs. A. G. Mabry, H. Backus, C. J. Clark, F. A. Ross, A. J. Reese, and W. P. Reese. In addition to the six former members, there were fourteen new members. Dr. F. A. Ross was president. Here again we see the guiding hand of Dr. Albert Gallatin Mabry. Dr. Mabry offered the following resolution:

> *Resolved*, That we, the members of the Medical Association of the State of Alabama, here assembled, do revive and reëstablish said Association, and invite the physicians present who are not members to join us in so doing and to become members of the association.[25]

The resolution was unanimously adopted, and Dr. Mabry was elected president. Among the officers elected was a newcomer, Dr. Jerome Cochran of Mobile, who served as secretary of the reorganized Association and was to have considerable impact on its future course.

The next annual session was held in Mobile on March 2–4, 1869. Ten counties were represented with a total attendance of forty. Dr. Mabry presided. Dr. Barckley Wallace Toole (1835–1898) of Talladega stated that this was the third time Dr. Mabry was so honored. Dr. Mabry's presidential address was about the medical profession; he presented another paper during the same meeting, which was entitled "Miasmatic Fever."[26]

After its reorganization, the State Association grew steadily. It met in Montgomery, March 15–17, 1870, with Dr. R. F. Michel as its president. Considerable discussion was held on the disease of malaria, particularly the hemorrhagic type. Dr. W. P. Reese said he was not satisfied with the name "hemorrhagic malarial fever" and preferred to call the disease "malignant jaundice."

A movement was begun (probably at the instigation of Dr. Cochran) at this meeting to rewrite the Association's constitution. There was, however, strenuous opposition to the formation of a strong central organization. Even so, it became obvious to most members that such a move was necessary if the profession was to properly influence the practice of medicine in the state. Dr. Cochran's first attempt to implement his plans met with failure.

From the time of his first involvement with the Medical Association of the State of Alabama, Dr. Cochran had hoped to change its constitution in order to make it a more disciplined and organized body. In his words, the prewar organization "was a simple convention of doctors, very loosely bound together with very few duties, and no penalties which were ever enforced." He believed that the medical profession should have more dynamic objectives in view.

> The first as relates to the influence of the proper organization over the profession itself, over the profession as a whole, and over every one of its individual members, in the upholding of a high standard of medical education and of medical ethics, and in the promotion of professional brotherhood and high-toned, chivalric emulation in the elevation of professional character, and the advancement of professional interests.
>
> The second relates to the influence of proper organization over public opinion and state legislation, and involves such questions as the protection by provisions of law of the medical profession in its legitimate privileges, and the protection of the general public against all the demoralizing and destructive agencies of medical ignorance and quackery.
>
> The third relates to the influence of proper organization over the advancement of medical science and medical art, by the systematic elucidation of the climatic, endemic and epidemic influences at work in the different sections of the state, together with the development of our indigenous therapeutic resources, and such contributions to the practical medicine as our physicians may be able to discover.[27]

Dr. Cochran was an outstanding leader of the profession in Alabama during the years following the Civil War and was the author of major parts of the constitution for the Association and a prominent proponent of its adoption. Indeed, the constitution that he proposed remains today substantially as originally written.

The Mobile Medical Society served as a model for the organization of the State Association. It was founded in 1841, and in order to combat more effectively the yearly visitations of yellow fever, it was granted a charter that gave the local society the right to act as both the Medical Licensing Board and the Board of Health of the City of Mobile.[28] This association had been so effective that it undoubtedly impressed and influenced Dr. Cochran.

In 1871, the Association met in Mobile with Dr. Frank Armstrong Ross (1821–1885) as president. The friends of reform were again present and presented a draft of the new constitution.[29] It was brought up for discussion, but no final vote was taken. Instead, the proposed constitution was to be published in the *Transactions*, and further discussion was postponed until the next meeting. This was to give the entire membership of the Association an opportunity to read and study implications of the proposed constitution.

In 1872, the annual Association meeting was held in Huntsville with Dr. Thomas Childress Osborn of Hale County as president. The new constitution was freely discussed, but some opposition still remained. In an effort to secure cooperation of as many members as possible, the vote was again postponed until the following annual session. Dr. Cochran felt a favorable decision was needed and was willing to wait.

The Association met in Tuscaloosa in 1873 with Dr. George Ernest Kumpe (1818–1887) of Leighton as president. The new constitution was discussed, section by section, and voted on separately. Finally, with the help of a strong North Alabama contingent led by Dr. Kumpe, the constitution was adopted. This process took two days, but the entire document with some minor amendments was finally adopted by more than two-thirds of those members present. The new constitution thus established the fundamental organizational structure of the Medical Association of the State of Alabama.

The new constitution provided for an executive body with a president, two vice-presidents, a secretary, a treasurer, and a board of five censors (ten after 1877). The president was given general supervisory authority over the Association, while the vice-presidents, one each for the northern and southern parts of the state, were in charge of county medical societies. The board of censors constituted the general executive committee.

The board of censors' role was one of the most distinctive features of the organization.

> All the business of whatever character, which is presented to the association, is referred to them [board of censors] without debate and without motion, to be reported back to the association with their recommendations and the reasons, after which said business is discussed and voted upon by the association.[30]

The constitution was adopted; and the following were chosen members of the first board of censors: Drs. Jerome Cochran of Mobile, for five years; James Guild, Sr., of Tuscaloosa, for four years; A. G. Mabry of Selma, for three years; R. F. Michel of Montgomery, for two years; and George E. Kumpe of Leighton, for one year.

The democratic principle in the organization was implemented by a legislature composed of a College of Counsellors and delegates from the county medical societies. The College consisted of a group of 100 physicians "who had won their places through service and merit."[31] The counsellors were elected for life by the State Association, and all the officers and censors were selected from their membership. In this manner, Dr. Cochran made certain that some future "Young Turks" could not reorganize or effectively alter the format of the organization of the Association. The members of the county medical societies were the rank and file of the organization. These societies were chartered by the Association, and their members were *ipso facto* members of the State Association. As far as possible they were organized according to the same plan as the State Association (officers, censors, counsellors): each society had the right to send two delegates to all of the State Association meetings.

The Cochran constitution thus provided for a strong, centralized organization. As a result, in Cochran's words, "[the Association's] constitution, regulations, and . . . enacted ordinances, are vigorously enforced—are enforced certainly, promptly, inexorably and without either fear or favor."[32] This fact, apparently, enormously increased the confidence of the medical profession in the Association. Membership rose from twenty in 1868 to some 1,100 in 1893; and the number of county societies rose from four to sixty-six, one for every county in the state. With fees set at ten dollars annually, the Association's financial condition reached a degree of stability that the prewar society had never attained.

Each of the county societies received its charter from the State Association. When the new constitution was adopted in 1873, only about half of the counties in the state had nominally organized medical societies, and only fourteen of these were represented at the 1873 meeting. It was not until 1888, fifteen years after the adoption of the constitution, that all the counties had organized medical societies chartered by the State Association.[33]

Among the first county medical societies to apply for a charter were those of Autauga, Butler, Dallas (which succeeded the Selma Medical Society in 1874), Hale, Perry, and Talladega in 1875; Lowndes, Mobile, Morgan, Sumter, and Walker in 1876; Elmore, Jefferson, Lamar, Lawrence, Limestone, Madison, Marengo, Monroe, Shelby, and Tuscaloosa in 1877; and Barbour, Blount, Etowah, Montgomery, Pickens, Pike, Randolph, St. Clair, and Wilcox in 1878.[34]

The General Assembly passed a law implementing the Association's organizational plan in 1875. One of the stipulations of this law was that the State Medical Association would constitute the Board of Health of the State of Alabama with authority and control over county boards. County medical societies were likewise given the duties and powers of county boards of health. By an act of the State Legislature approved September 29, 1919, the boards of censors of the county medical societies, rather than the society as a whole, constituted the county boards of health. Thus, private skill and initiative were channeled to meet public needs and were implemented by law.[35]

The General Assembly's second Medical Practice Act, February 9, 1877, marked the culmination of earnest effort on the part of the Association over a number of years. It specified that no person would be permitted to practice medicine in any of its branches or departments unless a certificate of qualification had been obtained from an authorized Board of Medical Examiners. Even irregular practitioners found it necessary to procure a diploma or certificate of qualification in anatomy, physiology, chemistry, and the mechanism of labor.

Of greater importance was the law's designation that the state and county boards of censors serve as the authorized boards of medical examiners. The law also provided that the qualifications required of persons desiring to practice medicine would be determined by the Medical Association of the State of Alabama.

County medical societies proved to be unsatisfactory licensure boards, so in 1907, this regulation was amended, and a state licensing board was created. The law regulating the practice of medicine was incorporated in the Code of Alabama in 1923.[36]

Thus, despite the terrible ordeal of the Civil War, almost insurmountable transportation problems, epidemics, dissensions within the organization itself, and various other internal troubles, Alabama was eminently successful in its formation of a state medical association. This Association met not only the problems of the people's health but became a model for similar organizations in other states.[37] The motto of the Association is *Nos Etiam Sperarumus Meliora*: "we also have hope for better things."

In the early years of the twentieth century, when the American Medical Association (AMA) was struggling to bring about uniformity of structure in the various state medical societies, Dr. Cochran's organizational plan was freely studied and drawn upon. In 1901, Dr. Charles A. Reed, then president of the AMA, referred to the Alabama State Medical Society as "the incomparable Alabama plan." In 1902 Dr. Edwin Lesley Maréchal (1850–1909) of Mobile, president of the Alabama Association, stated that "the American Medical Association, in its plan of reorganization, adopted the fundamental principles underlying our system." This was probably due to the Alabama Association's appraisal by Dr. George H. Simmons, secretary of the AMA, "as the best medical organization in the world."[38]

The Association in the 1880s

An act "to provide for the supervision of the public health . . . in the several counties of the State of Alabama," was approved by the General

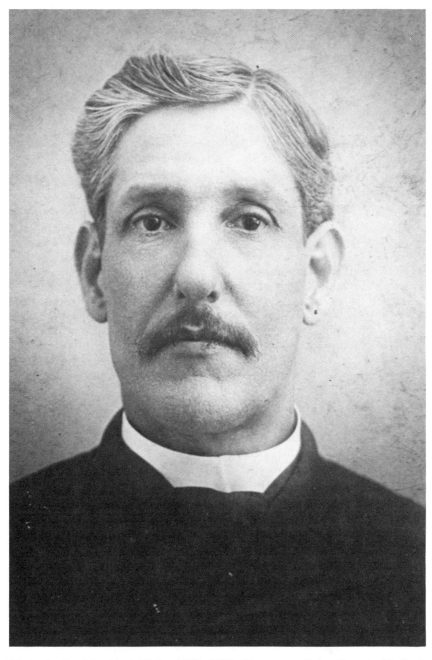

Edwin Lesley Maréchal, M.D., 1850–1909 (Courtesy of the Heustis Medical Museum, Mobile, Alabama)

Assembly on February 28, 1881. This act assigned certain duties to county boards of health and granted them authority to elect a county health officer for their respective jurisdictions and fix his term of office. Thus, another link in the organizational chain that had been envisaged by Dr. Cochran was shaped.

Attending the annual session of 1886, Anniston, April 13–16, was Dr. William A. Love of Atlanta, appointed by the president of the Medical Association of Georgia to "look thoroughly into the workings of the Alabama Association." The president was anxious to have the Alabama Association's organizational plan understood by the profession of Georgia. Dr. Love reported:

> that the Medical Association of Alabama is a representative body, that its working is at once unique and complex, its very complexity giving it strength. It has united the profession of the State as one man; its influence for good is felt throughout its jurisdiction. From irregular [practitioners] it has met [strenuous] opposition. These for a time played upon the prejudices, the credulity, and gullibility of the people, and brought what at times seemed to be formidable opposition to it, but its intelligent officers . . . have so far guided it safely to a condition of prosperity and power that would seem to vouchsafe a successful future . . . They are united in peace, they are working in harmony, and their social and political standing and influence is such that it is a sufficient guarantee that in the future, as in the past, they will be amply sustained by the enactments of the General Assembly in all their efforts for the common good of a confiding community.[39]

At the 1888 meeting, the organization of all county medical societies in the state was completed.

> Four new county societies have been organized, . . . which completes the organization of the whole State . . . This [has been the goal] of twenty years of assiduous and persistent effort. Without doubt the . . . Association . . . of Alabama is now by far the most powerful medical organization in the United States, and so far as we know, the most powerful in the world . . . Our past history is a continuous record of successful effort; and our future is bright with the promise of better things.[40]

The Association in the Nineties

On April 18–21, 1893, the Association convened in Selma. Dr. James Thomas Searcy (1839–1920) of Tuscaloosa, president of the Association, made reference in the following statement to Dr. Peter Bryce, who died August 14, 1892.

> At his death the sense of a great loss pervaded the whole State. In accordance with the general sentiment, and as a mark of public respect,

the Governor ordered the flag at half-mast on the Capitol at Montgomery, and the people and the press of the State uniformly mourned his loss. Bryce Hospital will ever remain an enduring monument to him who died with his mind clear to the last, and with his hand still on the machinery of that much loved institution, the product of his life work.[41]

Dr. Jerome Cochran, state health officer, died in Montgomery on August 17, 1896. The expression of the State Board of Censors was appropriate:

> During the last year a great calamity befell us in the death of our leader (Jerome Cochran), the man who conceived this organization, and, above all others, built it up and made it what it is. Let us hope that his work was so well done that, although he is no longer here to guide us with his wisdom and to animate us with his courage, we may be able to push on and reap that splendid fruition for which he so earnestly worked and eagerly longed.[42]

In January, 1903, an opinion was handed down by Justice Tyson, and concurred in by the other four distinguished jurists who composed the Alabama Supreme Court. This decision established beyond doubt the constitutionality of the 1877 Medical Practice Law as enacted. It fully upheld the Association's right, under the law, to examine the qualifications of all applicants desiring to practice medicine in the state.

Moreover, on February 26, 1903, when Dr. Russell McWhorter Cunningham (1855–1921; acting governor of Alabama from April, 1904, to March 18, 1905) of Birmingham was lieutenant governor, the chief executive of Alabama approved an act defining the branches of medical learning upon which applicants had to be examined to practice medicine in the state. The law specified in part:

> Any applicant for a certificate of qualification to treat diseases of human beings by any system whatsoever, shall, according to rules prescribed and standards established by The Medical Association of the State of Alabama, be examined . . . in the following branches of medical learning, to wit: Chemistry, anatomy, physiology; the etiology, pathology, symptomatology, and diagnosis of diseases; obstetrics and obstetrical operations; gynecology, minor and major surgery; physical diagnosis; hygiene, and medical jurisprudence.[43]

That same year other legislation was approved in response to an accusation: "That the chapter of health laws as written in the code is illogically construed, faulty in sequential arrangement, and ambiguous in verbiage." A general bill designed to correct these deficiencies was offered by the Honorable E. S. Starr, representative from Dallas County; and on October 9, 1903, an act was passed "to amend, reconstruct and provide for the enforcement of the laws relating to public health."[44]

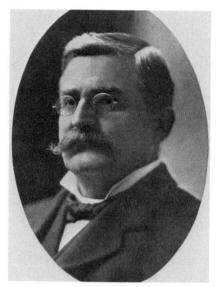

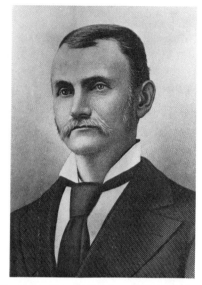

Russell McWhorter Cunningham, M.D., 1855–1921 (Courtesy of the Alabama State Department of Archives and History)

Mortimer Harvie Jordan, M.D., 1844–1889 (Courtesy of the Alabama State Department of Archives and History)

In 1906, a new constitution for the State Medical Association was adopted; but there was no fundamental change in the basic principles of the constitution of 1873.

The Medical Practice Act was amended on August 9, 1907. The new act required that all examinations for certification to treat diseases of human beings be held in Montgomery. Also, the State Board of Censors (the Board of Medical Examiners) was granted authority to establish reciprocity with similar boards of other states requiring examination upon substantially the same branches of medical learning as those enumerated in the statutes of Alabama. It was not until 1917 when rules governing reciprocity were adopted that this privilege was exercised.

On February 6, 1893, the General Assembly confirmed, amended, and extended the charter of the Association. The organization "conferred upon the State Board of Censors the right to prepare for issuance [of] new charters for all County Medical Societies." In 1912, Dr. W. H. Sanders, chairman of the Board of Censors, informed the State Medical

Association: "the original charters, . . . were very short and incomplete . . . written on paper . . . not especially prepared for the purpose, . . . it is highly proper that new charters should be issued in proper form." The president of the Association, assisted by the secretary and Dr. Sanders, issued charters to each of the sixty-seven county medical societies. Houston County had been organized in 1903.[45]

In Birmingham at the 1915 annual session, representation in the house of delegates was changed from two members for each county to the number corresponding to the county's representatives in the lower house of the State Legislature, but in no case would this number be less than two.

On March 5, 1915, the State Legislature gave the Association the right to alter, amend, or extend the charter of the Association by a vote of two-thirds of those present at an annual or other lawful meeting of the Association.

The momentous days of 1917 and 1918 saw Alabama physicians respond to the call to aid their country in World War I. Just as their forebears did at another period in the history of the Association, they "were found exchanging their pleasant reunions for the camp and bivouac, confronting danger amid the carnage of the bloody battle field, or ministering at the bedside of the wounded and suffering in hospitals and infirmaries."[46] A muster roll, which is thought to be incomplete, listed 454 physicians from sixty-seven counties who served in the Army, the Navy, and the United States Public Health Service. When they returned, the Association welcomed them at the annual session in Mobile on April 16, 1919. But some were beyond reach of this praise; those who gave their lives were: Drs. Bryant C. Rudder, Paul Lee Cocke, Mortimer H. Jordan, Philip M. Kyser, James D. Atkins, and Robert C. Goldthwaite.[47]

A monthly journal, which had been under discussion as far back as 1885 under the presidency of Dr. Benjamin A. Riggs, was first published on July 15, 1931. The forty-four–page journal had long been advocated by such prominent physicians as Dr. Seale Harris of Birmingham and Dr. W. W. Harper of Selma.[48] (See Chapter 9, "Medical Journals in Alabama.")

Summary

The Medical Association of the State of Alabama has remained the bastion against poorly trained practitioners, ill-advised health laws, and nonethical practitioners. It has freely fulfilled the dreams of Dr. Jerome Cochran and his colleagues who formulated the basic constitution more than a century ago.

Notes

1. Emmett B. Carmichael, "Albert Gallatin Mabry," *J.M.A. Ala.* 38 (1969): 1018.

2. This letter, sent by Dr. Mabry at the direction of the Alabama Medical Society, is on file in the Minutes of the Mobile Medical Society and is used with their permission.

3. Carmichael, p. 1018.

4. Ibid.

5. Emmett B. Carmichael, "The Medical Association of the State of Alabama," *J.M.A. Ala.* 30 (1961): 587.

6. Ibid.

7. Barckley W. Toole, "The Annual Message of the President (Historical Sketch of the Medical Association of the State of Alabama)," *Trans.* (1897), p. 18.

8. Carmichael, "The Medical Association," pp. 587–88.

9. *Alabama Tribune*, 3 December 1847, p. 2, col. 1.

10. Dr. Johnson's name does not appear on the Association's rolls after 1850. Apparently, he moved out of the state.

11. Jerome Cochran, "The Medical Profession," *Memorial Record of Alabama: Historical and Biographical* (Madison, Wisconsin: Brant and Fuller, 1893), 2: 118.

12. William H. Brantley, Jr., "Alabama Doctor," *Ala. Lawyer* 6 (1945): 257.

13. Cochran, p. 118.

14. Ibid.

15. Ibid.

16. The editor of the *New Orleans Medical and Surgical Journal* in a commentary upon the receipt of the 1852 Proceedings of the Medical Association of the State of Alabama had the following to say about the Medical Association in Alabama: "All honor to Alabama! She has neither a medical college nor a Journal, but her students are educated in the best schools of the country and her physicians enrich the pages of the Medical Journals of both North and South."

17. Cochran, pp. 118–19, 135–36.

18. Ibid., pp. 119–20. There is no listing of a Dr. Denney in the membership rolls for this year. Other records, however, give Dr. A. Denny of Suggsville as president in 1854.

19. Cochran, p. 119.

20. The looming sectional crisis resulted in the proposal of and funding of "States' Rights" Medical Schools. John Duffy, ed., *The Rudolph Matas History of Medicine in Louisiana* (Baton Rouge: Louisiana State University Press, 1962), 2: 95–98.

21. Cochran, pp. 119, 134–35; and Brantley, pp. 262–63.

22. Cochran, pp. 119–20.

23. Ibid.

24. Dr. Albert G. Mabry stated in his presidential address to the reorganized Association in 1869 that yearly meetings were held until the outbreak of the Civil War. There is some evidence for this as the slate of officers for the year 1859 are known, but no *Transactions* were printed after 1855.

Officers of the Alabama Medical Association in 1859 were:

J. C. Nott, president

M. G. Meriwether, Line Creek, Montgomery County, first vice-president

G. W. Files, Gosport, Clarke County, second vice-president

W. C. Ashe, Demopolis, Marengo County, third vice-president

F. A. Ross, Mobile, corresponding secretary

R. Miller, Mobile, first recording secretary

A. H. Smith, Summerville, Sumter County, second recording secretary

W. H. Anderson, Mobile, treasurer

A. F. Alexander, Eutaw, Green County, orator

J. M. Williams, Montgomery, alternate

25. "Annual Session of 1868," *Trans.* (1869), pp. 5–7.

26. Toole, p. 23.

27. G. A. Ketchum, "Memorial Meeting," *Trans.* (1897), p. 99.

28. Acts of Alabama, 21 December 1841, p. 74.

29. Cochran, pp. 120–22.

30. Ibid., p. 124.

31. Carey V. Stabler, "The History of the Alabama Public Health System" (Ph.D. diss., Duke University, 1944), p. 58.

32. Cochran, p. 125.

33. D. L. Cannon, "Alabama's Eighty-Nine Years of Medical Organization: A Brief History of the Association, Part 2," *J.M.A. Ala.* 5 (1936): 348–56.

34. Ibid., p. 349.

35. Ibid., p. 348.

36. D. L. Cannon, "Alabama's Eighty-Nine Years of Medical Organization: A Brief History of the Association, Part 3," *J.M.A. Ala.* 5 (1936): 387; and *Code of Alabama 1923*, chap. 52, "Physicians," Article 1 (Atlanta: Foote and Davies Co., 1923), pp. 1279–89.

37. William H. Brantley, Jr., "An Alabama Medical Review," *Ala. J. Med. Sci.* 4 (1967): 185–207.

38. *A Compend for the Members of the Organized Medical Profession of Alabama* (Montgomery, Ala.: Brown Printing Co., 1928), pp. 4–5.

39. Cannon, Part 2, pp. 353–54.

40. Ibid., p. 355.

41. Ibid.

42. Ibid., p. 356.

43. Ibid., Part 3, p. 386.

44. Ibid.

45. Ibid., p. 388.

46. Ibid., p. 391.

47. Ibid.

48. Ibid., p. 392.

Chapter 8

Regional Organizations

The Southern Surgical Association

Drs. J. D. S. and W. E. B. Davis made several joint resolutions at the beginning of their professional careers. One of these was to "organize a state society of surgeons and gynecologists, upon which it might prove possible some day to build a regional or Southern association."[1]

In November, 1886, the office of the *Alabama Medical and Surgical Journal,* which the Davis brothers had founded, was used for a meeting of Birmingham physicians who were interested in forming a state surgical and gynecological association. At this meeting, Dr. H. N. Rosser of Birmingham was elected president and Dr. W. E. B. Davis was elected secretary; the organizational meeting for the Alabama Surgical and Gynecological Association was set for December 15, 1886.[2]

At this December meeting, approximately twelve leading southern surgeons were elected honorary members with the idea that they would be a nucleus for a proposed southern association. Some of the honorary members were in favor of organizing a southern association immediately. However, Dr. W. E. B. Davis felt that it was more important to first organize a state association. He won his point, and the first annual meeting of the Alabama Surgical and Gynecological Association was scheduled for October 11–12, 1887.[3]

Prior to this meeting, Dr. Davis had written to a number of the honorary members of the association about the possibility of organizing a southern association. He received favorable support from eighty physicians, among whom was Dr. W. D. Haggard of Nashville, Tennessee, whose "services proved of inestimable value to the Society during its earliest formative years."[4]

The Southern Surgical and Gynecological Association was founded October 12, 1887—on the second day of the Alabama Surgical and Gynecological Association's first and only meeting. Dr. W. D. Haggard was elected president; Dr. W. E. B. Davis, secretary; Dr. J. S. Cain of

Nashville was made chairman of the Judicial Council; and Dr. J. D. S. Davis, chairman of the Committee on Arrangements for the first meeting of "The Southern." The meeting was to be held in Birmingham on the second Tuesday in November, 1888, but had to be postponed until December 4–6, 1888, due to an outbreak of yellow fever.[5]

Dr. W. E. B. Davis made many suggestions that still remain an integral part of the association. He recommended that representative surgeons from other parts of the country be included in the membership of "The Southern." In 1916, the Southern Surgical and Gynecological Association changed its name to the Southern Surgical Association, and gynecologists were no longer affiliated with it.[6]

The Southern Medical Association

The Southern Medical Association was founded by a group of physicians from the Tri-State Medical Association (Alabama, Georgia, and Tennessee) who met in Chattanooga, Tennessee, at the Read House Hotel on October 2–3, 1906.[7] These physicians felt there was a need for a regional association so that southern physicians could keep abreast of recent developments in medicine. The purpose of the Southern Medical Association was "to develop and foster scientific medicine and medical fraternalism." Therefore, the founding fathers wanted the association to be strictly a scientific organization that would promote scientific medicine in the South.[8]

In order to qualify for membership, the physician had to be a member of the state and local societies of either Alabama, Florida, Georgia, Louisiana, Mississippi, or Tennessee. These states were all represented originally in the Southern Medical Association.[9]

At the organizational meeting of the association, the officers elected were: Dr. H. H. Martin, Savannah, Georgia, president; Drs. J. B. Cowan, Tullahoma, Tennessee, Mack Rogers, Birmingham, Alabama, and J. R. Tackett, Meridian, Mississippi, vice-presidents; Dr. Raymond Wallace, Chattanooga, Tennessee, secretary; and Dr. J. L. Abernathy, Chattanooga, treasurer.[10]

The first annual meeting was held in Birmingham on September 24–25, 1907. The headquarters were at the Hillman Hotel, and the meetings were held at the city hall.[11]

In 1915, the Southern Medical Association established its headquarters in Birmingham. Mr. Clyde Loranz was employed by the Association for many years and served as secretary, treasurer, and general manager.[12] He contributed greatly to the building and strengthening of the Association. Mr. Loranz gave untiringly of his time and energy for the betterment of the Southern Medical Association.

Alabama has had four physicians who served as president of the Southern Medical Association. These physicians were Drs. B. L. Wyman, 1907–1908; Seale Harris, 1921–1922; M. Y. Dabney, 1945–1946; and J. Garber Galbraith, 1965–1966.[13]

Notes

1. Robert M. Moore, "The Davis Brothers of Birmingham and the Southern Surgical and Gynecological Association," *Trans. South. Surg. Assoc.* 74 (1962): 1–2.

2. Ibid., pp. 2–3; and W. E. B. Davis, "Annual Address of the President," *Trans. South. Surg. & Gyn. Assoc.* 15 (1902): 1.

3. Davis, p. 5; and Moore, p. 3.

4. Moore, p. 4.

5. Davis, pp. 5–6.

6. "Report of the Council," *Trans. South. Surg. Assoc.* 29 (1916): liii.

7. "Golden Anniversary, Southern Medical Association," *J.M.A. Ala.* 26 (Sept. 1956): 76.

8. C. P. Loranz, *Golden Anniversary—Fifty Years of Service to Physicians of the South—Southern Medical Association, October 2–3, 1906–1956* (Birmingham: Birmingham Printing Co., September 1960), p. 3.

9. Ibid.

10. Ibid.

11. Ibid.

12. Seale Harris, "Clyde Porter Loranz and The Southern Medical Association," *South. Med. J.* 42 (Jan. 1949): 1–2.

13. *The Southern Medical Association Yearbook, 1979–80* (Birmingham: Southern Medical Association, 1979), inside back cover.

Chapter 9

Medical Journals in Alabama

In the first issue of the *Alabama Medical and Surgical Journal*, an editorial pointed out that although the South had produced many great physicians during the nineteenth century, it had had few medical journals.[1] This was particularly true of Alabama, where physicians depended either on the *Transactions of the Medical Association of the State of Alabama* or on out-of-state journals for all medical news—whether local, national, or international. Such out-of-state journals as the *New Orleans Medical and Surgical Journal* could only devote limited space to contributions from Alabama physicians; and the *Transactions*, because of the time necessary to edit, print, and distribute, were out of date by the time they reached the physician.

Another problem with local publications was that they often had little influence outside their own region. For example, Dr. J. Marion Sims of Montgomery felt it necessary to report his famous surgical cure for the vesicovaginal fistula, not in a southern publication, but in the older and more prestigious *American Journal of Medical Sciences* of Philadelphia (1852).[2]

The success and proper functioning of the Medical Association of the State of Alabama, which acted as the State Board of Health, depended on well-informed members to implement recommendations. Therefore, the need for better communication among Alabama physicians was acute.

Alabama Medical and Surgical Journal

In 1886, Drs. J. D. S. and W. E. B. Davis founded the *Alabama Medical and Surgical Journal*, the first medical journal published in the state. Objectives were to "advance the knowledge of medicine and surgery; to promote a higher appreciation of medical ethics; and to improve medical literature in the South and the West, especially in Alabama."[3] The Davis brothers, known throughout the country for their experimental surgery on dogs, contributed articles that enhanced the journal's prestige.[4] All physicians in the state were invited to contribute material. Each issue included four or five such articles as well as book reviews, reprints from other medical journals, editorials, and a section dealing with Alabama medical news.

Unfortunately, from the beginning, the *Alabama Medical and Surgical Journal* was in dire financial straits. Because complimentary copies were sent to potential subscribers, many were slow in paying and frequently did not subscribe at all.

Of a more serious nature was an acrimonious editorial disagreement between the Davis brothers and Dr. Jerome Cochran, state health officer and an influential member of the State Medical Association.[5] The Davis brothers favored a central state board for licensing physicians. Dr. Cochran felt that an examining board in each county would serve the medical profession more efficiently. In March, 1887, the State Medical Association voted in favor of county boards, and the Davis brothers lost more than just an editorial disagreement. For after the May, 1887, issue, eleven months after its inauguration, the *Alabama Medical and Surgical Journal* ceased publication.[6]

The Alabama Medical and Surgical Age

The Alabama Medical and Surgical Age was founded in 1889 by Dr. J. C. LeGrande. Although *The Age* was similar in format and ideals to the journal sponsored by the Davis brothers, it was not a continuation of the *Alabama Medical and Surgical Journal*. However, Dr. W. E. B. Davis did serve as editor of its gynecological section. *The Age* was a completely independent venture, owned wholly by Dr. LeGrande, and although initially published in Anniston, it was published in Birmingham after 1895. (Dr. J. C. LeGrande moved to Birmingham and helped to found the Birmingham Medical College in 1894. He served as the college secretary.) In 1900, when *The Age* became the official organ of the Medical Association of the State of Alabama, the name was changed to *Alabama Medical Journal*.[7] After the death of Dr. LeGrande in 1906, a committee of collaborators, including Drs. L. C. Morris and B. L. Wyman of Birmingham, J. T. Searcy of Tuscaloosa, E. D. Bondurant of Mobile, and W. W. Harper of Selma, continued to publish *The Age* until the end of that year. In December, 1906, with volume 19, number 1, Dr. W. H. Bell became the editor and proprietor. This arrangement continued until early 1911 when the journal ceased publication.

Southern Medical Journal

A third Alabama medical journal, the *Mobile Medical and Surgical Journal* was initiated by Dr. E. L. Maréchal in 1902. An editorial

Mobile Medical and Surgical Journal.

VOL. I.   JANUARY, 1902.   No. 1

Original Articles.

WOUNDS OF THE HEART. *

By L. L. Hill, M. D., Montgomery, Alabama.

In 1881 John B. Roberts of Philadelphia, conceived the idea of suturing the heart, and Billroth said, "no surgeon who wished to preserve the respect of his colleagues would ever attempt to suture a wound of the heart," but the wand of progress had touched the art of surgery and the *ipse dixit* of this arcangel of the operating amphitheater staggered but could not stay its onward march.   In 1882 Block closed a wound in a rabbit's heart, and in 1894 Del Veochio of Naples demonstrated the feasibility of suturing the heart before the Eleventh International Medical Congress in Rome, by his experiments on dogs. In 1896 the human heart was sutured by Farrina and Cappelen, and in 1897, successfully, by Rehn.

Wounds of the heart may be either non-penetrating or penetrating—injuring the cardiac wall or opening a cavity. The chief dangers from the former are shock and injury to a coronary artery.   Ninety per cent. are penetrating, and of these only nineteen per cent. are immediately fatal.   The right ventricle is most frequently injured, and the left auricle is least so.   Auricular wounds are more fatal than ventricular, and injuries to the apex are less dangerous than either.   A needle puncture will rarely cause hemorrhage from a ventricle, but excessive bleeding, which is mostly systolic, is liable to follow a like injury to an auricle.   A wound inflicted during diastole is less dangerous than a similar injury during systol, perpendicular wounds are more fatal than diagonal, and those of the right heart bleed more profusely than those of the left. The presence of the foreign body in the heart, the size of the wound, the location of the wound, the number of wounds, the connecting of cavities, the attending syncope, the involvement of Kronecker's co-ordination centre, are important factors in determining the outcome.   Pericardits, myocardits, endocar-

*Read before the Elmore county Medical Society at Wetumpka, Alabama, Nov. 20, 1901.

The Mobile Medical and Surgical Journal was the third Alabama medical journal. It was begun in 1902 by Dr. E. L. Maréchal. The title of this journal changed in March 1909 to the *Gulf States Journal of Medicine and Surgery and Mobile Medical and Surgical Journal*. (Courtesy of the Alabama Museum of the Health Sciences, Lister Hill Library, Medical Center, The University of Alabama in Birmingham) outlining objectives of the journal stated that the journal proposed to keep readers informed of the latest advances in medicine, to promote a high standard of ethics and to make efforts "toward safeguarding the entrance of the profession, so that none but the competent men need aspire to its honours and its emoluments."[8] This statement expressed a growing concern throughout the state and the nation that many physicians entering practice were not adequately trained and that more stringent laws, together with improved medical schools, were needed to maintain high standards in the profession.

Dr. Seale Harris purchased the journal and became editor in February, 1909, (vol. 14, no. 2). In March of the same year, the name was changed to *Gulf States Journal of Medicine and Surgery and Mobile Medical and Surgical Journal*. The new title reflected the regional aspirations of the journal. Since 1902, it had been the official organ of the Mobile Medical Association. Actually, its influence was much greater than that associated with the local medical society. Throughout 1910, Dr. Harris conducted negotiations for the purchase of the *Southern Medical Journal*. This journal had originated in Nashville in July, 1908, with Dr. J. A. Witherspoon as editor-in-chief, together with over fifty other physicians from Nashville and other parts of the South as collaborators. In December, 1910, the *Southern Medical Journal* (vol. 3, no. 1) merged with the *Gulf States Medical Journal*, with Drs. Seale Harris and H. A. Moody as editors and Dr. Harris as publisher. It then became the *Journal of the Southern Medical Association*. For the next few years it was published monthly, both in Nashville and Mobile. In 1916, it was moved to Birmingham, where it is still published today. In that same year, Dr. M. Y. Dabney of Birmingham became associate editor. In 1921, he took over editorial control when the Southern Medical Association purchased the journal from Dr. Harris.[9]

Journal of the Medical Association of the State of Alabama

With the failure of the *Alabama Medical and Surgical Age* and the transformation of the *Mobile Medical and Surgical Journal* into a publication for the whole South, Alabama was again left without a medical publication of its own other than the annual *Transactions*. This occurred at a time when rapid strides were being made in public health and medicine. It was imperative that communications be maintained among Alabama physicians if the State Medical Association was to successfully function as the State Board of Health. The State Medical Association decided the need was too great not to have a journal of its own.[10] In July, 1931, the first issue of *The Journal of the Medical Association of the State of Alabama and of the State Board of Health* appeared. It was published

THE JOURNAL

OF

The Medical Association of The State of Alabama

AND OF

The State Board of Health

Vol. 1, No. 1   Montgomery, Alabama   July 1931

THE PRESIDENT'S MESSAGE*

W. G. HARRISON, M. D., Birmingham

The average physician is in active practice less than three and a half decades. It is no insignificant distinction to be one of thirty-five chosen from its entire membership to preside at a meeting of the State Medical Association. I am fully conscious of the honor accorded and beg you to accept every assurance of my genuine appreciation.

On this occasion inclination persuades, and custom seems to command, that we praise our past achievements and magnify our present pre-eminence.

Our Constitution directs that the President shall deliver "a message devoted to a discussion of the interests, organization, objects or business of the Association." What a gracious forethought by the authors of our Constitution. They evidently knew the garrulous weakness of all men beyond the fifth decade and were familiar with the physician's "bent for counsel." What privilege more precious than to force on his own profession advice hitherto imposed on his helpless patients! It was this tendency referred to by old Robert Burton in his "Anatomy of Melancholy":

"Who can not give good counsel?
'Tis cheap; it costs him nothing."

*President's address before the Association at the Sixty-fourth Consecutive Annual Session, Birmingham, April 21, 1931.

> ## "BON VOYAGE"
>
> Deal kindly, gentle reader and fellow member, with this our maiden effort. The field of journalism is for us still an uncharted sea. May we ask that you carefully scrutininize your "first born" from cover to cover and send in to its "god-parents" such constructive suggestions as will speed up a lusty growth.

Cochran planted; Sanders watered, and Welch witnessed a glorious increase. What of the present? I congratulate the Association upon its selection of a health officer last year and sincerely believe the future will demonstrate his achievement as equal to that of his predecessors. Alabama's experience amply illustrates the fact that success of a public health officer depends upon character, culture, intelligence, tact and sympathetic understanding of our system, rather than upon a narrow technical training.

I have spent one day in the offices of the State Health Department at Montgomery, have attended seven divisional meetings, have earnestly interviewed about a hundred physicians throughout the State, and have tried to appraise some of our present problems. After mature deliberation, I have reached only two definite convictions. First, the more one studies these problems the less dogmatic are his conclusions; and second, physicians should more frequently and frankly discuss the affairs of purely professional as well as scientific interests, and should constantly consider public health problems. In its broader aspects public health touches nearly every phase of human activity and we should feel ourselves burdened with the duty of integrating and stimulating the many factors that help, and of curbing those that hinder. In harmony with the idea of helping, I have deliberately placed upon our program five papers

---

The Journal of the Medical Association of the State of Alabama and of the State Board of Health first appeared in July 1931. This was due to the failure of the *Alabama Medical Journal* and the changing of the *Mobile Medical and Surgical Journal* to one publication for the South. (Courtesy of the Alabama Museum of the Health Sciences, Lister Hill Library, Medical Center, The University of Alabama in Birmingham)

monthly in Montgomery and, initially, editorship was shared among members of the Board of Censors. These ten physicians also served as the State Board of Health. With the May, 1932 issue, Dr. Fred E. Wilkerson became editor-in-chief. At the same time, "and of the State Board of Health" was removed from the title of the journal. Apparently, most out-of-state physicians, not being familiar with the dual role of the State Medical Association, thought that two separate organizations were responsible for publishing the journal.[11]

The publication contained several original articles, usually papers previously read at annual meetings of the State Medical Association and authored mostly by Alabama physicians. In addition, there were sections dealing with the news of county medical societies, editorials, and book reviews. But what made this journal unique in the history of Alabama medical literature was the section dealing with the State Public Health Department. In it the heads of the Departments of Laboratories, Vital Statistics, Preventable Diseases, and Child Care discussed the current duties and future plans of their departments. Thus, even the physicians who were not directly involved with the Public Health Board came to learn of this important function of the State Medical Association. The information that they gained was then passed on to the people of the state, and the Medical Association could more efficiently implement the mission assigned it by the State Legislature.

Alabama Journal of Medical Sciences

The *Alabama Journal of Medical Sciences* was established in September, 1962, at The University of Alabama in Birmingham Medical Center. The first issue of the journal appeared January, 1964. The journal has four issues a year. Dr. Emmett B. Carmichael, Emeritus Professor of Biochemistry and then assistant dean of the School of Medicine and Dentistry, was editor until December 31, 1973. Dr. Walter B. Frommeyer, Jr., served as editor until his death January, 1979.[12] In June of 1979, George T. Smith, M.D., a pathologist and former dean of the University of Nevada, became editor of the *Journal*. The *Journal*, as a publication of the Medical Center of The University of Alabama in Birmingham, is designed to serve the needs of medical communities throughout Alabama.

Notes

1. Velimir Luketic, "Early Medical Journals in Alabama," *Ala. J. Med. Sci.* 6 (1969): 422.

2. W. Fisher, "Physicians and Slavery in the Antebellum Southern Medical Journal," *J. Hist. Med. & Allied Sci.* 23 (1968): 46–48.

3. Luketic, p. 422.

4. Robert M. Moore, "The Davis Brothers of Birmingham and the Southern Surgical and Gynecological Association," *Ann. Surg.* 157 (1963), 665–67.

5. The state health officer was the presiding officer of the State Board of Health, and the only board member devoting his full time to the Board of Health. The Board was elected by The Medical Association of the State of Alabama.

6. Moore, p. 658.

7. W. H. Bell, "Announcement," editorial, *Ala. Med. J.* 19 (Dec. 1906): 51–52; and Luketic, p. 423.

8. E. L. Maréchal, editorial, *Mobile Med. & Surg. J.* 1 (Jan. 1902): 32–33.

9. C. P. Loranz, *Golden Anniversary of the Southern Medical Association, 1906–1956* (Birmingham, Ala.: Southern Medical Association, 1960), pp. 8–10.

10. Board of Censors of the Medical Association of the State of Alabama, "Our New Venture," editorial, *J.M.A. Ala.* 1 (July 1931): 20.

11. T. Gaines, "The President's Message," *J.M.A. Ala.* 1 (June 1932): 446.

12. Emmett B. Carmichael, Emeritus Professor of Biochemistry, TS, "The Alabama Journal of Medical Sciences," 22 October 1979.

Part III
The Regulation of the Medical Profession

Chapter 10

Irregular Practice of Medicine

In the pioneer territories of Alabama and Mississippi, conditions were not conducive to the traditional practice of medicine. Communications were poor or nonexistent. Roads were little more than trails and frequently impassable during winter and spring. The settlements were far apart, and physicians were usually unavailable to the rural areas. Family medical manuals found in surviving plantation libraries provide evidence that many lay people, including self-trained nurses, midwives, or trusted slaves, practiced medicine in nineteenth-century America. Self-medication was commonplace. Sometimes the advice of an Indian "herb doctor" was sought. Such conditions invited an invasion of irregular practitioners whose quackery and charlatanism went unchallenged for years.

Furthermore, the medicine practiced by regular physicians was often no more scientific than that of irregular practitioners. The "heroic" principles of treatment—well known to this day—consisted of bleeding, blistering, purging, and administering large doses of dangerous and ineffective drugs. These obviously met with little success in the day-to-day struggle against common complaints and failed utterly in such diseases as yellow fever, cholera, typhoid fever, malaria, and tuberculosis—the great killers in nineteenth-century America. The proliferation of proprietary or profit-oriented medical schools after 1820 and the strong competition among these schools rapidly made a farce of medical education. To add to the confusion, there were frequent and embarrassing exchanges among the profession's outstanding practitioners over a host of divisive issues, which ranged from rival medical practices and political differences to petty personal problems. The resultant loss of public confidence caused in part a major revolt against traditional medicine.[1]

Irregular practitioners had been part of American life from the earliest days, but sectarian medical systems that threatened traditional medicine did not appear until the early nineteenth century. The first half of the century saw Americans turn in varying degrees to several medical sectarian beliefs: Thomsonianism, eclecticism, homeopathy, hydropathy, and chrono-thermalism.[2]

Thomsonians or Steam Doctors

In early nineteenth-century Alabama, the Thomsonians, a sect founded by Samuel Thomson, appeared to be the most formidable threat to regular medicine. Thomson himself was a remarkable individual. Born in 1769 to a poor pioneer farm family in New Hampshire, he had little opportunity for formal education. He was lame and began his working life prosaically as custodian of the family livestock. His interest in the therapeutic properties of plants developed during his association with a female herb doctor whom he aided in gathering herbs. It was during this time that he was introduced to the plant, *Lobelia inflata* (campanulaceae), a powerful emetic that became the cornerstone of his future therapeutic regimen. He stated in the years following his discovery, that his herb extracts had saved the lives of members of his family after they had failed to respond to traditional methods of treatment; he was, therefore, convinced of his gift of healing.[3]

One writer has stated that "the Thomsonian theory of disease was not unlike that of Galen's humoral pathology of the second century A.D."[4] According to Thomson's explanations,

> all animal bodies are formed of four elements, earth, air, fire and water. Earth and water constitute the solids, and air and fire, or heat, are the cause of life and motion [while] cold, or lessening the power of heat, is the cause of all disease. [On the other hand,] a state of perfect health arises from a . . . balance . . . of the four elements.[5]

Thomson thought the loss of natural heat was caused by obstructions in the system and in the stomach in particular. The duty of the physician was simply to rid the body of these obstructions and restore the delicate balance of the four elements.[6]

At the outset of his practice, Thomson confidently proclaimed that lobelia was a cure-all and, indeed, the only medication anyone needed. When it failed to live up to this high claim, he unhesitatingly supplemented it with other botanic remedies as well as steam baths and enemas. A regular Thomsonian regimen was rigorous. For several days the patient was given oral doses of pennyroyal and cayenne pepper. When the patient was considered ready, the regimen began with a steam bath that continued until sweat "as thick as your finger" rolled off his body. A cold bath followed. The shivering victim was put to bed immediately with hot bricks "to bring back his heat." If the patient survived this ordeal of contrasts, a potent emetic was administered so that nothing would remain in the stomach. This emetic consisted of bayberry, cayenne pepper, and lobelia mixed with forty-proof brandy. The "victim" was then required to drink warm water until vomiting occurred. A second steam bath, followed by a cold bath, more hot bricks, and two enemas of pennyroyal, cayenne pepper, and lobelia had to be endured before the first day's treatment was completed.[7]

Thomson's practice flourished despite accusations of quackery by the regular medical profession. In the fall of 1809, he was accused and stood trial for having caused the death of a patient with his method of treatment, but was acquitted for lack of evidence. Still believing in the superiority of his "treatment regimen," and no doubt sensing that financial rewards might ensue, he was determined now to put himself above state laws governing the practice of medicine. National patent laws were lax in the early nineteenth century, and Thomson was able to obtain a patent on his system.[8]

Armed with his patent, Samuel Thomson launched an extensive campaign to advertise his method of therapy—now referred to as Thomsonianism—and to accrue a substantial profit in the process. He skillfully used all existing promotional techniques, including advertisements, agents, testimonials, and personal appearances. The goal of his campaign was to entice laymen into paying twenty dollars for the right to teach the Thomson system to prospective patients. Those who subscribed were familiarized with the principles of Thomsonianism and were organized into "Friendly Medical Botanic Societies" for the purpose of sharing information. They were forbidden to disclose the sect's secrets to nonsubscribers.[9]

By the 1830s, Thomson was claiming three million followers. Without a doubt, this was an exaggeration; however, between 1822 and 1839, his *New Guide to Health* went through thirteen editions and more than 100,000 copies were sold. This was an astonishing accomplishment when we consider that in 1839 the population of the United States was less than seventeen million and that a copy of Thomson's book cost twenty dollars. Undoubtedly, a very large percentage of the populace adhered to his doctrine of botanic medicine. In 1835, the governor of Mississippi stated that in his opinion half of the people in his state practiced Thomsonianism; and it was conceded in Ohio that one out of three used this regimen. It was also popular in Boston where it was estimated that by the late 1820s, one-sixth of the city's inhabitants were taking steam baths and lobelia.[10]

In the beginning, Thomsonianism had been popular in Massachusetts, New Hampshire, and Vermont. From there it spread first to New

York and then to the rest of the nation, finding special acceptance in the West and South. Thomson's son, Cyrus, carried his father's doctrines through western New York into Ohio and the West where its appeal was greatest. At the height of the movement, vast sections of New England, the South, and West had been won over to Thomsonianism. There were Thomsonian medical schools and infirmaries; botanic journals were published; and national conventions of delegates from the Friendly Medical Botanic Societies were held annually.[11]

The Reformed (Thomsonian) Medical College of Georgia was the first sectarian school in the South. Originally the college was to be located in Macon, the capital of Georgia. In 1839, Dr. Lanier Bankston, the Alva Curtis of the South,[12] obtained a state charter for the Southern Botanico-Medical College, which was opened in Forsyth, Georgia. This school was the first irregular medical college to attract funds from a state legislature. It received $5,000 in grants in 1842 and 1844. Dissension in the faculty led to the discharge of the dean, Dr. William Fonerden, a clergyman and a botanic doctor who spread Thomsonianism in the South. Dr. Bankston replaced him. In 1845, the college was moved to Macon. But shortly thereafter another schism occurred; and dissenting faculty members moved to Wetumpka, Alabama, where they joined the staff of the Alabama Medical Institute, which had received its state charter in 1844. The Alabama Medical Institute faculty then was composed largely of dissenters from the Forsyth school. The Wetumpka school closed in 1845 after only one session, and the seemingly itinerant faculty then moved to Memphis, Tennessee, and joined the staff of the newly chartered (1846) Botanico-Medical College of Memphis.[13]

The funds appropriated by the Georgia Assembly not only aided the school in Macon financially, but enhanced its prestige in the South before the Civil War. As a result of mounting sectional hostilities, Southerners began patronizing the Macon school in the 1850s, but its student population was never large.[14] In 1854, the school was renamed Reformed (Thomsonian) Medical College of Georgia. Although the Civil War caused its closure in 1861, it was revived in 1867 under the name of the College of American Medicine and Surgery. In 1881, it was removed to Atlanta and merged with the Georgia Eclectic Medical College and became the Georgia College of Eclectic Medicine and Surgery.[15]

The Thomsonians, quick to exploit the regular physicians' inability to effect cures, exaggerated claims of their own success. Indeed, they heralded Thomsonianism not only as a veritable cure-all but as a gift of God. The accuracy of these claims is questionable. Certainly the Thomsonian treatment was scarcely more humane than an ordeal of bloodletting and calomel.

Given the state of traditional medicine, the Thomsonians may have been as effective as the regular physicians. Moreover, their claims of cures must be taken in the context of the crude and semi-scientific state of medical science at the time. A favorite ploy of the Thomsonians and regular physicians alike was to diagnose a mild disease as a severe one, thus increasing their prestige when the disease remitted.[16]

In the end the regulars won, but only after a long, uphill fight. Although the Thomsonians were a formidable foe, their existence probably created a salutary demand for less drastic treatment. Unfortunately, the scarcity of sources precludes any in-depth portrayal of the extent of Thomsonian influence in Alabama medicine. It is only through its impact on the medical practice laws passed by the General Assembly that we can trace this influence.

The Alabama Medical Licensure Boards established under the "1823 Law" were particularly hostile to the irregular practitioners.[17] As a result of friction between the Thomsonians and the regular medical fraternity, the General Assembly amended this law in 1832, thereby permitting Thomsonians to practice and to collect pay without being licensed by the medical boards. The amendment said that if the Thomsonian practitioners bled, applied blisters, administered calomel or any of the mercurial preparations—antimony, arsenic, tartar emetic, opium or laudanum—they would be subject to the penalties of the law.[18]

Exceptions to legal restrictions obtained through special interest legislation were not uncommon. In 1847, a special act of the General Assembly granted Jesse Tyre of Walker County permission to practice botanic medicine without a license.[19] Legislative records reveal that exceptions of this sort were granted on other occasions.

Alabama's first published code of law became effective on February 5, 1852, and it reaffirmed the Medical Licensing Board and societies already established.[20] The new code, by merely stating that the section concerning "Physicians" did not apply to Thomsonians, left the latter without a license to practice. In effect, the new code implied that these practitioners were not physicians. As a result, at the next session of the General Assembly, the Thomsonians introduced a bill of their own drafting. It was passed and became effective on February 15, 1854.[21] This act provided for the creation of licensing boards in each county. These boards were to be composed of not less than three and not more than five Thomsonians or botanic doctors, and were to have power to examine and license applicants who wanted to practice the botanic system. The board members were to be selected by the judges of probate and commissioners of revenue in their respective counties.[22]

The Thomsonians in Alabama were thus independent of regular medicine and its restraints. They had a local organization and were recognized and governed by a law of their own. Yet, they failed to flourish in Alabama. The group appears to have reached the height of its popularity in 1856 when the General Assembly created a "Board of Botanic Physicians in the State of Alabama."[23] There is no record that the board ever functioned.

Thomsonian medicine persisted in one form or another for decades after 1865; and many Americans continued to dose themselves with herbal remedies and to consult herbal practitioners. These practitioners no longer cared to invoke the name of the unlettered Thomson and soon dropped the name Thomsonians, choosing instead to call themselves "Botanico-Medicals" or "Physico-Medicals." Some of these practitioners were self-taught; but many were graduates of the twenty-odd botanical schools that continued to function in the United States in the latter part of the nineteenth century. The medical historian Alexander Wilder estimated that at the turn of the century several thousand botanic, reformed physiopathic, and physio-medical doctors were still practicing in the United States. Interestingly enough, he stated that most of these were still treating patients much along the lines laid down by Samuel Thomson more than eighty years before.[24]

After 1900, the use of herbal medicines declined. Although they continued to compete with calomel, they were completely outclassed by newer treatments based on exciting discoveries in human physiology and the nature of disease. These discoveries ushered in a new era of medicine beginning with the chemotherapeutic agents of the 1930s.

Most botanic practitioners gradually disappeared from the American scene, but the idea persists among some Americans that simple herbal remedies are inherently superior to the powerful drugs prescribed by physicians today. This idea has been advanced in a book first published in 1939 and popular today entitled *Back to Eden; The Classic Guide to Herbal Medicine, Natural Foods and Home Remedies* (latest revision in 1972). The publisher, Woodbridge Press, Inc., describes the book as a "million-copy best seller." It is frequently displayed in health food stores. Its author, Jethro Kloss, has devoted a good deal of space to lobelia, describing it as "a most efficient relaxant, influencing mucous, serous, nervous, and muscular structures." He also recommends its use for treatment of "cough, bronchitis, asthma, whooping cough, pneumonia, hysteria, convulsions, suspended animation, tetanus, febrile trouble, etc."[25] Continuing, Kloss avows that "lobelia possesses most wonderful properties"; he argues, "[It] is a perfectly harmless relaxant. It loosens disease and opens the way for its elimination from the body. Its action is quick and more effective than radium." Nonpoisonous herbs like lobelia, Kloss concludes, will do everything that conventional physicians try to do

with "mercury, antitoxin, serums, vaccines, insulin, drug preparations."[26]

Botanic medicine is alive and doing well!

Homeopathic Medicine

In 1810, a German physician, Samuel Hahnemann, published the
Organon of the Homeopathic Art. This book stated that disease or symptoms
of disease could be cured by those particular drugs that produced
similar pathologic effects upon the body. Thus, he proclaimed the
doctrine (not a new one in the history of medicine) that "like cures like,"
meaning that drugs causing certain symptoms could cure disease which
exhibited those same symptoms. Hahnemann further asserted that the
way to achieve better results with similar diseases was to give minute or
diluted doses of a drug. These could be administered in such pleasant
forms as in water or sugar pills.

Hahnemann's theory found wide acceptance, especially in America
after the 1850s, when a popular revolt had begun against excessive
bleeding and purging. While the "allopaths" (regular physicians) did
violence to nature with their heroic doses, homeopaths sought only to
strengthen the natural tendency of the body to restore itself.

Homeopathy had little impact in Alabama. There is only one instance
in which homeopathy is mentioned in the acts of the Alabama General
Assembly; but unquestionably this type of medical practice occurred in
several sections of the state. On February 10, 1852, the General Assembly approved a charter of the Homeopathic Medical Society of Montgomery whose members consisted of Drs. G. A. Ulrich, John H. Henry,
Gustav Allbright, P. McIntyre, George Singer, Julien Sampson, a Dr.
Angle, and a Dr. Hunley.[27]

Wilder cites a lawsuit brought in 1889 against a homeopathic doctor
who had refused to undergo an examination by the Alabama State
Board of Medical Examiners. The Alabama Supreme Court ruled
unequivocally that he had violated no statute that would subject him to
criminal prosecution. Wilder also states, inaccurately, that this decision
put an end to further prosecution of recusant practitioners and to the
enforcing of licensure examination by the Board of Censors in Alabama.
The Medical Licensure Statute of 1877 required that no person be
permitted to practice any system of medicine without a certificate of
qualification in anatomy, physiology, chemistry, and the mechanics of
labor granted by the Board of Censors of the State Medical Association.[28]

A close relative of homeopathic medicine was that represented by the Eclectic Medical Association of Alabama. It had been organized in 1884 by Drs. J. W. Raleigh Williams of Opelika, R. J. Thornton, William H. Lamar, and others of like sentiment. The association, according to Wilder, proclaimed its hostility to "State Religion, State Medicine and a State Medical Priestcraft." After the enactment in 1877 of laws governing licensing of practitioners in Alabama, the Eclectic Association appointed a Central Protective Committee to test the validity of the provisions of the new laws, which they found obnoxious.[29] In 1892, the eclectic and homeopathic doctors of Alabama made an attempt to have the General Assembly radically change the regulatory statute itself. They wanted to secure protection from what they saw as invidious persecution, but this effort failed. There are no records of further activity by these irregular practitioners.

Osteopathy

The American School of Osteopathy was chartered in Kirksville, Missouri, on May 10, 1892. This school purported "to improve [the] system of surgery, midwifery, and treatment of general diseases [by] the adjustment of the bones." The founders of the school were Dr. Andrew Taylor Still and Dr. William Smith. Dr. Still, who supposedly had cured a case of "flux" in 1874 in this manner, founded a journal devoted to osteopathy. Reviewing the state records of Alabama, the osteopaths appear not to have been a threat to the regular practitioners of medicine. They were allowed to take the licensing examinations that had been set up by the State Medical Association in 1877. Although osteopathy changed very little for many years, during the last two decades the training of osteopathic physicians has moved more into the mainstream of regular medicine, and schools of osteopathy are subject to accreditation by the American Medical Association.[30]

Chiropractic Practice

The chiropractic or hand practice was originally described as a new science of healing by Dr. Daniel David Palmer of Davenport, Iowa, in 1895. Dr. Palmer gave his first treatment or adjustment in 1895. In 1900, he founded a school, named for himself, to teach this new method of treatment. The underlying philosophy is explained as being the same as that of osteopathy, except there is a wider range of possibilities for both operator and patient. The chiropractor uses one specific "movement" for each disease, while the osteopath employs many. Dr. Palmer stated that disease was caused by a mechanical obstruction of the natural functions. "The human mechanic can remove and adjust that cause by his knowledge of Anatomy and a highly-cultured sense of touch—accomplishing with the hands what the medical men could do with drugs and the scalpel." In order to obtain a license to practice in Alabama, it was necessary for chiropractors to fulfill the requirements established by the State Licensing Board for physicians set up by the State Medical Association in 1877. This licensing law effectively kept the number of chiropractors practicing in the state to a minimum.[31]

Medical Practice Act of 1959

As a result of a persistent and effective lobby by the chiropractic practitioners, the Alabama State Legislature passed the Medical Practice Act of 1959.[32] With this law, a State Board of Basic Science Examiners and a State Licensing Board of the Healing Arts were established. This statute changed the system of licensing that had been in effect since 1877 so that chiropractors could be examined by a council of their peers and licensed to practice in Alabama. (See Chapter 11, "Regulation of Medical Practice.")

Miscellany of Sure Cures

The newspapers of Alabama, particularly the rural weeklies and agricultural monthlies, carried numerous advertisements for a miscellany of "sure cures," patent medicines as well as irregular healers. Treatments for deafness, palsy, rheumatism, and various chronic diseases were expounded by highly touted itinerant lecturers. Cure of dropsy, leg sores, cancer, and consumption was freely promised. Many of these expositors touted remedies for all types of pulmonary diseases. Pills of pine gum rolled in clay were frequently a stock-in-trade as was a weak alcoholic solution of bitters. The more repulsive the taste, the more efficacious the remedy. One quack who extolled his own virtues acknowledged that "to feel pulses is smaller business than to feel purses."[33] Rabbits feet found a steady market in America, at prices ranging from a dime to five dollars. Charms, voodoo bags, and love potions brought in millions of dollars annually from residents of Alabama.

The practice of medicine was probably regulated more effectively from 1825 to 1860 than during the early years following the Civil War. The extensive poverty of the state during reconstruction aided the persistance of quackery. Irregular practitioners supplied a large part of the medical care in Alabama following the war. Among the most colorful of these doctors were the omnipresent "Indian Doctors" who frequently advertised with enticing testimonials and exaggerated claims for cures of illnesses ranging from "fits" to cancer. The name "Indian," which was applied to a host of patent medicines, gave those medicines sufficient mystery to render them desirable to the general public. Advertisements for highly touted patent medicines and nostrums of one sort or another were to be found in most types of news media well into the twentieth century.

Cures for venereal diseases were frequently advertised. The secrecy surrounding sex in the nineteenth century resulted in an almost hopeless position for victims of these diseases. Public censure and personal guilt made the victims afraid to consult their family physicians; they were drawn to the quacks who assured them that they could be cured in complete confidence and privacy. Frequently, a dispensary for the treatment of "private diseases" was advertised, where a cure could be accomplished without the use of mercury, exposure to friends, or hindrance from business. The advertisement would warn the public not to trust "mercurial physicians," whose remedies might "produce the most horrible deaths." This no doubt referred to treatment of syphilis with mercury salts. Indeed, there were claims that "clap" or gonorrhea, could be cured within 24 to 48 hours. A related, but equally hyperbolic, claim was that virility could be restored and, "weakness of the organs" could be cured.[34]

Rheumatism or arthritis has always been a fertile field for all types of quacks and nostrums. The continual pain from this disease and the empirical nature of some of its most popular remedies have nurtured the quack use of copper bracelets, buckeyes, and orange juice and cod liver oil.[35] Pain is unusually adept at sweeping aside intellectual defenses.

The Persistence of Quackery

Why is quackery more prevalent in medicine than in other areas of science? Probably it is due to the fact that the irregular practitioner imputes to himself cures that are frequently those of nature. Nature cannot build a bridge or road, but it can and often does cure diseases. Irregular practitioners have harvested countless testimonials from customers whose gratitude was misplaced. The quack not only lauds his own alleged miraculous cures but also criticizes reputable medicine. Here, too, he finds an eager hearing from some individuals.

There will always be believers in quackery but hopefully its zenith has passed.

> Ever stronger federal regulation, more rigorous state laws better enforced, education more appropriately aimed than in the past, an increasing

adequacy of sound medical care for a larger portion of the population, these forces might be expected eventually to reduce in some measure quackery's enormous toll in wasted dollars and frustrated hopes for health.[36]

Conclusion

This is not, nor could it be, the full story of irregular medical practice in Alabama. Such an account would be virtually impossible due to unavailability of necessary sources. Rather, this has been an attempt to use existing material to provide insights into the sect of Thomsonianism as well as other irregular practices at the state and local levels. Perhaps this chapter will direct researchers to other topics for a more complete understanding of the history of irregular practice of medicine in Alabama.

Notes

1. James O. Breeden, "Thomsonianism in Virginia," *Va. Mag. Hist. Biog.* 82 (April 1974): 150–80; H. B. Shafer, *The American Medical Profession, 1783 to 1850* (New York: Columbia University Press, 1936), cited in Breeden, p. 150; and Richard H. Shryock, *Medicine in America: Historical Essays* (Baltimore: The Johns Hopkins Press, 1966), pp. 49–70.

2. Richard H. Shryock, "Quackery and Sectarianism in American Medicine," *Scalpel* 19 (May 1949): 91–96, cited in Breeden, p. 150.

3. Samuel Thomson, *A Narrative of the Life and Medical Discoveries of Samuel Thomson* (Boston: E. G. House, 1822; reprint ed., New York: Arno Press & The New York Times, 1972), pp. 14–19.

4. Breeden, pp. 150–80.

5. Thomson, p. 43.

6. Ibid.

7. F. G. Halstead, "A First-Hand Account of a Treatment by Thomsonian Medicine in the 1830's," *Bull. Hist. Med.* 10 (1941): 681–82.

8. Thomson, pp. 95–104, 121–23.

9. Ibid., pp. 124–26, 145; Alex Berman, "The Thomsonian Movement and Its Relation to American Pharmacy and Medicine, Part I," *Bull. Hist. Med.* 25 (1951): 416–18; and J. H. Young, *The Toadstool Millionaires: A Social History of Patent Medicines in America Before Federal Regulation* (Princeton: Princeton University Press, 1961), pp. 51–52.

10. Spencer Klaw, "Belly-My-Grizzle," *Amer. Heritage* 28 (June 1977): 98.

11. J. F. Kett, *The Formation of the American Medical Profession: The Role of Institutions, 1780–1860* (New Haven: Yale University Press, 1968), p. 106; F. C. Waite, "Thomsonianism in Ohio," *Ohio State Archeological and Historical Quarterly* 49 (Oct.–Dec. 1940): 327, cited in Breeden, p. 154; and S. C. Gholson, "Quackery in Ohio—Medical Heresies," *Stethoscope* 2 (Oct. 1852): 546–49, cited in Breeden, p. 154. The *Southern Botanic Journal* was published in Charleston,

South Carolina, 1837–1839. After this time, it was moved to Augusta, Georgia. J. I. Waring, *A History of Medicine in South Carolina, 1825–1900* (Charleston: South Carolina Medical Association, 1967), pp. 109–10, 114.

12. Alva Curtis was a rebel from the traditional Thomsonian school. He migrated to Ohio where he had his greatest success combining Thomsonianism and traditional medicine in what became known as neo-Thomsonianism.

13. Alex Berman, "Neo-Thomsonianism in the United States," *J. Hist. Med. & Allied Sci.* 11 (1956): 139–40; and Alexander Wilder, *History of Medicine* (New Sharon, Maine: New England Eclectic Pub. Co., 1901), pp. 525–28. In 1841, botanic doctors from Georgia and Alabama held a convention in Columbus, Georgia. They organized the "Southern Botanico-Medical Society" whose purpose was to promote harmony and further the interest of the Southern Botanico-Medical College. Alexander Wilder, p. 526.

14. F. C. Waite, "American Sectarian Medical Colleges Before the Civil War," *Bull. Hist. Med.* 19 (1946): 153; and "Reform Medical College of Georgia, Macon, Ga., Catalogue of the Officers, Graduates and Students," *Southern Medical Reformer* 6 (April 1856): 1–7, and 7 (April 1857): 125–26, cited in Breeden, p. 173.

15. Wilder, pp. 527–28.

16. See Note No. 4.

17. Acts of Alabama, 22 December 1823, pp. 45–47; and William H. Brantley, Jr., "Alabama Doctor," *Ala. Lawyer* 6 (1945): 252. This was the first law enacted by the General Assembly regarding the practice of medicine in Alabama.

18. Brantley, p. 252.

19. Acts of Alabama, 4 March 1848, p. 394.

20. *Code of Alabama 1852*, title 13, chap. 2, sect. 971, "Physicians, Surgeons, and Dentists" (Montgomery: Brittan and DeWolf, State Printers, 1852), p. 233.

21. Acts of Alabama, 15 February 1854, pp. 58–59.

22. A charter for the "Blount County Medical Board of Botanic Physicians" was approved in 1860. It is of interest that for the first time the lawmakers used the word "medical" in reference to this group of practitioners. Acts of Alabama, 21 February 1860, pp. 450–51.

23. Acts of Alabama, 11 February 1856, pp. 72–73.

24. Klaw, p. 105.

25. Jethro Kloss, *Back to Eden*, 5th ed. (Santa Barbara, Calif.: Woodbridge Press Publishing Company, 1975), p. 271.

26. Ibid., p. 281.

27. Acts of Alabama, 10 February 1852, p. 259.

28. Acts of Alabama, 9 February 1877, pp. 80–82.

29. Wilder, pp. 752–53.

30. J. N. Kane, *Famous First Facts—A Record of First Happenings, Discoveries and Inventions in the United States*, 3rd ed. (n.p.: H. W. Wilson Co., 1964), pp. 371, 451.

31. Wilder, p. 882; and Kane, p. 157.

32. *Code of Alabama 1975*, vol. 18, title 34 (Professions and Businesses), chap. 24, "Physicians and Other Practitioners of Healing Arts," (Charlottesville, Va.:

Michie Company, Bobbs-Merrill Law Publishing, Law Publishers, 1977), pp. 474–540.

33. J. I. Waring, *A History of Medicine in South Carolina, 1825–1900* (Charleston: South Carolina Medical Association, 1967), pp. 115–16.

34. John Duffy, ed., *The Rudolph Matas History of Medicine in Louisiana* (Baton Rouge: Louisiana State University Press, 1962), 2: 40–42.

35. Dan Dale Alexander, *Arthritis and Common Sense*, 3rd ed. (Hartford, Conn.: Witkower Press Incorporated, 1954).

36. J. H. Young, *The Medical Messiahs* (Princeton: Princeton University Press, 1967), p. 433.

Chapter 11

Regulation of Medical Practice

The "1823 Law"

Alabama was made a part of the Union in 1819. The state was open to anyone who wanted to practice medicine and surgery, regardless of education, training, or experience. In as much as there were no laws regulating the practice of medicine, quacks, charlatans, and impostors were everywhere. Because of this unrestrained "irregular" practice of medicine it is understandable that the first demand for laws to regulate the practice of medicine came early and directly from the people.

During the first session of the Territorial Assembly of Alabama in February, 1818, at St. Stephens (Alabama's first capital), the heroic scout, soldier and Indian fighter Sam Dale, as representative from Monroe County, petitioned the legislature to establish a board of physicians to examine and license applicants to practice medicine in that county.[1] He hoped that a strong licensure act would cause the irregular physicians to close shop and leave. Apparently, nothing resulted from this early petition.

In a new country with poor transportation and communication, members of the medical profession were less inclined to emigrate than individuals engaged in farming or business. However, some physicians did come. Among Alabama's pioneer physicians were those educated in Eastern schools. A few of these had training in the great medical centers in Europe. The first governor of Alabama, William Wyatt Bibb (1781–1820; governor of Alabama, 1819–1820), was a physician. Although he never practiced medicine in Alabama, his qualifications for the times were among the best in the area.

Among early leaders in the profession of medicine in the state was Dr. Henry Chambers (1790–1826) of Madison County. In addition to being an able physician, he was also a member of the 1819 State Constitutional Convention and a member of the Alabama House of Representatives. He was later elected United States Senator from Alabama, only to die on

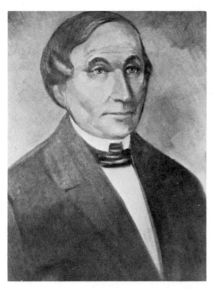 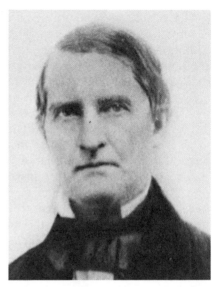

John Watkins, M.D., 1793–1853
(Courtesy of the Alabama State Department of Archives and History)

Henry Chambers, M.D., 1790–1826
(Courtesy of the Alabama State Department of Archives and History)

his way to Washington, D.C., where he was to have been sworn into
office.[2]

Other prominent physicians who settled in the state, contemporaries
of Dr. Chambers, were: Dr. Thomas Fearn, also of Madison County; Dr.
Clement Billingslea of Montgomery County; Drs. Richard Inge and
Robert L. Kennon of Tuscaloosa County.[3] These physicians had considerable influence upon political development in the new state. It was
fortunate that men of such stature in the field of medicine were also
mindful of the public welfare. Probably because of the interest of these
pioneer physicians, the urgent need for early regulation of medical
practice was brought to the attention of the lawmakers.

The result was a law passed December 22, 1823, "To regulate the licensing of Physicians to practice."[4] It forbade practicing medicine without a license and provided for medical boards in the five leading communities of the state at that time—Huntsville, Tuscaloosa, Cahaba, Claiborne, and Mobile. Cahaba had been the capital of Alabama, but after the removal of the state capital to Tuscaloosa in 1826, Cahaba's medical board was moved to Selma.

This first statute for regulating the practice of medicine was referred to as the "1823 Law." It was in this act that the seeds of control of medical licensure and regulations pertaining to health were planted in Alabama law. This basic law placed in the hands of physicians control over their profession in their respective communities. Certainly, these were the men best qualified to judge the ability of an applicant to practice medicine; and this fact was early recognized by authorities in the new state. It is this principle that has been the bedrock of legal regulations of the medical profession in the state of Alabama for over 150 years. Indeed, it has met and survived every challenge presented. Chief provisions of the "1823 Law" were:

1. No person shall be allowed to practice physic or surgery for fee or reward unless he shall be licensed to do so.
2. That all charges made to any person not licensed for services rendered as a physician or surgeon for cure of diseases shall be null and void.
3. That there shall be five boards of physicians, to consist of three members each, to be elected by joint vote of both houses of the General Assembly; which boards shall meet annually for the purpose of examining all applicants for license to practice medicine.
4. These boards shall receive five dollars for every examination and five dollars for each license.
5. This money shall be applied to the purchase of a medical library for the use of the board.[5]

To implement the "1823 Law," the General Assembly met in joint session on Christmas Eve, 1823. The voting was held in the hall of the House of Representatives at seven o'clock, in the town of Cahaba. The room was lit by candles, and in the large open fireplace at the end of the hall, a bright fire from fat pine kindling kept off the chill of evening. The only business of this session was the election of members for the newly established medical boards, as authorized in the law passed two days before. Any vacancies were to be filled by an election by remaining members of the board in which the vacancy occurred. It was recognized that it was of utmost importance that responsible men be chosen as members of the first boards regulating medical practice. Despite the late hour, the time of year, and no doubt the love of conviviality and hard liquor by the pioneer Alabama representatives, when the General Assembly was called to order, the members promptly left their comfortable positions by the fireplace and sixty-nine answered roll call. They were there to do their best for the people and for the profession of medicine in Alabama.

Medical boards were elected for Huntsville, Cahaba, Claiborne, Tuscaloosa, and Mobile. Henceforth, the destiny of the medical profession in Alabama was to be guided by the physicians of the state; and Alabama physicians proved themselves equal to the challenge. Later, as the population of the state increased, additional boards were created, such as those for Montgomery and Demopolis in 1835, Livingston in 1836, and Talladega in 1845.[6] The General Assembly elected the first members of each board, and that board then became self-perpetuating.

In 1845, the duty of the Talladega Medical Board was to examine all applicants who did not hold a diploma from a regular medical college and to grant them a license to practice if found qualified. Another of the board's duties was to examine for fitness and ability all persons who applied for road duty, military duty, or patrol duty and to make judgments in cases of insanity. Drs. James C. Knox, Henry McKenzie, William Sommers, Edward Adolphus Pearson, Abner Faut, and Benton W. Groce served on this examining board.

The plan set out in the "1823 Law" was a bold one, but from the beginning it faced a number of insurmountable problems. Frontier conditions made policing the profession extremely difficult, and attempts at enforcing the law were feeble.[7] It was not until 1889 that an illegal practice case reached the Alabama Supreme Court.

Amendments and exceptions directed by the legislature also weakened the law. The original act exempted all those already practicing in the state before 1823, those who had practiced in another state for two years, and all the graduates of "regular" medical colleges. Some of these exemptions were at best a dubious proof of competency. There was also a tendency to pass special acts exempting specified individuals from provisions of the law. Particularly damaging was an amendment passed in 1832, exempting practitioners of the "botanical system of Dr. Samuel Thomson," provided they did not "bleed, apply a blister of Spanish flies, administer calomel . . . opium or laudanum."[8]

The board examinations at times seemed to have been rudimentary, if one can judge from the following spoof on medical examinations published in a Cahaba newspaper in 1853.

Professor of Anatomy—How many bones are there in the human body?

Student—That depends upon what one has for dinner. In hard times there are generally more or less.

Professor—Where is the heart situated?

Student—Commonly in the left side of the thorax; but the majority of the students lose theirs altogether before they leave college.

Professor—Where are the carotid arteries?

Student—They arise on each side of the neck, and pass up as high as the shirt collar, then down the insenate [sic] canal, and terminate in both boots.

Professor of Chemistry—Of what is the atmosphere composed?

Student—Oxygen, nitrogen, and four other gases; depending somewhat upon the inhabitants and the filth of the street.

Professor—Give an example of the non-electrics.

Student—[Resin], feathers, hoops, old bachelors, and lightning rods.

Professor of Materia Medica—Name some of the emetic agents.

Student—[Ipecac], warm water, too much liquor and sea-sickness.

Professor—What is considered the maximum dose of opium?

Student—One drop of the millionth dilution of one-half of the smallest possible quantity is a powerful dose for a homeopathic; but we have been advised to give it as long as the patient can swallow and repeat the dose.

Professor of Surgery—How would you distinguish a dislocation from a sprain?

Student—The safest way is to twist the injured limb until we are sure it is dislocated, then set it. All concerned are better satisfied.

Professor—What is the treatment for enlargement of the tonsils?

Student—That must depend upon circumstances. If I had a tonsil instrument I should remove them, but otherwise treat them rationally.

Professor of Theory and Practice—Give us the best treatment for intermittent fever.

Student—Give quinine until the patient is blind, and then send him to an eye surgeon.

Professor—Would not the warm bath be good in connection with the quinine?

Student—Certainly, and the warmer the better.

Professor—How long would you keep the patient in it?

Student—Until the skin slips, and then sweat him off with hot stuff.

Professor of Obstetrics—Have you any experience in the lying [in] department?

Student—Certainly, sir; I was noted for—*lying* in our town, and came near being laid for it.

The student was allowed a license.[9]

Under these circumstances, it is not surprising that at least one board, the one in Mobile, ceased to exist through neglect and had to be reinstituted.

In 1849, an American Medical Association (AMA) report claimed that Alabama's licensure act had been repealed.[10] This report was vigorously denied by the Alabama delegates to the AMA but there was certainly an element of truth in the report.

In 1850, the State Medical Association directed a county survey of licensed doctors in the state. A published account of the census is given below.[11]

Dallas County	
Having diplomas	36
Licentiates	2
[Thomsonians]	4
Clairvoyant	1
Bibb County	
Having diplomas	4
Licentiates	7
[Thomsonians]	2
Botanico-Eclectic	1
Mobile County	
Regular Practitioners	40
Homeopathists & Hydropathists	2
Root Doctors & [Thomsonians]	3
General Quackery	3
Idio-Eclectopathist	1
Clarke County	
Having diplomas	8
Licenses	8
[Thomsonians]	2
Monroe County	
Having diplomas	7
Licenses	7
[Thomsonians]	3

Baldwin County
 Having diplomas   4
 Licenses   1
 [Thomsonians]   0
Washington County
 Having diplomas   4
 Licenses   0
 [Thomsonians]   1
Perry County
 Having diplomas   27
 [Thomsonians]   4
 Special license   2
Wilcox County
 Having diplomas   23
 Uncertain   5
 Licentiates   1
 [Thomsonians]   1

The local examination boards created by the "1823 Law" continued to function throughout the years prior to and during the Civil War up until the passage of the Licensure Law of 1877.

The State Licensure Law of 1877

In 1873, Dr. Jerome Cochran's plan for organization of the State Medical Association was accepted by the members at an annual meeting in Tuscaloosa.[12] Cochran's constitution, which governed the State Association, stipulated that an executive committee of ten censors (a committee of five from 1873 to 1877) would exercise the principal executive, legislative, and judicial powers of the Association. It was officially known as the Board of Censors. The constitutional provisions for the organization of the county medical societies, which received their charters from the State Association, were similar to those of the State Association regarding the executive committee or Board of Censors. The organizational arrangement approved by the General Assembly in 1875 provided a framework for the new Medical Practice Act of 1877.

The law of 1877 set aside the previously existing local examining boards and established the Medical Association of the State of Alabama as the body responsible for setting the standards and qualifications required of persons desiring to practice medicine in the state. It also established the Board of Censors of the State Medical Society as the duly authorized Board of Medical Examiners. Although the Board of Censors of the state society serving as the State Board of Medical Examiners had the ultimate responsibility for issuing certificates to practice medicine, each county Board of Censors established its own examination, and the license it issued as a result of the exam was valid throughout the state.[13]

There was agitation around the turn of the century to remove licensing of physicians from the county Board of Censors and to substitute a standard examination given at the state level. Thus, in 1907, the Medical Practice Act was amended in such a way as to require all examinations for certification of qualifications to treat diseases of human beings to be held in Montgomery. This eliminated the county Board of Censors as the primary licensing body and standardized the examination for practitioners throughout the state. Thus, the Board of Censors of the State Medical Association served as the State Board of Medical Examiners with the chairman of the Board of Censors also serving as head of the Board of Medical Examiners.

This individual also served as state health officer under the Cochran devised plan of 1875 where the Medical Association of the State of Alabama served as the State Health Department. Thus, this one individual, elected by a single majority vote of the Medical Association, became the most powerful member of the medical community serving in the triple capacity of state health officer, chairman of the State Board of Censors and chairman of the Board of Medical Examiners. This situation existed with one exception until the death of Dr. D. G. Gill (state health officer).

When Dr. Baker was elected state health officer on April 18, 1930, he preferred to devote his time exclusively to administering the health department and was not elected chairman of the State Board of Medical Examiners or of the State Board of Censors.

When Dr. Ira Myers became state health officer in 1963, the duties of the Board of Medical Examiners were removed from the State Board of Health and rested in a separate board. By separating the position of state health officer from that of executive head of the medical examination boards, a very significant precedent was established. The head of the Department of Health was relieved from many duties, and many of his great powers were withdrawn. No longer the most powerful figure in the medical organization, the state health officer became the principal agent of the State Board of Health.

State Licensure Laws

In 1959, the Alabama Legislature passed a law revising the licensing procedures for all aspiring practitioners of the healing arts in the state.[14] The law established a basic science examination and a State Licensing Board of the Healing Arts. Thus, medical and chiropractic applicants were placed on the same footing: all had to pass the State Basic Science Examination. Those successful were then certified to their individual licensing boards. The chiropractic applicants were examined by a State Board of Chiropractic Practitioners and medical applicants by the Alabama Board of Medical Examiners.

The law for licensing was revised for United States, Canadian, and foreign medical graduates in 1975. To be licensed, a physician must have a year's AMA internship and be licensed in a state other than Florida by written examination, or be a diplomate of National Boards. To be licensed in Alabama, this written examination is either the State Board Examination, or the Flex examination given in Atlanta, or all three parts of the National Board of Medical Examiners examination. Osteopaths may be licensed under the same law by serving a year's internship and by taking the State Board Examination, or the Flex, or by passing an examination given by the National Board of Osteopathic Physicians and Surgeons. The Alabama Board of Medical Examiners then issues a certificate of qualification to the Healing Arts Board, which then issues the license.

Thus, the successful applicant, whether a chiropractor, osteopath, or physician, is licensed by the same State Board of Healing Arts. These licensing procedures instituted in Alabama have effectively given physicians some control over their profession, and have given medicine in Alabama the strength it requires to play a role in national and world medicine.

Notes

1. William H. Brantley, Jr., "Alabama Doctor," *Ala. Lawyer* 6 (1945): 248–49.

2. Of the forty-four delegates to the Alabama Constitutional Convention that met in Huntsville on July 5, 1819, there were four physicians: Dr. Henry Chambers of Huntsville, Madison County; Dr. George Phillips of Shelby County; Dr. John L. Tindall of Tuscaloosa County; and Dr. John Watkins of Burnt Corn, Monroe County. Drs. Chambers, Watkins, and Phillips were on the committee of fifteen elected by the Convention to draft the State Constitution. M. C. McMillan, *Constitutional Development in Alabama, 1798–1901: A Study in Politics, the Negro, and Sectionalism* (Chapel Hill: University of North Carolina Press, 1955), p. 34.

3. Brantley, p. 249.

4. Ibid., pp. 249–52.

5. Howard L. Holley, "Medical Education in Alabama," *Ala. Rev.* 7 (1954): 246. It was hoped that the resulting medical library would be of assistance to members of the profession in improving their knowledge by further study.

6. D. L. Cannon, "Alabama's Eighty-Nine Years of Medical Organization, A Brief History of the Association, Part 1," *J.M.A. Ala.* 5 (1936): 314.

7. Brantley, p. 270.

8. Cannon, p. 314.

9. "A Medical Examination," *Dallas Gazette*, 30 September 1859, p. 1, col. 5.

10. "The Legal Requirements Exacted of Medical Practitioners in the Several States of the Union (and in other Countries)," *Trans. Amer. Med. Assoc.* 2 (1849): 330.

11. J. C. Marks, "Report on the Number, Character, etc., of Practitioners of Medicine in Dallas County," *Trans.* (1854), pp. 147–48; J. W. Crawford, "A Report on the Number and Character of Physicians of Bibb County," *Trans.* (1854), p. 148; and "Report on the Number, Character, etc., of Practitioners of Medicine," *Trans.* (1852), pp. 163–66.

12. D. L. Cannon, "Alabama's Eighty-Nine Years of Medical Organization, A Brief History of the Association, Part 2," *J.M.A. Ala.* 5 (1936): 348.

13. Acts of Alabama, 9 February 1877, pp. 80–82.

14. *Code of Alabama 1975*, vol. 18, title 34 (Professions and Businesses), chap. 24, "Physicians and Other Practitioners of Healing Arts," (Charlottesville, Va.: Michie Co., Bobbs-Merrill Law Publishing, Law Publishers, 1977), pp. 474–540.

Part IV
The Development of the Various Health Fields

Chapter 12

The Development of Public Health in Alabama

From the beginning, there existed in Alabama a tradition of governmental involvement in the health field. In part, this tradition was inherited from the European paternalistic attitudes of various colonial governments in the territory that later became Alabama. But it was also due to encouragement by the more responsible individuals within the medical profession who saw state and local governments, with their fiscal and coercive powers, as allies in the fight against disease, inadequate medical care, and poorly trained medical practitioners.

Colonial Origins

In an attempt to reduce the number of inadequately trained practitioners, the French colonial council in the 1720s decreed that all physicans must pass an examination to be licensed to practice medicine.[1] In addition, at least one member of the French Superior Council acted as supervisor of government hospitals in the colony of Louisiana.[2]

Insofar as public health activities were concerned, the most advanced were instituted after the British acquired Mobile and the surrounding territory in 1763. Under the direction of General Frederick Haldimand, British commander of the Mobile Colony, the swamps around Pensacola were drained and the fort (probably Fort Barrancas) was rebuilt, making it a much healthier place in which to live. Similar steps were proposed for Mobile: in 1767, Dr. John Lorimer was sent to study health conditions there and to make suggestions for improvement. After a six-month study, he recommended that the trees close to Fort Charlotte (formerly Fort Condé, circa 1763) be removed so the marshes could dry out; the area surrounding the fort be leveled to prevent water from stagnating; an additional story be added to one-story barracks to increase ventilation; and a creek be diverted through the town to make a clean supply of water available at all times.[3]

Due to the withdrawal of the British forces (1783), this plan was never executed; but the tradition of governmental interest in public health was continued by the newly created territorial government of the United States. The territorial governor was empowered to enforce health laws and to authorize county and town officials to deal locally with health problems. A law passed in 1798 empowered the governor of the Mississippi Territory to take any measures necessary to prevent the spread of contagious diseases.[4] The law was invoked on at least one occasion during a smallpox epidemic in Natchez in 1802.[5] Alabama, once it had become a separate territory (1817), continued to enforce these measures. In addition, there was also "An Act to promote Health by preventing the Sale of Unwholesome Liquors and Provisions," although it was probably poorly enforced.[6] According to C. V. Stabler in his thesis, "The History of the Alabama Public Health System," these laws were later incorporated in the first Alabama Code.[7] Thus, a base for public health legislation had been established by the authorities of the Mississippi Territory from which Alabama was formed.

Preventive Medicine from 1820 to 1875

A state system of public health could not be realized until the medical profession discarded the idea of a single cause for all infectious disease, recognized the germ theory, and understood that epidemic diseases could be transported from one locality to another. It was difficult for people to accept the idea that all physical suffering was not a result of God's will, in which instance no amount of precaution could prevent a city or its citizens from a preordained attack.

Prior to 1850, only a small number of Alabama physicians accepted the more advanced ideas about the cause and spread of disease. One of these was Dr. Josiah Clark Nott. Dr. Nott, a native of South Carolina, graduated from South Carolina College in 1824 with an A.B. degree. In 1825–26, he attended a course of lectures at the College of Physicians and Surgeons, New York and in 1827, he graduated from the University of Pennsylvania with an M.D. degree. From 1829 to 1834, Dr. Nott practiced in Columbia, South Carolina. The following year he went to Europe to study medicine and natural history. Dr. Nott considered medicine to be his professional interest and natural history his hobby. He gave his remarkable intellect to both medicine and natural history; and by so doing, left them much further advanced than he had found them. In 1836, Dr. Nott returned from Europe and moved to Mobile where he entered the practice of surgery. He lived in Mobile until 1861, with the exception of one year when he was a member of the medical faculty of the University of Louisiana. In 1861, he joined the Confederate States Army.[8]

Dr. Nott was never physically strong, and the effect of his Civil War experiences seriously impaired his health, forcing him into early retirement. For a time he lived in New York City, but because he believed the Gulf Coast's environment to be healthy, he returned to his home in Mobile.[9]

Dr. Nott postulated three important factors concerning disease: (1) diseases could be imported; (2) many were transmissible; and (3) they could be caused by germs. He believed that yellow fever and malaria were *sui generis* diseases, but he was, apparently, the only Alabama physician before 1850 who subscribed to the theory of insects as a vector. In the 1840s, most medical men refused to accept the idea of importation, the germ theory, or even a specific cause of disease. The theory of insects as a vector was thought to be "utterly fantastic."[10] Dr. Nott's scientific knowledge and his common sense approach helped lay a firm foundation for public confidence in the medical profession, a confidence that later helped establish a viable public health system.

Dr. Nott was a regular contributor to the professional journals, and his most original writing and logical thinking was on the subject of the cause and transmission of disease. In 1848, Dr. Nott published an article on the insect theory, which he believed best explained the cause of yellow fever and other diseases. The physicians of the state were soon to debate these theories and eventually to agree upon them.[11]

Believing that various types of fevers could be attributed to various causes, Dr. Nott stated:

> [Identity for all malarias appear incorrect to me] . . . I am by no means sure that all these types may not be most rationally explained by attributing them to various insect species, . . . it would be a strange anomaly in nature, should it be proven that but one morbific cause of fever is generated over the broad surface of our variously compounded globe . . . the difficulty will probably be found to be in false 'hypothesis' and not in false facts. May not these contradictions be more rationally reconciled by *supposing a plurality of morbific causes to exist?*[12]

Dr. Nott argued further that the insect theory was as applicable to periodic malarial fever as it was to yellow fever. After he had reviewed many leading bacterial experiments, he reached the conclusion that each disease had a specific cause. Therefore, he could find no reason why a specific remedy could not be found for yellow fever as well as for other diseases.[13]

It was Dr. Nott's opinion that disease could be transportable as a germ and at the same time not be contagious. He further theorized that a disease could spread as though it were contagious without being contagious, insisting that there were a thousand instances of ships going up the Alabama River that carried yellow fever without spreading the disease.

> I am equally strong in the opinion that there exists no conclusive evidence, that the *germ or malaria morbific* may not be transported from one locality to another . . . no reasonable man, in the present state of facts, can assert positively that yellow fever may not under peculiar circumstances be transported. . . . I have no idea that the gaseous emanations from . . . vegetables or animal substances could produce yellow fever.[14]

Having destroyed the accepted theory of the cause of disease, Dr. Nott proceeded to construct a tenable one. The insect, in his opinion, was the only explanation of the manner in which yellow fever and malaria spread. Dr. Nott had formulated a clear concept of the insect as an intermediate host.

Dr. Jerome Cochran, also from Mobile, is known as the "Father of the Alabama Public Health System." He, like Dr. Nott, held similar opinions in the 1860s on the etiology of disease. Dr. Cochran's pursuit of knowledge was remarkable, and early in his career he became widely recognized as a scholar.[15] He served on the faculty of the Medical College in Mobile.

Dr. Cochran also expressed his views regarding the spread of communicable disease, especially malaria and yellow fever. In 1869, he outlined the three main contemporary schools of thought concerning the source of infectious disease: (1) the school that thought that factors causing diseases were offsprings of climatic agencies such as heat, humidity, and vegetable decomposition; (2) the school that admitted that malaria was not caused by the same type of poison as yellow fever but argued that malaria was the result of climatic conditions; and (3) the school that endorsed the germ theory of communicable diseases. Dr. Cochran supported the latter theory.[16]

Considering malarial fever to be a specific disease that would yield to the wise application of known preventive measures, Dr. Cochran concluded that:

> the generation of malaria is entirely independent of vegetation and its decay. If we were to go to work and remove all vegetation from our malaria districts, our sanitary improvements would certainly result in woeful disappointment. We know that it is only when water is confined, imprisoned, held in bondage, that it gives birth to any such malignant offspring. It may be carried by the wind, but usually not more than a few miles.[17]

Concerning the relationship between yellow fever and malaria, he emphasized:

> Yellow fever is a special infectious disease, propagated by a . . . poison composed of organic material particles which live and grow . . ., and which can be transplanted . . . from place to place. Yellow fever poison is not indigenous to the soil of Alabama. . . . Whether sporadic or epidemic in form, it is always due to importations from abroad of the specific disease germs which are necessary to its production. . . . It has no relation whatsoever with malaria which is endemic.[18]

Opponents of his ideas had demonstrated that diseases could be transmitted although no contact whatsoever had occurred between the infected patients and the individuals developing the disease. Dr. Cochran termed this "aerial propagation" and described it as another method of spreading disease. He admitted, however, that knowledge concerning this was lacking. He was firm in his belief that diseases were invariably spread by organic germs.[19]

Dr. Cochran was a member of the committee that created the American Public Health Association. The purpose was to promote public health interest in the nation. In 1879, at the seventh annual meeting of the American Public Health Association, Dr. Cochran was asked to discuss a series of papers that were read on yellow fever. During his discussion, he summarized his ideas on the etiology of this disease. His uncomplimentary remarks included the following:

> I must be allowed to express my surprise at the character—crude, undigested, and often antiquated and exploded—of the doctrines that have been maintained by a majority of those who have spoken upon this question. While we have still much to learn as to the natural history of yellow fever, I am obliged to hold that there are some things about it that are already positively known. Amongst these I think that we may claim to know—1), That yellow fever is a specific disease, caused by a specific poison. 2), That this poison is material, and therefore may be transported from place to place. 3), That this poison is not akin to our ordinary marsh malaria. 4), That this poison is not in any way the product of ordinary filth, and has no necessary association with filth as such. 5), That when the yellow fever poison is brought into a healthy community it sometimes gives rise to an epidemic, and sometimes, for reasons of which we have no knowledge, fails to do so. 6), That the only prophylactic that can be depended on is nonintercourse with infected persons, infected places, and infected things.[20]

Early Measures to Control Infectious Diseases

Yellow Fever

The spread of yellow fever was largely controlled by quarantine. Mobile constantly maintained maritime quarantine in order to prevent yellow fever from being brought into the harbor by ships' crews. This procedure was effective, but it was found to be unnecessarily rigid.

During the 1870s, Dr. Jerome Cochran, who served as quarantine officer of Mobile, was able to reform the quarantine system at the Port of Mobile. There were many who believed in "foamites" through which diseases were supposed to be transmitted by cargo and personal articles. Dr. Cochran disproved the doctrine of foamites, and was then able to place restrictions on the crew itself. Commerce was allowed to continue, and tropical products were traded year-round.[21] His drastic reforms benefited and encouraged commerce without increasing the danger to Mobile's citizens.

Once yellow fever had penetrated the barriers at seaports and appeared inland, a number of measures were taken to prevent its spread. This plan of control usually included commercial nonintercourse and isolation and disinfection of patients.

As soon as the presence of yellow fever was officially recognized in the city, a feeling of panic spread over the population. Everyone who could leave the city did so, even if they only camped near the outskirts of town. These camps were poorly constructed, and the refugees were exposed to all the elements as well as to poor sanitation. Frequently, the fugitive sick only spread the epidemic faster and farther. The railroad station was piled high with the baggage of fleeing citizens; and every train leaving the city was packed to standing room only. The paramount purpose was to get away from the peril, and, indeed, there was need for haste if they were to escape at all. It was general knowledge that, as soon as the city officially acknowledged the presence of yellow fever, every town or hamlet along the lines of the railroads would establish a strict quarantine; and no train would be allowed to stop there. Lines of quarantine were drawn with the greatest severity. No train leaving Mobile was allowed to go more than ten or twelve miles before it was stopped and its passengers required to get off and undergo medical examination. If found physically well, they were required to walk to another train standing some distance down the track. Nothing but handbags could be carried, and most of the time these were fumigated. Frequently, two such changes in trains had to be made between Mobile and Montgomery or Mobile and Meridian.[22]

A quarantine was invoked both by land and sea. The embargo resulted in a cessation of trade and commerce. On all the highways leading out of Mobile, a shotgun quarantine was quickly invoked and strictly enforced.[23] Mail and express matter were fumigated, and letters postmarked from Mobile to other places were perforated and disinfected before leaving Mobile. These stringent measures added to the suffering of the inhabitants of the stricken city.

One story, revealing the general terror and desperate attempt to escape, has survived:

> It was a special train of refugees, made up at Mobile and booked over the Louisville and Nashville, straight through to the high grounds [presumably North Alabama], without a stop; but the train did stop at Montgomery, for the engines had to be changed. Long before that city was reached the drinking water had given out, and one can imagine what it was [like] in the crowded train, with all the windows closed, and the September sun shining on it the livelong day. At Montgomery, a desperate passenger took a desperate step. He opened the window on the far side of the car and bribed a guard in the station to bring him a bucket of water. The feat was performed; the water was brought, and the passenger was just lifting it through the window when a supervisor caught sight of the commission of the crime. Not only had a window been opened at Montgomery, thus permitting the fever bugs to jump out upon the defenseless inhabitants, but actually a bucket of water was being introduced through the opening. It might have taxed the ingenuity of the supervisor to say what harm the going in of the water would do, after the window had been opened, but he took no broad view of the situation. He commanded in a tremendous voice the water be handed out again, and spread on the ground; which was done. The window was caused to be closed, and the train pursued its journey, with its load of thirsty, waterless passengers.

> . . . what happened when any passenger showed signs of illness [was another tragedy of the journey]. It did not matter what the illness was. All sudden sickness was classed as yellow fever, and so, the ill person, for the safety of the well and to assure the further progress of the train, had to disembark, and on the spot, it might be in the woods, and generally was; and the sick [individual] was [left there] to his or her own devices; and also to the mercy of the [elements and] the inhabitants, who regarded a sick person from the [stricken] city as worse than a mad dog. Each settlement held the sick at gunshot distance and the order was: "Move on!" The rest of the story needs no detailing.[24]

Malaria

Malaria was the most widespread and fatal of the diseases occurring in early Alabama.[25] Dr. Jabez W. Heustis of Mobile, writing about malarial fevers in the early 1820s, stated:

> In 1821, '22, '23 many flourishing towns upon the rivers, which had risen up, as it were, by the hand of enchantment, received a sudden check, and became suddenly almost totally abandoned, from death and desertion. . . . There were [no] well persons to attend the sick and dying. It was my greatest experience of calamity.[26]

Dr. Benjamin Franklin Riley, Jr. (1879–1958), another practicing physician in the state, wrote of the panic that resulted from the widespread bilious and malarial fever in early Conecuh County.[27] The deaths caused by malarial fever during the summer seasons reached as high as 12 percent of some towns' populations.

Malaria reached epidemic proportions in some areas in Alabama almost every year and was present in varying degrees during every month of the year.[28] This disease was widely disseminated after 1820 in Alabama. Dr. P. H. Lewis, an early medical historian, wrote concerning congestive malarial fever:

> To ascertain that malady, which, from its malignancy, constitutes the outlet of human life in this section during summer and autumn . . . that malady which most excites the fears of the people, and absorbs the attraction of the medical man, it is only necessary to be brought to the bed-side of one laboring under congestive fever, and the search is at an end.[29]

The following statement described the situation as seen by members of the medical profession:

> Malarious affections constitute, undoubtedly and preeminently, the most familiarly-known. . ., of the endemic diseases. . . . Intermittents and remittents of every known type and intensity, and with almost every imaginable mask and complication, may be found somewhere within the county [or state], in almost every sickly season.[30]

Even though the leading physicians did not know the specific manner of transmission of malaria, they could predict where and when it would spread, the places that should be avoided, and the limit and extent of the infectious regions. A number of speakers at the annual sessions of the Alabama Medical Association from 1847 to 1855 advocated draining swamps and ponds for prevention of disease, especially yellow fever and malaria.[31] A committee was formed to address the planters of the state to inform them of the dire need for a proper drainage system.[32] (See Chapter 5, "Medical Practice After the Civil War.")

Dr. Nott observed that if good drainage systems were implemented, large portions of cottonlands could be freed from malaria, and therefore the proportion of the land unsuited to white habitation and labor would become minimal. Farmers, as well as inhabitants of cities and towns, were persuaded to spend relatively large sums of money and labor in instituting proper drainage of their land. The medical profession argued that as drainage improved, disease would decrease, transforming an unhealthy place into a veritable "health resort," and preventing practically all diseases.[33]

By 1850, only a few physicians of the state would have disagreed with the observation of Dr. G. A. Ketchum of Mobile: "The first and most important step would be a perfect system of sewage and drainage . . . underground or covered and daily flushed. . . . Sanitary [measures are] the path pointed out by experience and by all sound reasoning."[34] (For further preventive measures see Chapter 5, "Medical Practice After the Civil War.")

Smallpox

The measures to prevent and control smallpox, such as vaccination and isolation, were used in the early nineteenth century, but their enforcement required organization.

In 1862, an act of the General Assembly permitted the governor to appoint, and the state to pay, an agent to store sufficient amounts of smallpox vaccine virus for innoculating the inhabitants of Alabama. The state furnished the vaccine to an agent in each precinct, and a physician in each city or area was designated to administer it.[35] The disease continued to occur sporadically throughout the state, but no epidemic was reported.

Typhoid Fever

After 1840, typhoid fever was one of the most dreaded diseases; and its occurrence increased rapidly.[36] Many physicians believed that typhoid fever was a type of malarial fever rather than a *sui generis* disease. After 1850, there was some success in preventing the spread of typhoid fever due to the systematic institution of several practices, including an investigation of milk supplies, condemnation of existing water supplies, and location of new water supplies. A general sanitation program was set up in the area, and special attention was given to living quarters, even to the extent of moving inhabitants from suspected sites. Due to these health measures, typhoid fever reached epidemic proportions only in rare instances, but the disease remained a serious challenge well into the twentieth century. It proved less "amenable and submissive" than some physicians would have believed. (See Chapter 5, "Medical Practice After the Civil War.")

Diphtheria

Diphtheria, like typhoid fever, was recognized in Alabama around 1847 and again in 1850.[37] General sanitation measures used to control and eliminate epidemic diseases usually kept diphtheria from becoming epidemic. However, in its sporadic form, diphtheria remained severe and ofter fatal. (See Chapter 5, "Medical Practice After the Civil War.")

Intestinal Diseases

Early physicians observed that most diseases had a disposition, either primarily or secondarily, to involve the bowels. Diarrhea and similar infections were said to be caused by: (1) excessive heat, (2) rapid change in temperature, (3) food that was unsuitable and badly prepared and (4) the "misdirected vanities and kindnesses of a good mother." The most logical and effective way of helping new mothers was to educate them as to proper diet and the proper preparation of food. Some physicians in the state had an excellent understanding of this problem. They suggested a workable plan for sustaining and nourishing the mother and for providing the best scientific medical care of the newborn infant.[38] Unfortunately, no systematic, large-scale undertaking to accomplish this goal was attempted during the nineteenth century. *Cholera infantum* continued to be a common cause of death and disability in Alabama until the modern era of scientific medicine. *Cholera infantum* has been almost eliminated, and certainly the severity of this disease has been lessened, now that physicians know to replace fluids and electrolytes, and to use antibiotics and sanitation measures.

Infectious or bacterial diarrhea was apparently common in Montgomery in the 1840s.[39] Dr. J. Marion Sims refers to its widespread occurrence. Apparently, Dr. Sims was himself a victim; and his resultant precarious health caused him to move to New York City. At that time, no knowledge of the cause or spread of this type of diarrhea was known.[40]

Asiatic Cholera

Asiatic cholera was never widespread in Alabama, but there was an epidemic in 1873 that killed over 200 people in northern and central Alabama.[41] In the city of Birmingham, the water supply became contaminated and remained so because of ineffective public health measures. One physician from Montgomery, upon hearing that Asiatic cholera was in North Alabama and would soon be moving toward Montgomery, was not overly concerned as he thought that the people of Montgomery were safe from the disease due to their sanitation program. Many fancied themselves secure because "lime, carbolic acid and coal refuse were scattered freely over the surface of the city, and the soil was undisturbed, the cellars dry, and the offal hauled to the banks of the river."[42] Nevertheless, many cases of cholera and several deaths occurred in Montgomery. There were two other seasons in which forty to fifty fatalities occurred. It was not until the early 1900s when water supplies and sanitation were more rigorously controlled that cholera was eliminated in the state.

Respiratory Diseases

Between 1850 and 1875, respiratory diseases, particularly pneumonia and tuberculosis, were the principal causes of death in Alabama each year. Ten years prior to the Civil War, the State Medical Association expressed its faith in the prevention of "consumption" (tuberculosis) and its interest in enabling legislation that would make compulsory the physicians' ideas on prevention and treatment via rest, proper nutrition, and isolation. But the suggestions were not carried out, and there was very little community effort for the prevention of tuberculosis. It was only after a long difficult struggle that the antituberculosis campaign was finally successful. (See section, "The Antituberculosis Movement in Alabama.")

Public Health Becomes a Reality

Prior to 1850, only the more advanced observers agreed with Dr. Nott and later Dr. Cochran as to the causes of disease and its transmission. The middle of the century saw most Alabama physicians agreeing that the germ theory, transmissibility, and importation were indeed correct. In 1875, these physicians became the proponents of a State Health Department. As the etiology of disease was demonstrated, public health programs to control various communicable diseases became possible.

As early as 1816, the Mississippi Territory Legislature authorized Mobile to set up a board of health.[43] No particulars are known about this board, but there can be little doubt that from the beginning physicians were closely involved in its operations. A later document, the City of Mobile Charter issued in 1819 by the state of Alabama, required all appointed physicians to enforce the city's ordinances referring to the preservation of health.[44] Thus, the physicians of Mobile were involved closely with planning such public projects as drilling the first well for a city water supply, the construction of a sewer system (1819), and the yearly application of oyster shells to the streets (1829–1835). Dr. Henry Levert of Mobile believed the latter measure to be directly responsible for the absence of yellow fever during those years. Nothing further is known of this board.

An even more momentous event occurred in 1839 when a group of physicians, meeting at the office of Drs. J. C. Nott and R. L. Fearn, decided to form the Mobile Medical Society. The members of this organization petitioned the city of Mobile to grant the society authority to act as the City Board of Health. When the local government and the General Assembly were unable to cope with a severe yellow fever epidemic in that year, four physicians, all charter members of the Mobile Medical Society, were appointed to the Board of Health for Mobile. The members who served were Drs. Henry S. Levert, Josiah C. Nott, Solomon Mordecai, and John H. Woodcock.[45] The charter for the Board of Health, which was approved by the General Assembly in 1841, gave quasi-legal powers to the board.[46] The board's most important work was accomplished during actual epidemics. It coordinated the work of volunteers, such as the members of the Can't-Get-Away Club; ran hospitals that were set up to deal with the emergency; devised quarantine measures; and supervised such activities as the cutting and burning of weeds and spreading brine in gutters, privies, and yards.

For the next thirty-four years (except for a three-year period during reconstruction), the Mobile Medical Society selected and supervised all city health officials—that is, the city health officer, druggist, quarantine physician, sanitary inspector, and the supervisors of public institutions. Functioning as the Board of Health, these officials were required to investigate and control epidemic diseases; to devise and direct all quarantine and disinfecting measures; to inspect yards, houses, and streets; to insure the reporting of all births and deaths; and to superintend the city poorhouse, charity hospital, and dispensary.[47]

Later, the General Assembly granted similar board of health powers to the Selma, Montgomery, Huntsville, and Tuscaloosa medical societies. The activities of these local medical societies eventually led to the founding of the Medical Association of the State of Alabama in 1847.[48]

Organization of the State Public Health Department

The true claim to fame of the Mobile health plan is that it served as a model for the state in 1875, when the General Assembly made the Medical Association of the State of Alabama and the State Board of Health one and the same. In 1872, Dr. Jerome Cochran, having in mind the Mobile health department, had devised a plan in which the Medical Association of the State of Alabama would assume the responsibilities, functions, and powers of a state board of health. In this manner, public health responsibility was placed largely outside Alabama politics and under the control and management of physicians. The State Board of Health was so constructed that the state health officer held free rein over internal policy of the Medical Association. The state health officer was elected from and by a board of the Association's counselors and censors, who, as older, more prominent members, held lifetime positions of honor.[49]

This oligarchic power structure was repeatedly attacked from within and without the medical profession. There was no democracy exercised in the selection of the state health officer or in his use of his power. During its developmental stages, this system was justifiable when one considers the reactionary bent of the state government. In 1922, a *Montgomery Advertiser* reporter wrote that the state health officer was "a czar with self-perpetuating and autocratic power, but . . . he [was] a benevolent despot who decreed that lives should be saved."[50]

State Health Officers

DR. JEROME COCHRAN

Dr. Jerome Cochran served the state as its first state health officer from 1879 to 1896 and became the foremost medical figure in Alabama during the post–Civil War period. He came to Mobile in 1865 and

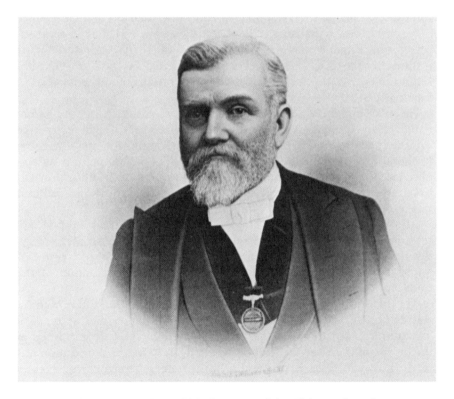

Jerome Cochran, M.D., 1831–1896 (Courtesy of the Alabama State Department of Archives and History)

immediately became involved in the work of the Mobile Medical Society and the City Board of Health. He gained a national reputation as a sanitation expert through his work as quarantine physician during a yellow fever epidemic in 1873. As city health officer in 1874, he led a successful fight against a smallpox epidemic that threatened to decimate Mobile's population. Later, he taught public hygiene at the Medical College of Alabama in Mobile and served on the National Yellow Fever Commission. As chairman of its subcommittee of "Experts on the Origin, Cause and Distinctive Features of Yellow Fever and Cholera," he almost single-handedly wrote the report on yellow fever presented to the United States Congress in 1878.[51] Through his experiences, Dr. Cochran became convinced that public health should be entrusted only to experts (physicians) and that a strong and united medical profession was essential to accomplish this goal.

As state health officer, Dr. Cochran received an annual salary of $1,500. Even though he spent most of his lifetime fighting outbreaks of yellow fever, smallpox, typhoid, diphtheria, and cholera, he did initiate some important activities in public health work, such as the maintenance of accurate health statistics. These statistics were essential to the concerted attack being made on the most prevalent diseases and to the institution of a program of preventive medicine. In 1881, the first law requiring registration of births and deaths in Alabama was enacted, but was ineffectual.

He encouraged each county to establish its own medical society and to employ full- or part-time public health officers. By 1882, thirty-nine counties had done so. In that same year, health authorities made the first proposal for compulsory smallpox vaccination, but the General Assembly chose to ignore the recommendation. It was not until 1906, after Dr. Cochran's death, that compulsory vaccination for school-age children was authorized.

Also during Cochran's administration, health officials became interested in sanitary conditions relative to public water supply, sewage disposal, food purity, house flies, and general filth. A direct result of improvements in health conditions was rapid industrialization of the state and the growth of its cities.[52]

The fifteen years following the 1868 reorganization of the Medical Association of the State of Alabama saw a veritable slate of medical legislation passed by the General Assembly. This was accomplished at the urging of the State Medical Association. In 1875, the Association was made the State Board of Health with general control over county boards, which, in turn, were controlled by county medical societies.[53] Two years later, a new medical practice act was passed, making the county societies the examining boards for licensing physicians to practice. This was enacted by the General Assembly on the recommendation of Dr. Cochran and over vigorous objections by some prominent members of the profession who preferred a state licensing board.[54]

In conjunction with his public health activities, Dr. Cochran continued the yellow fever research he had begun in 1873. Although the source of the disease was still unknown, he tentatively suggested the mosquito as a vector. Furthermore, he refuted those who believed yellow fever was "wafted by the wind" and insisted the disease was transmitted by insects. During a severe epidemic in the Mississippi Valley in 1888, in which 180,000 cases were reported, quarantine efforts of health officers were often hindered by business and civic organizations. Seemingly, they preferred yellow fever to the quarantine's interference in commerce. In 1887, a law was passed by the General Assembly regulating quarantine in the state; $5,000 was appropriated to enforce the law. A successful quarantine against commerce with Georgia and Florida probably prevented a yellow fever epidemic in Alabama during 1894.[55]

As the century drew to a close, the organization of a strong state medical association with its enabling legislation led to the establishment of a strong board of health. Of the many problems remaining, some probably came from Dr. Cochran's belief that "the best workmen were those who received no salary, but rather contributed time, effort, and money in meeting civic responsibilities willingly assumed."[56] Thus, the officers of the State Medical Association paid their own expenses. When the same principles were applied to the State Board of Health, it was found that it could not function effectively. Cochran was extremely reluctant to ask the General Assembly for additional appropriations. Consequently, aside from the state health officer who worked full time, the local public health authorities were expected to serve without pay. For many, this proved too great a burden.

County health boards were required to supervise all sanitary work, advise in health matters, inspect public institutions, educate the public concerning sanitation, administer vaccines and quarantines, investigate and prevent disease, and promote sanitary drainage. An even greater burden was placed on the county health officer, for in addition to carrying on his private practice, he was expected to join the health board in the performance of its duties. He was to issue and revoke midwife permits, supervise interments, and send regular reports on all epidemic diseases. In the event of an epidemic, he was to enforce all health regulations, declare quarantine, make sanitary surveys, regulate vaccinations, and even destroy property if he judged it dangerous to the general welfare.[57] Such duties often had to be carried out in the face of an unwilling and sometimes hostile public. Dr. Cochran's belief that serving the state without pay was a privilege must have seemed ludicrous to these men. A simple lack of time, as well as the requirements of their own professional and personal interests, caused many physicians in official capacities to neglect their duties as health officers. As a result, many laws were not properly enforced. In particular, collection of vital statistics was often neglected.

Among the duties of the county health officers was the supervision of the poorhouse, but inspections were usually perfunctory. One of the presidents of the State Medical Association declared that these poorhouses were indeed a "poor concern and a sad reflection on civilization and Christianity."[58]

After the State Board of Health repeatedly expressed concern as to the health among state prisoners, Dr. J. B. Gaston, then president of the State Medical Association, investigated the health conditions of prisons in 1882.[59] Thereafter he became active in promoting a program to prevent mistreatment of state prisoners.

The State Department of Health proposed a health education program for public schools to provide better health conditions for school children. Schools were required to conduct systematic and compulsory physical exercises; to provide adequate ventilation, lighting arrangements, and suitable desks; to plan for proper recreation; to require smallpox vaccination; to make available wholesome school lunches; to place sanitary supervision of private schools under the local board of health; to test the vision of all school children regularly; and to require all schools to teach physiology and hygiene.[60] In spite of this, little progress was made in improvement of health conditions in public schools.

In the 1870s, the need for a venereal disease control program was brought to the attention of the Alabama medical profession. Dr. Cochran believed that syphilis was not as bad as people were led to believe and that it was far more benign than generally thought. He described gonorrhea as "comparatively innocent." Because of his beliefs, he opposed all recommendations by those who wished to sponsor legislation. Consequently, the state morbidity report did not include venereal diseases.[61]

Several members of the State Board of Health recommended the establishment of a state institution for the rehabilitation of inebriates; this institution would be under the supervision of the superintendent of the Alabama Hospital for the Insane. However, Dr. Cochran was of the opinion "that the evils of strong drink were greatly exaggerated by the intemperate advocates of temperance." As a result of his opposition, the State Board failed to recommend a state prohibition law.[62]

Dr. Cochran's complacency or even obstinacy was a major factor in delaying the development of a progressive and comprehensive public health system in Alabama. His continued insistance that private physicians serve as health officers without compensation seriously impaired the collection of health statistics; without these the State Public Health Board could neither plan nor implement a program of disease control.

In spite of Dr. Cochran's apparent lack of insight into some of these problems, the physicians of the state recognized his outstanding leadership and organizational accomplishments. After his death in 1896, they sought to perpetuate his name and commemorate his life and service in various ways. The Jerome Cochran Annual Lecture of the State Medical Association was established in 1898.[63]

DR. WILLIAM HENRY SANDERS

At Dr. Cochran's death, Dr. William Henry Sanders (1838–1918) of Montgomery was named his successor. Dr. Sanders's tenure was from 1896 to 1917. Among the programs directly administered by Dr. Sanders were (1) public health education, (2) quarantine and epidemic control, (3) health programs among state prisoners, (4) establishment of a state laboratory, and (5) sanitary engineering.[64] During his administration, there was a marked increase of interest in county health work.[65] County health boards were organized and strengthened in several counties. Even though the industrial centers in the state had multiplied in size, the population was still predominantly rural; and hookworm, pellagra, tuberculosis, and typhoid fever were still the major health problems in Alabama.[66]

Dr. Sanders was not reticent about asking the State Legislature for money. In 1902, the annual appropriation was increased to $4,000; in 1907 to $15,000; and in 1911 to $25,000. With this money, Dr. Sanders was able to open a bacteriological and pathological laboratory and to appoint a full-time registrar of vital statistics.[67] He was also able to attract money from out-of-state health foundations. In 1910, an ambitious antihookworm campaign was instituted with funds donated by the Rockefeller Foundation. (See section, "The Fight for Eradication of Hookworm.")

Smallpox frequently demanded the attention of state and local boards of health, especially from 1897 to 1905. In 1898, ten counties were using control measures under Dr. Sanders's direction. A total of 3,638 cases of smallpox was reported that year. The disease persisted, but there was a much lower incidence after 1916.[68]

All proposed laws to make smallpox vaccination mandatory had failed to pass the State Legislature. As a result, the immunity of the general population remained low, and epidemics of this disease continued to be a possibility. In 1906, the State Board of Health "scarcely deemed it worthwhile to recommend that another effort be made to pass a bill

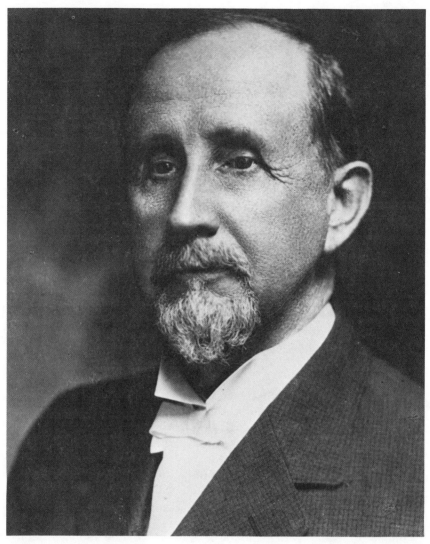

William Henry Sanders, M.D., 1838–1918 (Courtesy of the Alabama Department of Public Health)

requiring vaccination."[69] In 1907, a law was passed allowing a municipality to require vaccination of children entering public schools.[70] This was upheld by the Alabama Supreme Court in 1916.

The State Board of Health again investigated health conditions among state prisoners in 1911 and found that the death rate from all causes was three times as great among prisoners as in the general populace. Thirty percent of all deaths among prisoners was due to tuberculosis. The board advocated the construction of a separate state prison camp for all prisoners suffering from tuberculosis. In 1911, a tuberculosis hospital was built in Wetumpka for county and state prisoners.[71]

Pellagra continued to be a problem. The number of cases remained large and tended to increase, but no organized program for prevention and treatment was instituted. Although aware of national progress in the control of this disease, Dr. Sanders was apparently too involved with other problems to organize and conduct such a program. (See section, "Pellagra.")

Syphilis also continued to be widespread, and the incidence of gonorrhea was seldom reported. A number of speakers at the annual meeting of the State Medical Association described "how syphilis seriously impaired its victims' health; how widely prevailing the disease was in the state; how unpardonable was the indifferent attitude of the [physicians as well as the State Board of Health] and the Legislature; and [finally] how venereal disease could be prevented and cured."[72] No organized attack on these diseases was undertaken at this time.

Throughout Sanders's administration there were many proposals for constitutional changes to make the government of the State Medical Association and the State Board of Health more democratic.[73] From 1896 to 1916, Dr. Sanders controlled enough votes in the Medical Association to defeat every movement for change presented by his opponents.[74] Nevertheless, some changes were made in the organization of the State Medical Association.

DR. SAMUEL WALLACE WELCH

In 1917, Dr. Sanders retired; Dr. Samuel Wallace Welch became state public health officer and served from 1917 to 1928. Dr. Welch (1861–1928) was a native of Talladega and was educated at Tulane. Under Dr. Welch's direction, an attempt to strengthen the powers of the State Department of Health was begun.[75] The failures of public health activities were graphically depicted with the mobilization of troops in preparation for World War I. Alabama saw approximately 30 percent of its draftees rejected for health problems under the 1917 Selective Service Act and another 5 percent rejected by camp surgeons. Sixty percent of the Alabama National Guard detailed on the Mexican border suffered from hookworm. Of all the states in the Union, Alabama had the highest percentage of rejections during the draft from February 10 to July 10,

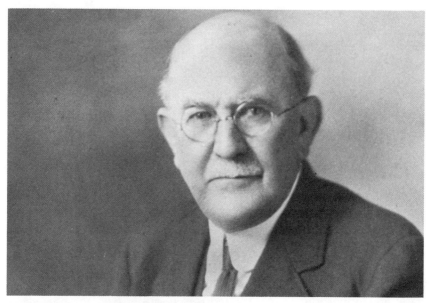

Samuel Wallace Welch, M.D., 1861–1928 (Courtesy of the Alabama State Department of Archives and History)

1918.[76] The public was now thoroughly alarmed, and much-needed public health measures were put into effect.

Dr. Welch realized that more funds were needed for the public health movement to be more effective. He was able to get state appropriations increased from $25,000 to $90,000 in 1919 and to $125,000 in 1920.[77] Dr. Welch acquired additional funds from the United States Public Health Service and the International Board of Health.[78] Bureaus of child hygiene, public health nursing, venereal disease control, and communicable diseases were added to the state public health service. Diphtheria antitoxin and typhoid vaccine were made available free of charge, and the number of laboratories was increased to meet the population's needs.[79] It was in this manner that a cooperative effort was made in the state to meet the health problems of its citizens.

Every effort that was made to establish fully funded local health departments throughout the state had the enthusiastic approval of the State Board of Health. Dr. Welch was able to persuade the State Legislature to partially finance such a program, and by the end of his administration, forty-six of the sixty-seven counties were able to maintain a permanent public health staff, consisting of a health officer, public health nurse, sanitation inspector, and laboratory technician or clinical worker.[80]

With the development of local health departments, the system originally designed by Dr. Cochran started to operate at peak efficiency and more than fulfilled the dream of the founders of the Medical Association of the State of Alabama.

In 1914, Walker County, the first Alabama county to institute a comprehensive health system, employed a full-time county health officer and staff. Dr. Carl A. Grote (1887–1964) was selected as county health officer. As he was not a native of Walker County, it was thought that he would be less likely to become involved in political or personal entanglements. Walker County received support for this project from many sources. The County Commissioners appropriated $3,000, but the United States Public Health Service financed most of the first year's work and even sent six men to aid in a sanitary survey. The State Anti-Tuberculosis Association apparently did not furnish any funds but gave aid in other ways. Dr. Grote's extensive program included a liberal amount of urgently needed health education. He saw to it that the county health office had health exhibits and sent bulletins on child care to all mothers of newborn babies. Also during the first year, Dr. Grote and his staff delivered 124 lectures on public health and published 147 articles in Walker County newspapers. Visiting agents distributed health bulletins throughout the county and inspected the sanitary conditions in approximately 8,000 homes.[81]

Even though Walker County's achievement in public health encouraged similar efforts throughout the state, progress was slow. Many Alabama counties could not participate because of lack of funds. Nevertheless, Alabama was the first state to have total county coverage even though it was not so covered until 1937. This was made possible by the financial support of the International Health Board and the United States Public Health Service.[82]

As previously mentioned, the State Bureau of Public Health Nursing was established in 1918 during Dr. Welch's tenure. Although Alabama was the first state to legally approve employment of nurses by local boards of health (1907), public health nursing was not routinely available until 1914, when the Walker County Health Service employed a public health nurse.[83]

However, several voluntary efforts were made to care for the sick-poor. Probably the earliest such effort came in 1910 when a visiting nurse service was organized in Birmingham by the Associated Charities in cooperation with the Metropolitan Life Insurance Company. This enterprise was discontinued after about one year but was followed by an independent Metropolitan Life Insurance Company nursing service and by a tuberculosis nursing service organized in 1912 by the Jefferson County Tuberculosis Association. Red Cross "Town and Country" nurses worked in 1913 in rural Chilton and Dallas counties.[84]

Public health nursing on a statewide basis began in 1918 when Miss Jessie L. Marriner, R.N., who previously worked for the Child Welfare Board, joined the Alabama State Board of Health as director of the Bureau of Rural Nursing. The Bureau later was called the Division of Public Health Nursing. The 1919 State Legislature approved funds for the Bureau. Under the able leadership of Miss Marriner, who served until 1933, the Bureau expanded from one primarily concerned with caring for the sick-poor in remote areas to a multifaceted, integral part of the State Health Department assisting in programs promoting the health and education of Alabama citizens.[85]

DR. DOUGLAS LAUNEESE CANNON

Dr. Douglas Launeese Cannon served as acting state health officer from August, 1928, to April, 1929.[86] Dr. Cannon (1892–1962) was a native of South Carolina. He was educated at the University of North Carolina at Chapel Hill School of Medicine and at Jefferson Medical College in Philadelphia, but spent most of his professional career in Alabama. On July 1, 1929, he resigned due to illness, but returned after six months to serve as the administrative assistant to the state health officer.

DR. JAMES NORMENT BAKER

Dr. James Norment Baker (1876–1941), a native of Virginia, was educated at the University of Virginia and served as state health officer from 1930 to 1941.[87]

A period of dissension and disagreement ended in 1930 when the State Public Health Board elected Dr. Baker. Dr. Baker had requested that he be allowed to devote his time exclusively to the public health problems of the state. The Board had had to reconsider the relationship between the state health officer and the State Medical Association. By his own wish, then, Dr. Baker was elected neither as chairman of the State Public Health Committee nor to the State Board of Censors as his predecessors had been. He did what he wanted to do: improve the state public health system and keep it intact during the economic vicissitudes of the depression. Under Dr. Baker, Alabama received aid from the federal government and from private organizations, without which public health would have suffered even more than it did during this time.

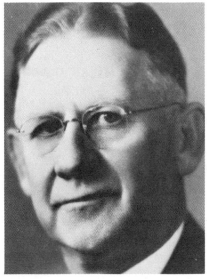

Douglas Launeese Cannon, M.D., 1892–1962 (Courtesy of the Alabama Department of Public Health)

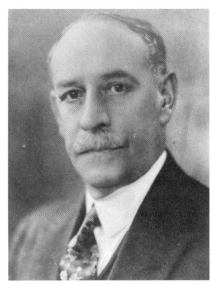

James Norment Baker, M.D., 1876–1941 (Courtesy of the Alabama State Department of Archives and History)

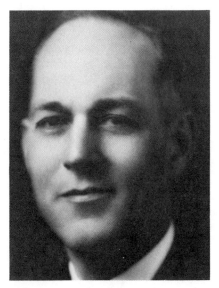

Burton Forsyth Austin, M.D., 1895–1970 (Courtesy of the Alabama Department of Public Health)

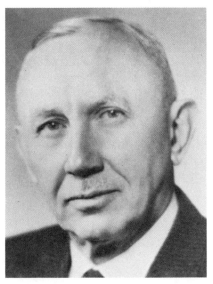

Daniel Gordon Gill, M.D., 1897–1962 (Courtesy of the Alabama Department of Public Health)

A division of mental hygiene was established under Dr. Baker; and the long planned goal of full-time county health officers was reached in 1937. Venereal disease control was emphasized, and large sums of federal money were expended in Alabama for control of syphilis and gonorrhea. Also the Tuberculosis Association and the physicians of the state cooperated with the health department to institute tuberculosis identification and control procedures. Eight modern tuberculosis sanatoria were built and equipped by 1939. Dr. Baker died on November 9, 1941.

DR. BURTON FORSYTH AUSTIN

Dr. Austin (1895–1970), a native of Alabama, was educated at the School of Medicine in Mobile.[88] He had served as the first county health officer of Morgan County. Dr. Austin received his Masters degree in Public Health at Harvard University. He became director of the Bureau of Maternal and Child Health in 1935 and served as the acting state health officer after the death of Dr. Baker from 1941 until 1947.

The economic boom and World War II resulted in an unprecedented demand on the Bureau of Vital Statistics and on the Laboratories of the State Health Department. These facilities were not equipped to respond fully due to inadequate funding by the state and the depletion of trained personnel in the war effort.

Programs that were emphasized during Dr. Austin's administration were in cancer research, tuberculosis, and syphilis control. During this administration, a Division of Venereal Disease Control was established. The internal friction that resulted from the increased work load, with little or no additional funding, was a major problem for Dr. Austin, and he resigned in the winter of 1946–1947.

DR. DANIEL GORDON GILL

Dr. Gill (1897–1962) was highly qualified for the position of director of Public Health programs in Alabama and served from 1947 to 1962.[89] He was a native of Canada and received his Doctor of Medicine and Doctor of Public Health degrees from the University of Toronto. He had been associated with the Rockefeller Foundation as an epidemiologist in the hookworm study in South Alabama. In 1928, he joined the State Health Department as a physician-epidemiologist and as the director of the Bureau of Preventable Diseases. Further fiscal problems were prevented in Alabama's health program due to the fact that Dr. Gill was an excellent fiscal manager.

As chairman of the Board of Censors, he was required to devote much of his time to the duties of the State Board of Medical Examiners. It was during his chairmanship that there was a long battle against the proposed system of licensing chiropractors in Alabama. A new licensing law was finally agreed upon, but the scars of the battle remained. Legislative attempts were made to abolish the State Board of Health, which was dominated by the Medical Association, and to replace it with a popularly elected one. Fortunately for medical care in Alabama, this proposal was defeated.

Financial support from the State Legislature for the health programs was minimal. Most of the funds available to the department were from federal health programs; therefore, the health department was compelled to develop according to guidelines set by the federal government. Most of the state money that became available was earmarked for the construction of health facilities and the operation of tuberculosis sanatoria. Local financial support for public health activities was less than adequate and did little more than meet the rising operating costs. During this period, the State Board of Health was program- rather than service-oriented.

One of the far-reaching programs established during Dr. Gill's administration was the federally funded Hill-Burton health facility construction program. Because of the Hill-Burton Act, a new central public health laboratory and forty-five new public health centers were built in fifteen years. For this reason, Dr. Gill's administration probably should be called the "brick and mortar era of public health in Alabama." In 1949, the state health officer was placed in a unique position by the State Legislature: he was made chairman of the Water Improvement Commission, the first health program in Alabama to receive direction outside the medical association.

During the Gill era, control of venereal disease was emphasized. There was a marked reduction in the number of deaths from measles, dysentery, malaria, and smallpox.

Dr. Gill died on December 3, 1962.

DR. IRA LEE MYERS

Dr. Ira Lee Myers was appointed state health officer after the death of Dr. Gill in 1962.[90] Dr. Myers (1924–), a native of Alabama, is as well trained as was Gill. He received his M.D. degree from the Medical College of Alabama in 1949 and his Masters of Public Health from Harvard University in 1953. Dr. Myers had been employed by the United States Public Health Service in the polio fly control project in Charleston, West Virginia. He had also been employed as an epidemiological officer in Erie County, Buffalo, New York, by the Communicable Disease Center of the Public Health Service in Atlanta. In 1955, Dr.

Myers returned to Alabama and joined the staff of the State Health Department as assistant to Dr. Daniel Gill, then state health officer.

Early in his administration, Dr. Myers asked that the affairs of the Medical Association and the Board of Medical Examiners be removed from the State Health Department. This was accomplished, leaving him more time to devote to public health matters. He has had unprecedented success in his liaison with the State Legislature. Two outstanding bills were passed early in his administration, both of which had a great impact on the progress in public health in Alabama. One changed the salary structure of the staff at the State Health Department to make the Department's salaries competitive. In the other bill, the State Legislature passed a new state tax to support public health work. By 1965, the Medicare program was on the agenda, and Medicaid was in the planning stage.

One of the most significant achievements of Dr. Myers's administration has been the extensive immunization programs, which have helped eliminate polio (the last case in the state was diagnosed in 1965), neonatal tetanus, and diphtheria.

During the 1960s and 1970s, with newer means of diagnosis and treatment, communicable diseases decreased in prevalence and severity; and the health department turned its attention more and more to degenerative diseases such as heart disease, cancer, and arthritis; home accidents; infant and maternal mortality; venereal diseases; and suicides.

The Fight for Eradication of Hookworm

The *New York Sun* announced in 1902 that the "germ of laziness" had been found in the South.[91] This statement referred to Dr. Charles Wardell Stiles's (1867–1941) discovery of an American species of hookworm *(Necator americanus)*. Dr. Stiles was a United States Public Health Service officer who believed that the abnormal human behavior of dirt-eating, clay-eating, and resin-chewing, observed in the "cracker" or "poor white" individuals was probably caused by anemia subsequent to hookworm infestation. He had proven this to be true through his investigations in the rural South where he found that widespread hookworm infestation caused anemia and poor health in the population. The parasite had been identified in an infected family of a South Carolina farmer and his wife who had five stunted children and ten more occupying premature graves, all victims of hookworm infestation. Unfortunately for Dr. Stiles, his findings only received public ridicule. The *New York Sun*, probably representative of Northern opinion, saw the discovery as a humorous way to rationalize Southern indolence. On the other hand, Southerners considered the findings to be a total fabrication or at the least one more example of "Yankee" derision and interference. Bewildered, Dr. Stiles consoled himself with the fact that the problem had received public attention.[92]

Dr. Stiles was by no means defeated. He began a one-man campaign in 1903—presenting his findings to medical and political leaders in the South. Among the many groups hearing his lectures was the Medical Association of the State of Alabama.[93]

Many a Southern physician's interest was aroused by Stiles's tour, but the states did not have the funds to finance the extensive eradication program that was necessary. Solving the problem began when Dr. Stiles was able to interest the Rockefeller Foundation in hookworm eradication. In 1908, John D. Rockefeller donated $1,000,000 for the elimination of hookworm disease in the South. The Sanitary Commission, which was established to distribute funds and offer advice, believed that the best way to gain the confidence of an already hostile and wary region was to work through the Southern leaders.[94]

Now that Alabama had the financial support necessary for a thorough investigation, its public health officials found cases of hookworm in all sixty-seven counties, and infections in the sandy soil areas of South Alabama in as much as 62 percent of the population.[95] The Alabama Hookworm Commission was organized in October, 1910, under the direction of the State Board of Health. This Commission instituted a campaign with two purposes in mind: (1) the eradication of the disease and (2) the education of the populace as to its prevention. The Commission sought financial help from the county and municipal governments. In addition to this, it worked within the county public health systems and enlisted the aid of charity organizations, women's clubs, and public-spirited individuals.[96] These groups set up free dispensaries, gave stereopticon-illustrated lectures, and distributed circulars. The success of this educational campaign was reflected in a report that one of these free dispensaries had treated 455 Alabamians in one day.[97]

Between 1910 and 1914, Alabama's share of the Rockefeller appropriations was $55,918.96. The State Board of Health supplemented this amount with $4,500, and fifty-seven counties contributed $7,863.25. In a total of fifty-three counties, 87,000 people were contacted through free clinics; and another 123,600 through public lectures during these four years.[98] However, an evaluation of the campaign indicated that it was not completely successful, for hookworm returned again and again to reinfect those previously treated and cured. Adequate control of this infestation was to come only after the economic status of the state improved. Proper disposal of human waste and the availability of shoes for the disadvantaged rural children eventually brought about a decrease in the incidence of the disease. The campaign did demonstrate that preventive medicine was feasible, especially when backed by public concern.

The medical societies, being relatively free from the prejudices created by sectionalism, eagerly vied for Northern financial backing. Alabama's projects, particularly work in rural towns and counties, continued to be financed by the Rockefeller Foundation, even though the new International Health Board had absorbed the Sanitary Commission, which had been funded by the Rockefeller Foundation.

The Julius Rosenwald Foundation was a private contributor to public health causes. The Rosenwald Foundation, prior to World War I, was interested in the promotion of education for blacks and was a major benefactor to the National Negro Health Movement. After World War I, the Foundation shifted its objectives to support the public health efforts of Tuskegee Institute, the Macon County Farmers' Institute, the Macon County Teachers' Institute, the Alabama Federation of Colored Women's Clubs, and the Mutual Aid Association of Mobile.[99]

Pellagra

Pellagra was second only to hookworm as a Southern "lazy disease" and was first diagnosed by Dr. George H. Searcy (1877–1935) at the Alabama Hospital for the Black Insane at Mount Vernon in 1906.[100] He very ably demonstrated not only that proper diet could prevent the disease, but also, when the disease occurred, that it could be eliminated by such a diet.[101] In 1914, extensive investigation into the cause of pellagra was begun.

Dr. Joseph Goldberger (1874–1929), who had worked for the United States Public Health Service since 1899, directed the experiments that were conducted by the United States Public Health Service among textile workers in Spartanburg, South Carolina, in patients at the Georgia Hospital for the Insane at Milledgeville, and in inmates at a prison farm in Mississippi. These experiments showed that pellagra was caused by a dietary deficiency that, in its advanced stages, could result in insanity.[102] Approximately 30 percent of the patients in Alabama's asylums were pellagra victims, a percentage that was similar to the number found in the other southern states.

Curing pellagra was fairly easy, but its prevention was almost impossible because of Southern socioeconomic conditions. Poverty was widespread among textile workers, but the plight of the tenant farmer was worse. He persisted in shackling himself to the one-crop system and refused to diversify or raise his own food. The sharecropper, who depended on precarious markets, prices, cotton futures, credit, and the elements, spent much of his life living marginally because of his ignorance of and inability to cope with dietary problems.

Even though it had been three years since pellagra had been recognized, it still claimed the lives of 1,073 Alabamians in 1,604 cases reported in 1909.[103] Until the quality of Southern rural life improved, efforts toward the prevention and cure of pellagra were to remain ineffectual. In the reports of the Alabama Hospitals for the Insane, large numbers of admissions and deaths of patients were attributed to pellagra. In fact, from 1900 until after World War I, pellagra was the single greatest cause of death at the Alabama Hospitals for the Insane. The work of Dr. Joseph Goldberger on the occurrence and prevention of pellagra did not go unnoticed in Alabama. However, Dr. Sanders and later Dr. Welch were so occupied with the control of hookworm and tuberculosis that they were not able at that time to mount a full-scale program against pellagra.

The year 1936 brought hope for relief from pellagra to both Alabama and the world. Dr. Tom Spies began his work at the Hillman Hospital in Birmingham, where he became director of the Nutrition Clinic in 1947. It was known that pellagra was a dietary deficiency that could be cured with eggs, milk, and meat. In 1937, Dr. Spies concluded that pellagra was caused by a deficiency of the vitamin, nicotinic acid. Thus, it was in Alabama that pellagra was first diagnosed by Dr. George Searcy, and it was in Alabama that Dr. Tom Spies made discoveries vital to its eradication. (See Chapter 5, "Medical Practice After the Civil War.")

The Antituberculosis Movement in Alabama

Virginia Brown and Jane Nabers stated in their typescript, "The History of the Anti-Tuberculosis Movement in Alabama," that tuberculosis, prior to 1900, was an enigma to the medical profession and that there were much more urgent and immediate problems to be solved: that is, yellow fever, malaria, smallpox, and cholera.[104] Therefore, the fight against tuberculosis had a fitful beginning, and no sustained effort for its identification and control was immediately forthcoming.

Dr. Ira Myers, state health officer, considers "tuberculosis to have been the single most important infectious disease in the state from the time the health department was organized until the early 1970s."[105]

Tuberculosis was usually chronic and most often deadly. Consumption, as tuberculosis was once known, was thought by many to be hereditary, as whole families often died of the disease. Dr. Jerome Cochran recognized that tuberculosis was infectious.[106] At the annual meeting of the Alabama Medical Association in 1872, he warned physicians that

we are on the verge of some important discoveries in tuberculosis which promise to revolutionize commonly conceived opinions . . . that most dreadful of all physical maladies from which humanity suffers, namely: consumption. It is more destructive than cholera or yellow fever. The investigation of its natural history through the aid of vital statistics and the comparison of great numbers of cases promises to lead to the discovery of its causes—that is to say, of the conditions under which it originates—and we may fairly hope that when these conditions are fully recognized they may be avoided.[107]

It took courage for this Alabama physician to stand before a group of medical men who, for the most part, believed tuberculosis to be hereditary, and tell them that it was instead a public health problem.

The controversy over the nature of tuberculosis raged annually in the meetings of the State Medical Association. As early as 1893, Dr. John Albert Pritchett (1849–1897) of Hayneville recognized the high susceptibility of blacks to tuberculosis. He recommended that health circulars describing the infectious nature of the disease and the means of disposing of sputum be given to physicians and to black preachers and teachers for distribution.[108]

"Prevention of Tuberculosis" was the title of a paper given before the Medical Association in 1900 by Dr. William Caswell Maples (1859–1919) of Scottsboro in which he deplored the scant consideration given to the prevention of tuberculosis as compared to other infectious diseases.[109]

Between 1900 and 1905, other papers presented at the annual meetings of the State Medical Association made specific recommendations for action against tuberculosis. In 1905, the entire program at the annual meeting of the State Medical Association was devoted to the tuberculosis problem. Association president Dr. Capers Capehart Jones (1846–1939) cited the need for education, for prevention through strict sanitary regulation, and for efforts to care for the tubercular poor in free dispensaries and hospitals. He earnestly recommended the appointment of a State Commission for the Prevention of Tuberculosis.[110] Dr. Jones's recommendation was not heeded. However, there was a special meeting in Montgomery, a Symposium on Tuberculosis held on Wednesday, April 19, 1905, to which the public was invited.[111] Enthusiasm kindled by this symposium resulted in the organization of an antituberculosis league.

Eugene DuBose Bondurant of Mobile, president of the State Medical Association, reported at the annual meeting in 1906 that at long last there was organized warfare against tuberculosis in the state. He recommended that a standing Tuberculosis Committee be created.[112]

The committee was appointed and held meetings in Montgomery in October and December of 1906. It adopted a specific statement of purpose that called for organization in each county to promote better understanding of tuberculosis. In addition, the committee directed the chairman to address the State Legislature as to the need for a state tuberculosis sanatorium.[113]

The result of this address was that Sam Will John, member of the House of Representatives from Jefferson County, introduced a bill to the Alabama Legislature to authorize construction of a sanatorium. The bill passed by the State Legislature provided $40,000 for obtaining a site and for constructing and equipping a facility. A sum of $10,000 was provided annually for maintenance. The bill authorized a board of seven trustees—including the governor, the state health officer, and three physicians of the Medical Association—to appoint a superintendent, purchase a site of not less than 160 acres, and construct the necessary buildings. A dairy farm was to be included.

The antituberculosis workers were greatly encouraged, but alas by the spring of 1908, the board of trustees had not been appointed. At the State Medical Association annual meeting of that year, Dr. Samuel W. Welch, president, deplored the governor's negligence in this matter.[114] Stung by the criticism, Governor Braxton Bragg Comer (governor of Alabama, 1907–1911) immediately complied by appointing Drs. Glenn Andrews of Montgomery, B. L. Wyman of Birmingham, G. T. McWhorter of Colbert County; and laymen H. T. Reese of Selma and David Marbury of Birmingham.[115] However, no further progress had been made and no funds had been released by 1910. By 1912, the funds had been made available, but the site had not yet been selected. Some years later, 400 acres of land were purchased in Cullman County. By this time, part of the act appropriating the funds had lapsed, so no buildings could be built. The state sanatorium, on which so many focused so much hope, was never built.[116]

Renewed agitation by the physicians of the state to inform the public that tuberculosis was an infectious disease resulted in still more legislation. In 1900 and 1903, respectively, Mobile and Montgomery passed antispitting ordinances. Birmingham followed suit in 1904, making it unlawful "for anyone to spit, throw hulls, peelings or other litter upon the sidewalks or . . . the floors of . . . public places over which ladies are accustomed to pass in walking through the city."[117] This seemed to be an elementary step forward. Yet Dr. C. L. Minor of Ashville, North Carolina, found it necessary to upbraid the physicians in an address at the State Medical Association in 1905 for their promiscuous spitting, reminding them how difficult it would be to teach others to refrain.[118] A comment by Dr. R. M. Cunningham indicated the public's lack of compliance up until at least 1912: "A few years ago when the city council passed an ordinance about spitting on the streets, a man would rare back and say, 'I have a right to spit where I please.' But now public sentiment is sustaining that ordinance."[119]

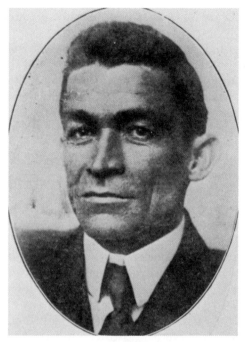

Glenn Andrews, M.D., 1862–1944
(Courtesy of the Alabama State Department
of Archives and History)

Education of the public concerning tuberculosis was a long, slow process. In 1903, Montgomery County designated tuberculosis a reportable disease; and in 1907, the State Legislature followed suit, reflecting the new public attitude.

The Great Awakening

The year 1908 marked the great awakening in the crusade against tuberculosis both in Alabama and in the nation. During that year, the National Association for the Study and Prevention of Tuberculosis sent an exhibit on this disease through the South. Local medical societies arranged for the exhibit to be shown in Montgomery, Birmingham, and Selma.

The dates of the traveling exhibit coincided with the annual meeting of the State Medical Association in Montgomery. Physicians from every part of the state witnessed a graphic presentation prepared by the nation's foremost authorities on tuberculosis. The exhibit, open to the public for ten days in the Old First Baptist Church in Montgomery, attempted to show the extent of tuberculosis—its ravages, causes, spread, and its means of prevention and cure.[120] To supplement the exhibit, the State Medical Association held a special symposium for the public on tuberculosis; the symposium emphasized the need for cooperation between government, the medical profession, and the public to combat this disease effectively.[121]

The Sixth International Tuberculosis Congress was held in Washington, D. C. in September, 1908. The Medical Association of the State of Alabama authorized the president-elect, Dr. Benjamin L. Wyman, to appoint fifty delegates to the congress. These delegates were selected from the medical profession and represented most counties.[122] The Alabama delegation was headed by Dr. R. M. Cunningham. Both Theodore Roosevelt, then President of the United States, and Sir Robert Koch, who discovered the etiological agent of tuberculosis, addressed the congress.[123]

The congress proved to be the most significant milestone in the progress of the antituberculosis movement in the United States. Its educational influence through those who attended and the resultant publicity throughout the country reached far into the nation's consciousness. In Alabama, Dr. B. L. Wyman continued the activities by inaugurating a drive to educate physicians and laymen together in the various counties on the problem of tuberculosis. These popular lectures were given before large audiences, and there was an increasing interest among people from all walks of life.[124]

Anti-Tuberculosis League of Montgomery

On May 27, 1908, the Anti-Tuberculosis League of Montgomery, the first of its kind in Alabama, was formed.[125] Under the enthusiastic leadership of Dr. Gaston J. Greil (1878–1932), the League immediately went to work educating the people. Information on prevention of the disease was distributed to every possible place in Montgomery County. Twenty-five thousand antituberculosis leaflets were distributed along with 8,000 copies of a small booklet entitled "The Key." This booklet described local health conditions in the city and county. Teachers were instructed in health rules, and lectures were given in every city school.[126]

The League cited the urgent need for a sanatorium in which to treat the tubercular patients of the county. Dr. Greil finally obtained a site on the Upper Wetumpka Road about three miles from the city of Montgomery. In 1911, the first cabin was built for $100, and eight small cottages, a dining hall, and a library soon dotted the shady hillside.[127]

In 1916, the capacity of the camp had increased to thirteen whites (one patient in a cottage) and ten blacks (two in a cottage). No charges for patients were made, but patients were encouraged to pay if they were able.[128] By 1925, twenty-five cottages lined the hillside.

In the same year, a modern one-story frame hospital with a fifty-two-bed capacity was erected, and the cottages were dismantled. The Fresh Air Camp became the Montgomery Tuberculosis Sanatorium.[129] At the cornerstone ceremonies, Dr. S. W. Welch, state health officer, noted that "Montgomery is the first city of Alabama to have such a modern hospital . . . Gadsden will shortly rebuild its fresh air farm destroyed by fire a few months ago. Birmingham's is in construction, and Mobile is planning." Alabama was at last awakening to the perils of this great killer.

Pioneer Antituberculosis Crusaders in Jefferson County

On May 31, 1910, a mass meeting was held in the Chamber of Commerce Auditorium in Birmingham to form an antituberculosis association in Jefferson County. One of the factors that brought about this action was a sermon on tuberculosis delivered in a downtown theater on Sunday night by the Reverend George Eaves, D.D., local Congregationalist minister.

Dr. Eaves (1858–1926) was a native of England and had been a missionary to Japan. In 1887, he became ill with tuberculosis and moved to the United States for his health. For several years he lived in the Colorado mountains. His health improved, and in 1907, he came to Birmingham where he exerted a marked influence on the religious and intellectual life of the community. A subtle sense of humor and a talent for a good story, combined with a profound humanitarianism, won him a host of friends. So great was his own enthusiasm and devotion to a cause that it won over his friends.

Soon after the organization of the Jefferson County Anti-Tuberculosis Association, a committee of three local physicians was appointed to survey Jefferson County for those who had or had had tuberculosis. The Association president, B. M. Allen, a Birmingham attorney and civic worker, initiated the establishment of a sanatorium. He appointed a committee, consisting of Representative Sam Will John, Dr. B. L. Wyman, and himself, to confer with the governor on a tuberculosis sanatorium for Jefferson County.[130] The committee selected the southeastern slope of Red Mountain as the site for a temporary camp and obtained a tract of land owned by the city of Birmingham. In July, tents were raised near the Rock House overlooking Shades Valley. In August, the first patient was admitted, and by September 1, 1910, ten patients

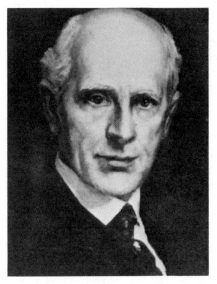

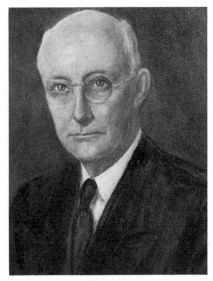

George Eaves, D.D., 1858–1926 (Courtesy of the Alabama Museum of the Health Sciences, Lister Hill Library, Medical Center, The University of Alabama in Birmingham)

Cabot Lull, M.D., 1874–1958 (Courtesy of the Jefferson-Shelby Lung Association, Birmingham, Alabama)

were in residence. Rates were twenty dollars a month for those able to pay.

Since the organization depended on public subscriptions, a group from the Association went before the Board of Revenue to plead for funds for the sanatorium.[131] Immediate financial assistance, however, came from another source. The Birmingham Chapter of the American Red Cross furnished $2,300 for the work of the Jefferson County Anti-Tuberculosis Association.[132]

A pavilion for patients with advanced tuberculosis was built with money from the sale of Christmas Seals. Wooden structures replaced the tents, and the rooms were furnished by various philanthropic individuals and societies. A dining pavilion, which could accommodate seventy-five patients, was built early in 1911. The sanatorium also owned three cows. All of this was accomplished in a period of less than one year by the unselfish and persistent efforts of a group of Jefferson County men and women.

The physicians of Birmingham responded with the same generosity that characterized the efforts of the laymen. From the inception of the organization, Dr. Cabot Lull (1874–1958),[133] Dr. James Alto Ward (1892–1943), Dr. Earle Drennen, Dr. Henry Silas Ward (1866–1950), and Dr. Enoch Marvin Mason (1878–1944) gave their services to the camp and to the dispensary. Among Birmingham physicians, Dr. Lull was considered one of the most experienced in the diagnosis and treatment of tuberculosis.

The Fresh Air Camp, renamed the "Red Mountain Sanatorium," greatly increased its facilities with the addition of two- and four-bed wards, a private care unit, a new recreation hall and office, a kitchen and storeroom, complete sanitation equipment, and steam heat for all the buildings. Important work was performed at the outpatient dispensary, which had been established by the Jefferson County Anti-Tuberculosis Association in 1910. It served outpatients six hours a week. Four physicians, who gave their services free, composed the first staff. The Graduate Nurses Association furnished nurses. More nursing service was needed, however, and church societies were asked to finance a dispensary nurse. In 1914, Bertha Clement was employed as a full-time nurse. Mr. Eugene Brown of the city paid her salary in full for the first six months and in part until 1932 when the Association became a part of the Community Chest.[134]

Dr. Eaves was especially concerned about preventive health work with children. In 1913, over two-thirds of the recorded deaths of children in Alabama were due to tuberculosis.[135] The funds for operation, referred to as the "Children's Fund," were raised by the sale of Christmas Seals and tin foil from wrappings of chewing gum, cigarettes, and candy. Beginning in 1915, the Children's Page of the *Birmingham News* conducted a yearly tin foil collection contest among the city and county schools. On George Washington's birthday, when the foil was brought to the *News* building to be weighed, a tin foil party was given at which the winning school received a United States flag. At these parties, the Anti-Tuberculosis Association nurses conducted educational programs, giving out literature and talking to mothers and teachers. The money value of the tin foil was small, but the programs taught health concepts and preventive medicine, particularly tuberculosis prevention.

Another important project of the Jefferson County Anti-Tuberculosis Association was an open-air school for children from homes in which tuberculosis existed. In 1916, the school opened at Green Springs Park with Mrs. Barnes Morgan as chairman of the project. Mary Rumph, a social worker and kindergarten teacher, was in charge. Thirty-one children were served a mid-morning lunch of milk and crackers, a hot lunch at noon, milk again after lessons, followed by a play period in the afternoon. This project continued until Miss Rumph's death in the influenza epidemic of 1918. In 1920, the Children's Fund became the Mary Rumph Memorial Fund, and a special committee was named for its administration.[136]

Dr. Eaves initiated a program for the identification and treatment of malnourished children in Birmingham schools. Five schools were designated for a program in which every child was weighed and examined for defects, and health classes were planned for undernourished children and their mothers. Out of the program grew a summer camp for undernourished children which was held for six weeks at the Shades Cahaba School. Eventually, the Independent Presbyterian Church of Birmingham assumed this work, which is today conducted as the Fresh Air Farm on Shades Mountain.[137]

Local antituberculosis associations recognized the need for an effective educational program on general health. Wherever sound bodies could be built with proper food, rest, and cleanliness, tuberculosis could be prevented or its advance arrested.

The prevalence of hookworm was of particular concern because it often contributed to the development of tuberculosis by lowering vitality and reducing resistance to infection. Hookworm films were shown widely over the state by antituberculosis workers, and under their direction, schoolchildren were examined for hookworm.[138]

The most ambitious project of the program had its origins at the national level. It was entitled the Modern Health Crusade, a pioneer system of nationwide health education inaugurated in public schools in 1917 by the National Tuberculosis Association. Charles M. DeForest of the Association staff had worked out for his young son such a successful health game based on the chivalric system that it was expanded into a national project. The schoolchild, as he was being taught basic health rules, kept a daily chart on which he marked his diligence in eleven daily chores, such as "I was in bed ten or more hours last night and kept my windows open." As he progressed in faithfulness to this program, his rank changed from Squire to Knight, etc., toward the goal of a seat at the Round Table. Fleta McWhorter, who had worked under Dr. Eaves as a volunteer, became the full-time director of the state program of the Modern Health Crusade. She traveled over Alabama promoting the program in the schools.

By the end of the 1925 school year, every county in Alabama was using Modern Health Crusade supplies, and 50,000 children were enrolled. Cho Cho, the Health Clown, visited Alabama twice in 1926. Named for the Child Health Organization for which he worked for many years, Cho

Cho interspersed his stunts with lessons on health, diet, personal hygiene, and recreation. His visits to thousands of children in Alabama were financed by Christmas Seal money.[139]

As material evidence of the gratitude of the people of Jefferson County for Dr. Eaves's efforts, the modern $35,000 clinic that the Anti-Tuberculosis Association of Jefferson County opened in 1938 was named the George Eaves Clinic.[140] The building, located at 19th Street and 6th Avenue South, was demolished in 1946 to make way for new Medical Center construction.

Founding a Statewide Tuberculosis Association

Enthusiasm for forming a state group to fight tuberculosis had been growing in Alabama since 1904. It was not until 1914, however, that the Alabama Anti-Tuberculosis League was formally organized. A state organization was brought about largely through the efforts of Dr. George Eaves, who believed that to be effective, an educational and preventive program must be extended throughout the state. He became the first executive secretary of the State League. The young organization, poor in funds and inexperienced in this field, reached out to embrace a multitude of activities. The general objectives of the group were prevention and control of tuberculosis and care of the tubercular patient. To implement these objectives, it initiated a program that included the formation of organized units in all parts of the state, a much-needed program of education, agitation for sanatoria and clinics, and exploration of the means of financial support for this program.[141]

Since 1908, the national Christmas Seal sale has been the principal source of income for the antituberculosis associations. The Jefferson County Anti-Tuberculosis Association first sold Christmas Seals in 1910. The Alabama Anti-Tuberculosis League, from the time of its formation in 1914, encouraged the sale of seals throughout the state. The sale of Christmas Seals has been valuable not only for the income it has generated but also as educational advertising.

State Anti-Tuberculosis Commission

The Anti-Tuberculosis Commission was established by an act of the State Legislature in 1915.[142] Its aim was chiefly to develop interest in the construction of a state network of sanatoria. Dr. Eaves served as field agent for the Commission. He traveled to every county seat in the state and met with any group who would listen to his plea. In 1922, he was forced to retire due to ill health. The Commission continued its work until it was dissolved by the State Legislature on September 29, 1923.[143]

For many years, letters from tubercular patients or their families had deluged the Alabama Tuberculosis Association office begging for information on hospitalization. The answer had always been the same: Alabama had no state sanatorium. In 1923, a campaign was conducted over the entire state to obtain the endorsement of civic organizations for a state sanatorium bill. Civic clubs, fraternal organizations, the Legislative Council of Alabama Women, Chambers of Commerce, and American Legion posts all passed resolutions endorsing the bill. They recognized that Alabama's need was genuine, as only about 100 beds for the hospitalization of tubercular patients were available in the entire state. These hospital facilities were located in Birmingham, Mobile, Montgomery, and Gadsden and were operated by the county antituberculosis groups for residents of those counties only. The Sanatorium Bill, appropriating $200,000 for building and $50,000 annually for maintenance, survived committee hearings and was passed in the House.[144] This bill (House Bill 21) was originally presented to the State Legislature on January 16, 1923, by a Mr. Howze. The bill was assigned to the Public Health Committee. It died in this Committee. The State Health Department was opposed to a state institution; therefore the Alabama Tuberculosis Association was forced to turn its efforts elsewhere.

A law enacted in 1945 provided for the construction of seven district sanatoria for treatment of tubercular patients. The state furnished three-fourths of the funds for constructing and equipping these facilities. However, the introduction of effective therapeutic agents for the treatment of tuberculosis rendered these sanatoria obsolete. The State Legislature passed an act in 1973 that allowed the State Health Department to negotiate a contract with general hospitals for inpatient treatment of tuberculosis. Between 1973 and 1975, the sanatoria were converted, for the most part, into mental health and rehabilitation facilities. Thus, the era of sanatorium treatment of tuberculosis came to a close.

Tuberculosis continued to be a major health problem in Alabama until effective antibiotics were introduced in the 1950s. Prior to that time, tuberculosis killed 90 percent of those reported stricken. It had accounted for approximately 3,000 deaths annually in Alabama and was two to three times more common among blacks.[145] Today, though new cases are frequently identified, hospitalization is often unnecessary. Modern methods of treatment have also made the isolation of tubercular patients unnecessary. It is now possible to treat effectively and relatively quickly those identified and render them noncontagious. Although the death rate has decreased, the problem is still with us. In 1963, over half of the funds allocated by the state for the Health Department was for tuberculosis treatment, testing, and control.[146] In 1965, 12.5 percent more cases were detected than in 1964.[147] The continued identification of patients with active disease seems to indicate that there remains a substantial infectious focus in the population; it is hoped that this can be eradicated.

In the late 1960s, the Alabama Tuberculosis Association decided to identify patients with emphysema and direct its efforts toward its causes and treatment. Air pollution received a great deal of attention. Alabama was deemed to have the least pollution control in the country. Air pollution studies were carried out in Birmingham over a period of years, and the results were overwhelmingly bad. In 1969, Governor Albert Brewer (governor of Alabama, 1968–1971) formed the Alabama Air Pollution Control Commission in order to deal with the problem. The Alabama Tuberculosis Association began a campaign to educate the public. In 1973 and 1974, thousands of people across the state were given a pulmonary function test. Classes for patients with emphysema, who required breathing therapy, were held to teach the victims how to live more comfortably with their disease. Here again, education played an important role in the Association's activities. Anti-cigarette smoking exhibits and smoking withdrawal clinics became part of the Association's attempt to protect lung health. In line with this approach to providing lung health care to Alabamians, the Alabama Tuberculosis Association changed its name to the Alabama Lung Association.

Other Voluntary Health Agencies

Other voluntary agencies were promoted by the Medical Association of the State of Alabama. For example, a state affiliate of the American Cancer Society, which had been founded in 1913, was established.[148] In 1900, cancer ranked tenth as a cause of death, and from this time forward, interest in this disease increased in direct relation to improved techniques of diagnosis. By 1933, cancer was the second most common cause of death in Alabama.

A voluntary agency was established in Alabama for promotion of child health as an outgrowth of the child labor movement. Other nationwide agencies established in the state were the National Safety Council, the National Society for the Prevention of Blindness, the American Heart Association, the American Eugenics Society, and the American Social Hygiene Association.[149]

Summary

In 1875, a number of programs were implemented in Alabama for promoting public health measures and as a means of preventing disease. The close alliance of the State Medical Association and these programs was unique in medical history. Such an arrangement served to make the Medical Association and Board of Health quasi-independent of government control. Now, more than a century has passed, but this linkage system, formed by the legendary Jerome Cochran, still serves the people of Alabama. The State Medical Association made available its expertise, and the General Assembly furnished a portion of the financial support. In addition, the federal government and private health foundations have been generous in promoting public health in the state.

Notes

1. Milo B. Howard, Jr., "Health Problems in Colonial Alabama," *J.M.A. Ala.* 39 (1970): 1051–52, 1055–57.

2. D. Rowland and A. G. Sanders, eds., *Mississippi Provincial Archives, French Dominion, 1704–1743* (Jackson: Press of the Mississippi Department of Archives and History, 1932), 3: 430, 440, 482–83.

3. Peter J. Hamilton, *Colonial Mobile, A Historical Study* (New York: Houghton, Mifflin and Co.; Cambridge: Riverside Press, 1897), pp. 206–07.

4. S. G. Schoonover, "Alabama Public Health Campaign, 1900–1919," *Ala. Rev.* 28 (1975): 218–33.

5. L. D. S. Harrell, "Preventive Medicine in the Mississippi Territory, 1799–1802," *Bull. Hist. Med.* 40 (1966): 364.

6. H. Toulmin, ed., *Digest of the Laws of the State of Alabama: Containing the Statutes and Resolution in Force at the End of the General Assembly in January, 1823* (Cahawba, Ala.: Ginn & Curtis, 1823), pp. 690–91. Act passed 27 December 1815.

7. Carey V. Stabler, "The History of the Alabama Public Health System," (Ph.D. diss., Duke University, 1944), pp. 13–14 (hereafter cited as Stabler, "Dissertation").

8. J. I. Waring, *A History of Medicine in South Carolina, 1825–1900* (Charleston: South Carolina Medical Association, 1967), pp. 278–79.

9. Stabler, "Dissertation," pp. 20–21.

10. Ibid., p. 18.

11. Ibid., p. 21.

12. J. C. Nott, "Yellow Fever Contrasted with Bilious Fever—Reasons for Believing It a Disease *Sui Generis*—Its Mode of Propagation—Remote Cause—Probable Insect or Animalcular Origin, etc.," *New Orleans Med. & Surg. J.* (March 1848), pp. 569, 573.

13. Stabler, "Dissertation," p. 22.

14. Ibid.

15. Ibid., p. 27.

16. Ibid., pp. 28–29.

17. Ibid., p. 29.

18. Ibid.

19. Ibid., p. 30.

20. Ibid., pp. 31–32.

21. Ibid., p. 34.

22. Caldwell Delaney, *Craighead's Mobile* (Mobile, Ala.: The Haunted Book-shop, 1968), p. 95.

23. Ibid.

24. Ibid., pp. 98–99.

25. Stabler, "Dissertation," p. 1.

26. Ibid., pp. 1–2.

27. Ibid., p. 2.

28. Ibid., p. 3.

29. P. H. Lewis, "Medical History of Alabama, Part 2," *New Orleans Med. & Surg. J.* (July 1847), p. 12.

30. E. D. McDaniel, "Report on the Topography, Climatology, and Diseases, of Wilcox County," *Trans.* (1869), p. 107.

31. No annual meetings were held from 1860 to 1868.

32. Stabler, "Dissertation," pp. 32–33.

33. Ibid., pp. 14–15.

34. Ibid., p. 15. Dr. Ketchum was one of the founders of the Medical College of Alabama in Mobile. He served as the second dean of the school.

35. Stabler, "Dissertation," p. 35.

36. Ibid., pp. 35–36.

37. Ibid., p. 36.

38. Ibid., pp. 36–37.

39. Seale Harris, *Woman's Surgeon, The Life Story of J. Marion Sims* (New York: Macmillan Company, 1950), p. 93.

40. In 1848, a three-year-old son of Dr. J. Marion Sims succumbed to *cholera infantum*. Harris, p. 93.

41. Stabler, "Dissertation," pp. 37–38.

42. Ibid., p. 38.

43. Ibid., p. 14.

44. Forest E. Ludden, *The History of Public Health in Alabama 1941–1968* (Ph.D. diss., The University of Alabama, 1970), p. 8, Alabama Collection, Lister Hill Library, The University of Alabama in Birmingham, Birmingham, Ala.

45. William H. Brantley, Jr., "Alabama Doctor," *Ala. Lawyer* 6 (1945): 253.

46. Ibid.

47. D. L. Cannon, "Alabama's Eighty-Nine Years of Medical Organization, A Brief History of the Association, Part 1," *J.M.A. Ala.* 5 (1936): 315. The dispensary, funded by the City Council, provided medicines and treatment for the indigent sick of the city.

48. Brantley, pp. 256–57.

49. Schoonover, pp. 219–20.

50. Ibid., p. 220.

51. G. A. Ketchum, "Memorial Meeting," *Trans.* (1897), p. 96.

52. Schoonover, p. 221.

53. Jerome Cochran, "The Medical Profession," *Memorial Record of Alabama: Historical and Biographical* (Madison, Wisconsin: Brant and Fuller, 1893), 2: 129.

54. Drs. J. D. S. and W. E. B. Davis of Birmingham were leaders in the movement for a state board of medical examiners.

55. Schoonover, p. 222.

56. Stabler, "Dissertation," p. 59.

57. Ibid., pp. 78–81.

58. Ibid., p. 100.

59. Ibid., p. 101. Dr. Gaston was instrumental in obtaining passage of the law in the General Assembly establishing the State Department of Health.

60. Stabler, "Dissertation," p. 102.

61. Ibid., p. 105.

62. Ibid., pp. 106–07.

63. Ibid., p. 107.

64. Ibid., p. 119.

65. J. M. Gibson, "Dr. Cochran's Dream and Your Health," transcript of radio talk, 6 December 1951, p. 3, Library of the Alabama Department of Public Health, Montgomery.

66. M. Sullivan, *Our Times, the United States, 1900–1925* (Chautauqua, New York: Chautauqua Press, 1931), 3: 290–99, 327. Typhoid vaccine was first made available in 1914. (Ira Myers, state health officer, letter, 20 September 1979.)

67. Ludden, pp. 23, 25. The State Laboratory was established in 1907 and became operational in 1908 when Dr. Sanders employed Dr. E. M. Mason as the first state bacteriologist. The diagnosis of typhoid fever was one of the services rendered at that time. In 1922, the State Laboratory began manufacturing typhoid vaccine for free distribution. (Ira Myers, state health officer, letter, 20 September 1979.)

68. Stabler, "Dissertation," pp. 122–23.

69. Ibid., p. 123.

70. *Code of Alabama 1907*, chap. 32, "Municipal Corporations," article 19, "Powers, Authorities and Duties of Municipalities," sect. 1289, "Diseases, contagious, vaccination, etc.," (Nashville: Marshall and Bruce Co. Printers and Binders, 1907), p. 619.

71. Stabler, "Dissertation," pp. 124, 139–40.

72. Ibid., p. 147.

73. Ibid., p. 148.

74. Ibid., p. 149.

75. Acts of Alabama, 29 September 1919, pp. 909–45.

76. Schoonover, pp. 231–32.

77. Ibid., p. 232.

78. S. W. Welch, "Public Health Administration in Alabama," *Trans.* (1918), p. 196. The International Board of Health was established and financed by the Rockefeller Foundation.

79. Albert Burton Moore, *History of Alabama and Her People* (Chicago: Amer. Hist. Soc., Inc., 1927), 1: 988–89.

80. Ludden, pp. 36–39.

81. C. A. Grote, "A Two Year Public Health Campaign in a Rural County," *South. Med. J.* 9 (1916): 320–24.

82. Schoonover, p. 227.

83. John J. Hanlon, *Principles of Public Health Administration* (Saint Louis: C. V. Mosby Co., 1960), p. 450; and Jessie L. Marriner, "History of Public Health Nursing in Alabama," MS. p. 1, Library of the Alabama Department of Public Health, Montgomery.

84. Marriner, pp. 1–2.

85. Catherine Conley, "The History and Trends of Public Health Nursing in Alabama," TS, lecture to the Jefferson-Hillman Nurses, 20 February 1952.

86. Ludden, pp. 43, 46.

87. Ibid., pp. 46–58.

88. Ibid., pp. 62–103.

89. Ibid., pp. 105–71.

90. Ibid., pp. 173–260.

91. Schoonover, p. 222.

92. Sullivan, pp. 324–25.

93. C. W. Stiles, "The Significance of the Recently Recognized American Hookworm Disease for the Alabama Practitioner," *Trans.* (1903), p. 300.

94. Sullivan, pp. 324–25. The Sanitary Commission was established by John D. Rockefeller.

95. Schoonover, p. 223.

96. Ibid., p. 224.

97. Ibid.

98. Ibid.

99. Ibid., pp. 224–25.

100. G. B. Tindall, *The Emergence of the New South, 1913–1945*, vol. 10 of *A History of the South*, Wendell H. Stephenson and E. Merton Coulter, eds., (Baton Rouge: Louisiana State University Press, 1967), pp. 277–78.

101. Schoonover, pp. 225–26.

102. Tindall, pp. 277–78.

103. Schoonover, p. 226.

104. Virginia Pounds Brown and Jane Porter Nabers, "The History of the Anti-Tuberculous Movement in Alabama," TS, 24 pages.

105. Ira Myers, state health officer, personal communication, July 1980.

106. Robert Koch (1843–1910) identified the tubercle bacillus in 1882.

107. "Dr. Cochran's Paper on Public Hygiene," *Trans.* (1872), pp. 20–21.

108. J. A. Pritchett, "Tuberculosis in the Negro," *Trans.* (1893), pp. 352–70.

109. W. C. Maples, "Prevention of Tuberculosis," *Trans.* (1900), pp. 369–87.

110. C. C. Jones, "The Message of the President," *Trans.* (1905), pp. 20, 22.

111. Program of the Annual Session—Symposium on Tuberculosis, *Trans.* (1905), pp. 5–6.

112. E. D. Bondurant, "The Message of the President," *Trans.* (1906), pp. 13–14.

113. Eli P. Smith, "The Prevention of Tuberculosis," *Ala. Med. J.* 19 (1906): 35–41.

114. S. W. Welch, "Annual Message of the President," *Trans.* (1908), p. 19.

115. B. B. Comer, "Address of Welcome," *Trans.* (1908), p. 13.

116. Thomas McAdory Owen, *History of Alabama and Dictionary of Alabama Biography* (Chicago: S. J. Clarke Pub. Co., 1921), 2: 1227.

117. *Code of Ordinances of the City of Birmingham (1905)*, sect. 914, p. 354.

118. "Discussion," *Trans.* (1905), p. 379.

119. W. L. Dunn, "Some Lessons To Be Learned From Results of Treatment of Pulmonary Tuberculosis," *Trans.* (1912), p. 503.

120. Welch, (1908), pp. 23–24; and "The American Tuberculosis Exhibition," Editorial, *Ala. Med. J.* 20 (1908): 301–02.

121. "The American Tuberculosis Exhibition," Editorial, *Ala. Med. J.* 20 (1908): 301–02.

122. "The International Congress on Tuberculosis," Editorial, *Ala. Med. J.* 20 (1908): 546–47.

123. Brown and Nabers, p. 7.

124. B. L. Wyman, "Annual Message of the President," *Trans.* (1909), p. 24.

125. Brown and Nabers, p. 9.

126. Ibid.

127. Ibid.

128. Ibid., p. 10.

129. Ibid.

130. Minutes of Jefferson County Anti-Tuberculosis Association, June 24, 1910, in office of Jefferson County Tuberculosis Assoc. (hereafter cited as Minutes).

131. Minutes, 19 October 1910.

132. Minutes, 17 January 1911.

133. Dr. Lull was honored in 1953 when the $30,000 Education Building at the Jefferson County Sanatorium was named for him. The Jefferson Tuberculosis Sanatorium was opened in 1920 and operated for the care of patients with tuberculosis for fifty years. The name was changed to the Lakeshore Hospital in August, 1972. The facility became a rehabilitation center for crippling diseases in 1973. *Birmingham News*, 5 & 6 Nov. 1973.

134. Brown and Nabers, pp. 14–15.

135. Ludden, table 23, p. 329.

136. Brown and Nabers, pp. 15–16.

137. Ibid., p. 16.

138. Ibid., p. 21.

139. Ibid.

140. Ibid., p. 17.

141. Ibid., p. 18.

142. Ibid., p. 22.

143. Ibid., p. 23.

144. Ibid., pp. 23–24.

145. Stabler, "Dissertation," pp. 138–39.

146. 1963 state funds allocated for tuberculosis $2,728,735.31. Total state allocations for the Health Department $4,347,537.73, *Annual Report, Alabama Department of Health* 1963, p. 5.

147. *Annual Report, Alabama Department of Health* 1965, p. 35.

148. B. B. Simms, "Annual Message of the President," *Trans.* (1915), p. 12.

149. Schoonover, pp. 230–31.

Chapter 13

The History of the Mental Health Movement in Alabama

Early Laws

In the early 1800s, mental illness was poorly understood by the physicians of Alabama. At that time no organization of physicians existed, and there were no medical publications to further communications about mental illness within the medical profession. It is interesting and probably unique to note that the problems of mental health helped contribute to the initial organization of the state medical society.

At the time that Alabama became a state in 1819, some public responsibility for the mentally ill and the mentally deficient was set down in the laws of the territorial government. These laws were first enacted in 1803 and later revised in 1807 while Alabama was still part of the Mississippi Territory. According to Katherine Vickery, who wrote *A History of Mental Health in Alabama*, every county probate court was empowered, "where any idiots, or lunatics shall be within the jurisdiction thereof, to appoint them a guardian, taking bond with approved security for the faithful administration of the trust reposed in such a guardian in the same manner as bonds are taken from the guardians of orphans."[1] This law also provided for trial by jury, and established the fact that the court was presided over by a county judge of probate. If the mentally ill individual was fortunate enough to recover from his mental disability, his property and rights were restored to him.

Patients could be brought to the court upon request of relatives or friends who would describe their illness and give their names, ages, sex, and residences. This application was to be accompanied by an affidavit that the petitioner believed these statements to be true. The county judge of probate then set a day for a hearing and directed the sheriff to summon a jury. The sheriff was to furnish transportation for the allegedly insane person to the place of trial. If the individual was found to be "an idiot, lunatic or *non compos mentis* and was indigent, the law provided that he be cared for in [county] 'poor houses' or 'poor farms' " where hundreds were left to languish and die.[2] These facilities, which operated in most counties, were supported from the counties' treasuries. Alternatively, patients with mental illness were frequently confined at home in cellars and attics, under conditions too inhuman for belief.

In 1822, no Alabama code of laws existed, so Henry Hitchcock, the attorney general of Alabama, compiled an abstract of such laws to be used by local justices of the peace. This abstract included all the duties, powers, and authorities of the office of the justice of the peace.[3] It defined a lunatic or *non compos mentis* by the common law as:

> *Non compos mentis* is of four kinds. First [Idiots], who are of non sane memory from their nativity, by a perpetual infirmity. Secondly, Those that lose their memory and understanding by the visitation of God, as by sickness, or other accident. Thirdly, Lunatics who have sometimes their understanding and sometimes not. Fourthly, Drunkards, who, by their own vicious act, for a time deprive themselves of their memory and understanding.[4]

Idiots were not held responsible under the law because they were "under a natural disability [for] distinguishing between good and evil."[5] On the other hand, drunkards were not allowed any privileges and were judged as though they were of sound mind. If a person who had committed a capital offense became insane before conviction, he was not tried or if he became so after conviction, he was not executed.

The improvement in medical care for the mentally ill was a matter of constant concern to early physicians in Alabama. There was no method of treatment other than confinement in jails, county poorhouses, or restraint in private homes. The medical profession concluded that a state-supported hospital for the insane was sorely needed and undertook the task of gaining public support for this endeavor.

It was not until after a hospital for the insane was established that a physician's affidavit was deemed necessary in determining the legal status of persons suffering from mental illness or disease, and then it was only necessary for the purpose of commitment to the hospital. The Act of 1852 establishing the Alabama Hospital for the Insane required the county probate judge, upon committing a patient, to have on file a "respectable" physician's statement together with that of at least one other disinterested person.*

Dorothea Lynde Dix Visits Alabama

Miss Dorothea Lynde Dix (1802–1881) of Boston was an early crusader for humane treatment of the mentally ill in this country as well as abroad. She pleaded their cause in almost all the state legislatures of this

---

*The actual name of the Alabama Hospital for the Insane was "The Alabama Insane Hospital." Acts of Alabama, 6 February 1852, p. 10.

country prior to the Civil War. She sought the establishment of hospitals where mentally ill patients could receive treatment. In most instances, she was successful.

Miss Dix made her first visit to Alabama in the spring of 1847. After traveling by river steamer to New Orleans and Mobile, she visited Selma, Alabama.[6] Miss Dix continued on to Tuscaloosa where she visited in the home of Henry W. Collier, chief justice of the Supreme Court of Alabama who was later elected governor of the state. During her visit she convinced Judge Collier of the worthiness of her cause.

Physicians in Alabama, principally Drs. Albert Gallatin Mabry and Drewry Fair of Selma, had long been aware of the problems of mentally ill patients and the need for a hospital for their treatment. This subject had been discussed at length at the local medical society in Selma. It was concluded that the cooperation of other physicians in the state would have to be enlisted. During the year of 1847, Dr. Mabry contacted the physicians of Mobile suggesting a convention for the purpose of obtaining support for the construction of a hospital for the care of the insane.[7]

As a direct result of this inquiry, the physicians from the southern part of the state assembled in Mobile and organized The Medical Association of the State of Alabama on December 1, 1847.[8] One of their avowed purposes was to petition the General Assembly for funds to establish a hospital for the insane. This facility did not become a reality until 1852.

Although the minutes of the early State Medical Association meetings are not available, Dr. Benjamin Hogan of Dallas County had been appointed by the Association in 1847 to attend the next meeting of the General Assembly.[9] He presented the recommendation of the Association for the establishment of such a hospital. These plans were not successful.[10]

In 1849, Miss Dix returned to Alabama to plead the cause of a hospital for the insane.[11] Miss Dix's plea was read to the General Assembly by Senator George N. Stewart of Mobile, inasmuch as it was not deemed proper for a woman to address an all-male legislature. Miss Dix's "memorial" cited a desperate need in Alabama for an institution to care for the mentally ill patients. She reported that one-half of such patients treated early in their illness could possibly return to a normal life. Two thousand copies of Miss Dix's "memorial" were printed and distributed to members of the legislature and to prominent individuals in the state.[12]

The General Assembly appeared favorably inclined to establish such a hospital. The retiring Governor Reuben Chapman (governor of Alabama, 1847–1849) endorsed the project. Therefore, a bill to establish a state hospital for the insane was introduced and was referred to a committee on November 26, 1849. The Committee considered using the building and grounds of the former capitol in Tuscaloosa for the

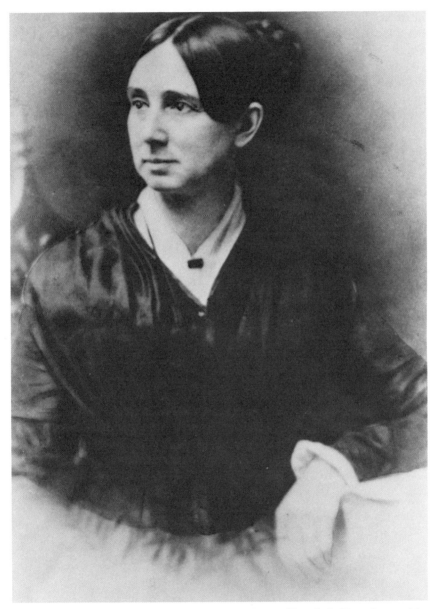

Dorothea Lynde Dix, 1802–1881 (Courtesy Bryce Hospital, Tuscaloosa, Alabama)

hospital, but abandoned the idea. Failing to pass the Senate on December 14, 1849, the bill was postponed for discussion until December 20. On the evening of December 14, 1849, the state capitol in Montgomery was destroyed by fire. This disaster almost sounded a death knell for the proposed hospital and a disappointed Miss Dix traveled on to Mississippi to continue her nationwide campaign.

In his inaugural address to the General Assembly on December 21, 1849, the new governor and friend of Miss Dix, H. W. Collier (governor of Alabama, 1849–1853), recommended the establishment of such a hospital facility, in spite of the disastrous fire. In 1850, a new committee was appointed by the State Medical Association to again petition the General Assembly for such a hospital. This committee was composed of Drs. A. Lopez, S. Holt, W. H. Anderson, H. V. Wooten, W. O. Baldwin, and William Boling. Their first efforts failed due to the strained financial status of the state treasury. However, later efforts were more successful, for two reasons. First, each physician had taken a census in his own county to determine the actual number of mentally ill, and the study revealed many more such individuals in the state than previous statistics had shown. Secondly, the physicians made an appeal directly to the governor to support the cause on the basis of moral duty.

Governor Collier, in his annual address to the General Assembly on November 11, 1851, again recommended the establishment of a state-supported hospital for the insane.[13] The bill was passed on February 6, 1852, and a committee was appointed to choose a building site.[14]

Miss Dix continued her interest in the hospital for the insane in Alabama; however, it is not known whether she ever visited the hospital after its completion.

The Hospital for the Insane Becomes a Reality

The Act of 1852 establishing the hospital stipulated that the place selected as a building site should have the following advantages:

1st. It shall contain at least one half section of land, one hundred acres of which shall be susceptible to cultivation . . .
2nd. It shall be . . . easily accessible . . .
3rd. It shall be in a healthy situation.
4th. There shall be upon the premises a supply of never failing water of good quality.
5th. It shall be so situated as to receive supplies of fuel, either wood or coal, . . .
6th. The site of the buildings shall be susceptibile of good underground drainage.
7th. It should command cheerful views.

8th. It shall open [on] such aspects as will admit the sun's rays a portion of the day into every [suite] of the building appartments.[15]

The General Assembly appropriated $100,000 for the construction of the hospital. This sum represented 5 percent of the net revenue of the state for the ensuing four years. Tuscaloosa County was selected for its location, and a 326-acre tract of land near the city of Tuscaloosa was purchased. Dr. Aaron Lopez was instructed by the legislature to collect information concerning the best type of building in which to house these patients. The building plan selected was known as the Kirkbride Plan and was prepared by Sloan and Steward, architects from Philadelphia, who worked under the direction of the famous Dr. Thomas S. Kirk-bride, superintendent of the Hospital for the Insane in Philadelphia. The plan consisted of a large center building, four stories high, with wings on each side three stories high and with accommodations for approximately 300 patients. The estimated cost was $250,000. The cornerstone was laid July 14, 1853.

In voting to place the hospital at Tuscaloosa, a medium-sized town in central Alabama, the General Assembly had been influenced by Senator Robert Jemison, Jr., from Tuscaloosa County.

Funds for the building were soon exhausted, and in 1856, the General Assembly appropriated $150,000 for its completion. Governor John A. Winston vetoed the bill, claiming that the funds already allocated had been improperly handled. Famous for his vetoes, Governor Winston stated:

I feel warranted in asserting that the [funds] then appropriated [had] been most shamefully perverted by those who have had the management of the planning of the building and the expenditure of the appropriation; . . .

The location is accessible neither by railroads or navigable streams, and only with delay and fatigue in any other manner. . . . The want of hotels for the accomodation of those who will be compelled to attend the inmates of the Asylum is also a consideration against the locality.

. . . We may expend half a million dollars in its construction, but it will never be fully occupied except by bats and owls.[16]

Stung by this criticism, Senator Jemison demanded that the Governor present proof that the funds originally appropriated for the hospital "had been shamefully perverted" by the people managing the selection of the site and construction of the hospital.

There is no evidence that Governor Winston altered his views. The appropriation bill was passed over the governor's veto and work pro-ceeded, albeit slowly. In 1858, an additional $5,000 was appropriated for furnishings for the hospital and fencing the grounds. In 1860, $24,000 was appropriated by the General Assembly for completion of the hospital and for the necessary expenses of operation.[17] In April of 1861, nearly ten years after the hospital was authorized, it was finally opened for patients.

The Hospital Begins Operation

A seven-member Board of Trustees, which was to oversee operation of the Alabama Hospital for the Insane, was appointed by Governor Andrew Barry Moore (governor of Alabama, 1857–1861) and submitted to the Senate for approval.[18] Dr. Reuben Searcy (1805–1887) of Tuscaloosa was a member of this first board and remained its president for a period of thirty years. Other members were Dr. James Guild, Dr. A. G. Mabry, Reverend Basil Manly, Judge A. S. Clitherall, Captain R. T. Nott, and Mr. Porter King.[19]

Dr. Peter Bryce (1834–1892) of Columbia, South Carolina, wrote the Board of Trustees on December 30, 1859, submitting his application for the superintendency. Miss Dix knew of Dr. Bryce's accomplishments and recommended him for this position.

Dr. Bryce had graduated from the Medical College of the University of New York in 1859. He had visited hospitals for the insane in Europe and served as assistant physician at the Hospital for the Insane of New Jersey and the State Hospital for the Insane at Columbia, South Carolina. Dr. Bryce was appointed superintendent by the board on July 6, 1860, at a salary of $2,000 annually in addition to his rent and household expenses. In its letter of appointment, the Board of Trustees stipulated that he must be married before assuming his duties. This was no problem for Dr. Bryce, as he brought with him his bride, the former Marie Ellen Clarkson of Columbia, South Carolina. He was twenty-six years old, and she was nineteen.[20] Mrs. Bryce, a talented and dedicated woman, exerted a profound influence on hospital life. She and Dr. Bryce had no children, and she devoted her life to the service of the hospital patients, conducting religious services, musical programs, and providing various forms of entertainment.

While the board had insisted that Dr. Bryce be married, his only request of them was that he be allowed to put his theories for treating mentally ill patients into practice without hindrance of any kind. The board readily agreed to this.

In an age when medication and other methods of treatment for the mentally ill were virtually unknown, Peter Bryce was far advanced in his thinking. He firmly believed in the following three principles, which he insisted should be started as early as possible: (1) tender loving care, (2)

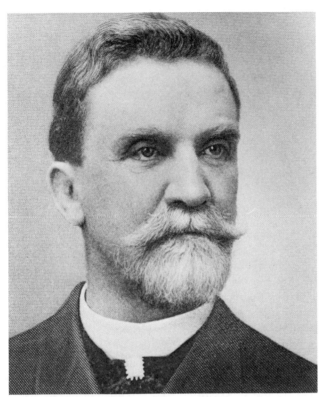

Peter Bryce, M.D., 1834–1892
(Courtesy Bryce Hospital, Tuscaloosa, Alabama)

occupational therapy, and (3) nonrestraint. These principles of treatment were to make him known and loved throughout the nation, and they were to bring high praise to the Alabama hospital for its humane treatment of the mentally ill. His conscientious adherence to these rules established a precedent for those who came after him. More than a century has passed and many new methods of treatment have been introduced, but the principles established by Peter Bryce are still in use in the mental institutions in Alabama.

Dr. Bryce engaged a nurse, Miss Ellen Barry, and two brothers, John and Patrick Kehoe, all from Mobile, to help administer affairs at the hospital.[21] John Kehoe was in charge of the building and grounds, and Pat Kehoe supervised the male patients. Miss Barry and the Kehoe brothers arrived in Tuscaloosa in April, 1861, on the riverboat *The John W. Wallace*. Dr. Bryce, Miss Barry, Pat and John Kehoe comprised the first staff of the Alabama Hospital for the Insane in Tuscaloosa.

Rules and Regulations for Employees of the Hospital

One of Dr. Bryce's chief concerns was to see that the patients received the best treatment possible. Therefore he was most concerned about the behavior of nurses and other employees toward the patients. He devised a system of rules and regulations for the employees, whereby fines were to be paid by those who could not or would not conform. Apparently, there were many infractions of the rules, for a total of $500 in fines was assessed the first year. Each employee was fined no less than twenty-five cents for an infraction of the rules. Two of the rules for which fines could be imposed were as follows:

1. Discourteous treatment, or impolite language to a patient.

2. Failure to keep the patients clean, neatly dressed, and properly attended at all times.[22]

Dr. Bryce realized that his system was rigid, but it enabled him to eliminate those who were not dedicated to their work. In this manner, he was also able to identify individuals who were genuinely interested in helping the mentally ill.

Dr. Bryce was a deeply religious man, outspoken in his views—particularly those on alcoholism. He felt that alcohol, tobacco, and opium were principal factors in the increased incidence of mental illness. It was his opinion that alcoholics should be confined in a separate hospital, disciplined, and given some form of employment. He believed that such an individual should be kept institutionalized for a period of five to ten years in order to regain self-control.

It was Dr. Bryce's belief that patients who were mentally deficient should be confined for life in a hospital or home suited for their particular needs. His philosophy of nonrestraint and kindness applied to these patients also.

The State Hospital During the Civil War and Reconstruction

The first patient admitted to the Alabama Hospital for the Insane was a forty-eight-year-old soldier sent from Fort Morgan on order of General Duff Green, Confederate States Army. He arrived April 5, 1861. The patient's illness was diagnosed as mania A. The alleged cause was political excitement.[23]

It is remarkable that the hospital survived the socioeconomic upheaval of the Civil War and the reconstruction era. Much to the dismay of Dr. Bryce, the recruiting officers for the Confederate Army were constantly attempting to enlist the employees of the hospital. Funds for care of the patients at the hospital were very limited as almost all available state funds went towards the war efforts. The Board of Resident Trustees granted permission for a portion of the building to be used as a hospital for the injured and sick Confederate soldiers, and after the Battle of Shiloh in 1862, the east wing was converted into a military hospital.[24]

One account of an historic event at the Alabama Hospital for the Insane has survived.[25] On the night of April 3–4, 1865, General John T. Croxton of the Union Army invaded Tuscaloosa with 1,500 mounted men. He had orders to burn the University of Alabama. Patrick Kehoe, supervisor for male patients, was in Tuscaloosa that night and gave the alarm that federal troops were approaching the University. The University of Alabama was burned, including its excellent library. Only token military resistance was offered. The next morning a detachment of Croxton's men went to the hospital for the insane and was met at the door by Dr. Bryce, Pat Kehoe, and C. W. Shedd, the steward. Shedd, who was from a Northern state, said, "Gentlemen, I am glad to see you." Dr. Bryce, however, told them that he was not pleased to see them, but if they wished to go through the building they could. The soldiers left the hospital unharmed probably because they decided it would be unkind and useless to disturb the patients. Meanwhile John Kehoe, in an effort to keep the horses and mules belonging to the hospital from being confiscated, led the animals to some dense woods about a mile from the hospital. His plan did not succeed as sometime that afternoon the federal troops discovered the animals and seized them. Except for the loss of its animals, the hospital suffered no direct damage from the enemy.

The resident trustees attended a called meeting on June 26, 1865, to consider Shedd's resignation. Shedd probably was not sympathetic with the difficulties Dr. Bryce had experienced as a result of the Civil War. He appeared before the trustees and presented a list of charges against Dr. Bryce's administration of the hospital. These were read and inquiries were made. The charges were dismissed "as unfounded and unworthy of further consideration."[26]

There was little or no money in the South immediately after the war. The majority of the white population had been ruined financially. Although the slaves were free, they were untrained and, therefore, unable to obtain work.

By 1865, the hospital was in considerable debt. The trustees made a complete report of the conditions to the governor in hope of obtaining assistance. However, no financial help was forthcoming. The hospital continued to have financial difficulty, and the board decided to ask the governor's permission to seek a loan from the United States Government in the amount of $15,000.[27] Dr. Bryce was authorized to negotiate the loan and was given power of attorney to mortgage the hospital and grounds as security for the loan, but he failed to secure any assistance from the federal government. The plight of the hospital was now desperate. The trustees decided that a petition on the subject should be drawn up and presented to the General Assembly. The state's financial situation was in a deplorable condition. Lewis E. Parsons, the provisional governor (June, 1865–December, 1865) appointed by President Andrew Johnson, pointed out in an address to the General Assembly of 1865 that there were many individuals who were impoverished due to the war and who must have food to tide them over the winter. Therefore, the hospital, as well as other state facilities, could not expect any financial assistance from the state.

Governor Parsons did appoint a Senate Committee with Senator J. T. Foster of Sumter and Choctaw counties as chairman to inquire about the conditions at the Alabama Hospital for the Insane as well as about those at the Deaf and Dumb Asylum in Talladega. The committee reported that the hospital continued to have a good reputation, but that the state had no financial means on hand to allocate for the institution.[28] Dr. Bryce was left to solve the hospital's problems in whatever way he could.

During that time, there were twenty-six black patients under treatment in the hospital. In 1868, $1,900 was made available to the hospital by the Freedman's Bureau for use in the care of black patients. Brevet Lieutenant Colonel Edwin Beecher, assistant commissioner of the Freedman's Bureau, also authorized agents to issue rations for the black patients.

Some individuals donated money to the hospital in this crisis. Miss Dix had not forgotten the hospital, and she sent a contribution of $100 and some books for the hospital library. She also obtained monetary contributions from other individuals. The exigencies of the reconstruction era forced the hospital to become almost self-sustaining. The patients and their attendants did the farming, gardening, and laundry.

In 1869, the State Medical Association recommended that the hospital be authorized to admit inebriates and "opium eaters." However, the Board of Trustees did not believe it practical or wise to admit these patients. Instead, they agreed to unite with the Association in recommending to the General Assembly that a suitable hospital be established for treatment of such patients.[29] No action was taken on this recommendation.

Dr. Bryce's reports and the minutes of the meetings of the Board of Trustees reflect the courage of the individuals responsible for the hospital during the first decade of its operation. They reveal not only the financial difficulties of the post–Civil War years but also the then-limited knowledge of psychiatric illness. They also reflect the exceptional intelligence, perseverance, and insight of Dr. Bryce and his board in meeting the needs of the hospital and the patients. Although Dr. Bryce lacked modern means of diagnosis and treatment, he was aware of the patients' need for kindness and understanding rather than restraint and punishment.

The Hospital After 1870

In Dr. Bryce's report of 1870, he reiterated that:

The old and very absurd [idea] that insanity is a disgrace and ought to be concealed, and that patients are abused or neglected in even the best conducted hospitals for the insane, are still entertained, . . . It seems, too, to have been forgotten or discredited in many quarters, that dungeons, cells, chains, cribs, showerbaths, and other appliances of cruelty, have long since been abandoned in the scientific treatment of insanity; and that, combined with judicious medication, systematic kindness, and undeviating candor, with firmness, are alone the great moral agents upon which the humane and enlightened physician relies for success.[30]

Dr. Bryce continued to be concerned with the number of deaths of patients suffering with "fevers." He complained that the mentally ill were being kept at home until hopelessly prostrated by disease and that the patients often reached the hospital in a moribund condition.[31] Many patients arrived by horse-drawn vehicle in all types of weather and were frequently malnourished. Certainly, distance and lack of suitable transportation were factors in the high mortality rate.

A description of the journey from Talladega to Tuscaloosa by Reverend Joseph Camp of Mumford, Alabama, a patient at the Tuscaloosa hospital, has survived.[32] The difficulties experienced on this trip probably best explained why patients in the more remote areas of Alabama frequently found it difficult to travel to the hospital. On Thursday, May 19, 1881, Reverend Camp, his wife, and son-in-law left Talladega at 2:30 P.M. via the railroad for Calera. They spent the night there and the next morning they continued on by train to Birmingham. They spent several hours in Birmingham and then boarded the train for Tuscaloosa, arriving late in the evening on May 20th. It can be seen that even with transportation by railway the trip proved to be quite arduous.

Public Attitude Toward the Hospital

Some idea of the attitude of Alabamians toward the hospital may be gained from the following article that appeared in the *Eutaw Mirror* on April 26, 1881:

we had the melancholy pleasure of going through the entire institution, and were much delighted at the exquisite neatness and order that pervaded every part of the building. The first floor which is used for the better class of patients, with its long carpeted halls, and many bed rooms opening in same, . . . like a well kept hotel. Save for the unfortunate beings grouped together, you would never know the difference. . . .

We were struck on being shown into a small dining parlor, for the use of the invalids, whose delicate constitutions refused substantial food and could only relish something light and dainty. . . . What a blessing such an institution is to the country. . . . No unkindness is ever practiced or permitted among its keepers, no harsh words ever spoken, to the unfortunate beings, while everything is done to make them comfortable and happy as they can be under the circumstances. Religious services are held on Sunday afternoon in the chapel, . . . morning prayer is conducted daily. . . . Mrs. Bryce, . . . has been organist and leader of the singing since the opening of the institutuion.

. . . Dr. Bryce has provided pianos, billiards, ten pens, croquet, etc. for the pleasure of his patients. . . .

The insane hospital at [Tuscaloosa], is conducted more economically than any building of [its] kind in the southern states.[33]

A different view was offered by Reverend Joseph Camp, the patient who made the railway trip and who was, as he expressed it, "incarcerated" in the Alabama hospital in 1881. In 1882, he privately published a book entitled *An Insight Into An Insane Asylum* in which he tells of his experiences in the hospital in Tuscaloosa. The stated purpose of the book was to let Alabamians know just how weak the laws governing the institution were. He was very critical of the fact that only one man was under bond to the state at the time "yet, the lives of hundreds of our husbands, wives, sons, and daughters and thousands of dollars are in their hands." He further stated:

Dr. Bryce has more power and apparently less to do than any king or potentate on earth, for all he does is to pass through the various wards twice a week—Tuesday and Friday mornings at nine o'clock—with his young officers, [B. L.] Wyman, the physician, who had just graduated and went there one month before I went, Mr. Perkins, the secretary, and Davis, the apothecary, who told me he had never been out of the county of Tuscaloosa. . . . On the first review after I arrived at the institution, when he [Dr. Bryce] reached the eighth ward where I was incarcerated, he approached me and said he had heard that I was at the Centennial [1876]. I told him I was. . . . The doctor then left with his retinue of officers. The next time I asked him how he could treat me without an examination. He answered that he looked at me. I wondered how it was possible by looking at me he or anyone else could tell the internal complaint.[34]

There are no known responses to Reverend Camp's exposé.

Dr. Bryce's Studies of Syphilis

In 1872, Dr. Bryce reported on a study of patients who had been admitted to the hospital with a diagnosis of general paralysis or paresis.[35] Syphilis had not yet been recognized as the cause of this mental illness. Inasmuch as the disease's chief manifestation was an increasing general weakness rather than a paralysis, Dr. Bryce coined the term "general paresis," rather than the term "general paralysis" by which it was then known. It was not until 1894 that Dr. Alfred Fournier (1832–1914) of Paris reported that 65 percent of such patients that he had studied had a history of syphilis; and it was not until 1913 that Dr. Hicleyo Noguchi (1876–1928) and Dr. Joseph Earle Moore (1892–1957) demonstrated the causative organism of syphilis in the brain cortex in patients with general paresis.

Dr. Bryce's Nonrestraint Methods

Dr. Bryce was recognized as one of the outstanding authorities on mental health in the United States as well as a leader in the medical circles in Alabama. He continued to remonstrate against a movement favoring restraint in the care of patients with mental illness. He reported his philosophy in the *Medico-Legal Journal* of March, 1891. In the same issue, there appeared an editorial praising Dr. Bryce for his methods and suggesting that perhaps if a physician could not control the insane patients without using mechanical restraint he should seriously reconsider his ability to function as superintendent of an asylum for the mentally ill.[36]

In 1882, Dr. G. A. Tucker, an Australian physician, made an extensive international survey of mental institutions and their methods of treatment. He visited more than 100 institutions in the United States and reported that the Alabama Hospital for the Insane was one of only five where he found the system of absolute nonrestraint in practice.[37]

Near the end of his life, Dr. Bryce elaborated on his theory of the use of occupational therapy in the treatment of the insane. He quoted Thomas Carlyle's saying that "work is the grand cure of all the maladies and miseries that ever beset mankind" and observed that if Carlyle "had been writing with special reference to the insane, he could not have made a truer observation."[38] He considered that a life of enforced idleness could destroy the peace and tranquility of the patients. He enforced a rule that all patients must work except the physically ill or the acutely insane. As a result, more than 90 percent of the women and more than 75 percent of the men were actively employed in duties at the hospital complex. The female patients did most of the cooking, sewing, and laundry for the hospital. The men cultivated and harvested vegetables, processed meat, poultry, and other farm products. Some of the surplus was sold, thus increasing the hospital income.

Recreational therapy also played a part in the hospital treatment. Dr. Bryce requested donations of books, pianos, billiards, and cards, and many responded. He encouraged the patients to have dances and to take long walks in the surrounding woods. Dr. Bryce endeavored to make the hospital a home for the patients. He even had pictures hung in the wards housing the most disturbed patients. These pictures were highly appreciated and rarely defaced.

Dr. Bryce died August 4, 1892, and by his own request was buried on the lawn of the institution he had so capably and faithfully served for thirty-two years. In 1900, the General Assembly honored this remarkable man by changing the name of the Alabama Hospital for the Insane to Bryce Hospital. The foundation for the treatment of the mentally ill in Alabama had been well laid by Dr. Peter Bryce.

Mount Vernon Hospital Established

After Dr. Bryce's death, Dr. E. D. Bondurant served temporarily as acting superintendent until Dr. James T. Searcy was elected superintendent of the hospital on October 6, 1892. Dr. Bondurant served thereafter as the hospital's first pathologist.

Dr. James T. Searcy had served as chairman of the Board of Trustees of the Alabama Hospital for the Insane following the death of his father, Dr. Reuben Searcy. He had also served as an assistant staff physician at the hospital. Dr. Searcy was a Phi Beta Kappa graduate of the University of Alabama and valedictorian of his medical college class at the University of New York City. During the Civil War, he had served in the Confederate Army Medical Department, and after the war, he practiced medicine in Tuscaloosa.

One of Dr. Searcy's chief concerns was the proper care of the black patients. As Bryce Hospital continued to be overcrowded, with 1,148 patients in 1892, this problem had immediacy. After the Civil War, blacks had been admitted to segregated facilities in Bryce Hospital, but the original building had become so crowded that a separate facility for black patients had been built in 1883. However, even this facility could accommodate only a limited number of patients.

Dr. Searcy petitioned Washington authorities for the use of an abandoned military reservation located north of Mobile at Mount Vernon.[39] He wanted to use it as a hospital for insane blacks. The federal government awarded this facility to the state of Alabama on March 1, 1895. A lack of funds resulted in a delay in its use as a hospital until December 11, 1900. The property consisted of 1,600 acres of land that could be farmed. Dr. Searcy felt that with proper renovations the existing building could be used as a hospital for 400 to 500 patients. The state appropriated $25,000 for this renovation.

Dr. Searcy realized that the greatest economy had to be exercised if these funds were to cover the cost of renovation. The patients and employees at Bryce Hospital made the windows and other prefabricated building materials, which were then shipped to Mount Vernon. The renovations took about a year to complete, and in May of 1902, 318 black patients and 25 employees were transferred to the new facility. It remained a segregated hospital for insane black patients until the mid-twentieth century.

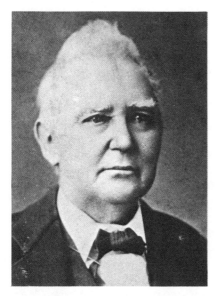

Reuben Searcy, M.D., 1805–1887 (Courtesy of Mrs. Leslie Dee, Jr., Great-Granddaughter, Tuscaloosa, Alabama)

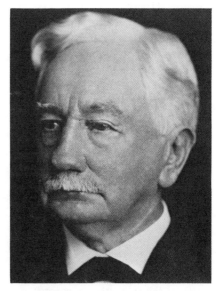

James Thomas Searcy, M.D., 1839–1920 (Courtesy of Mrs. Leslie Dee, Jr., Granddaughter, Tuscaloosa, Alabama)

Dr. Searcy's Definition of Insanity

It was Dr. Searcy's opinion that it would be far better to limit the term "insanity" to those individuals who showed an element of danger either to others or themselves. Also he felt that other derivations should be used to describe those individuals who were inoffensive and harmless. He believed that the incidence of insanity in the population was increasing, and because of this there would be a need for more hospitals for mental patients.[40]

Dr. Searcy deplored the large number of elderly, harmless, and senile individuals confined to the hospitals, but he also felt that the county poorhouses were ill equipped to care for these people. If they were discharged, they most likely would be confined to these unsatisfactory county facilities. He strongly recommended that the State Legislature aid in an effort to improve county care of paupers, which would in turn aid in decreasing the number admitted to the hospitals.

Revision of Laws Governing the Hospitals

In 1900–1901, the entire system of laws governing the Alabama Hospitals for the Insane was revised. Both Bryce Hospital and Mount Vernon Hospital were placed under the direction of one Board of Trustees and became known as the Alabama Hospitals for the Insane.* The Board of Trustees was made self-perpetuating. The new law specifically stipulated that the hospitals were to be maintained "solely for the care, treatment and custody of insane patients; no other class of patients shall be admitted."[41]

The laws governing the hospitals empowered the Board of Trustees to select a superintendent who would be accountable to them and would also serve as an executive member of the board. The superintendent was to be "a physician [with] good business capabilities, of a humane disposition, a graduate in medicine, and a man of good moral character."[42] He was to serve not less than eight years, and he could choose his own personnel. He also had the right to refuse admission to patients if the overcrowded situation warranted.

The law defined the insane individual much the way Dr. Searcy did as one "who, because of mental derangement, deficiency or defectiveness, is indecent in conduct or constantly troublesome to others; or who is a menace to the peace, welfare or safety of others; or who is dangerous to his (or her) own life or safety; or who is destructive of property."[43] In order for a patient to be admitted to the hospital, an elaborate questionnaire had to be completed and approved by the local county judge of

---

*The Alabama Insane Hospitals is the correct title.

probate. It also denied admission to "persons who [were] simply and permanently weak-minded, imbecile, idiotic, or otherwise demented, and [were] harmless" or patients whose mental derangement was due to intoxication.[44] However, every annual report revealed that a few such individuals had been admitted to the hospital.

Problems in the Hospitals

Pellagra Identified in the Hospitals

In 1906, the Board of Trustees of the Alabama Hospitals for the Insane met at the Mount Vernon Hospital. Dr. Searcy reported the occurrence of a new illness that was found in large numbers of patients at this facility. The Board of Trustees empowered him to do whatever he thought necessary to discover the nature of the disease and its control. Dr. Searcy discussed the clinical symptoms and findings of this new disease with his son, Dr. George H. Searcy (1877–1935), who thought

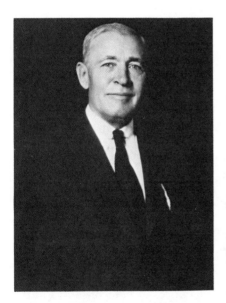
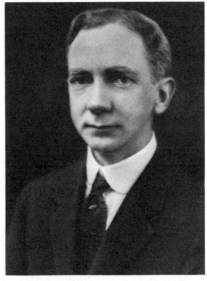

William Dempsey Partlow, M.D., 1877–1953 (Courtesy of Mrs. Margaret Partlow Pritchett, Daughter, Tuscaloosa, Alabama)

George Harris Searcy, M.D., 1877–1935 (Courtesy of Mrs. Harriet Searcy Murphy, Daughter, Chevy Chase, Maryland)

the disease might possibly be a condition previously identified in Italy as pellagra. Dr. George Searcy and the assistant superintendent, Dr. E. L. McCafferty, assembled data on these patients. In 1912, Dr. E. J. Wood published *A Treatise on Pellagra* in which this work was recognized.

> Nineteen hundred and seven saw the first real scientific work in this country, . . . for then it was that this great scourge, which has been [the] known curse of Italy for over a century and a half, became the problem of vastest importance equaling in the southern states the problem of tuberculosis. Probably no medical subject has ever produced such profound interest on the part of the medical profession as did pellagra at that time and ever since. The man whose name will be ever connected as the discoverer of the existence of the disease in this country is [Dr.] George H. Searcy, who reported an epidemic at the Mt. Vernon, Alabama, Insane Institution for Negroes. The cases were carefully studied by him, and also [Dr.] E. L. McCafferty of the staff of this hospital. They were assisted by [Drs.] E. D. Bondurant of [Mobile] and Isadore Dyer of New Orleans. This report embraced an account of eighty-eight cases with a fatality of fifty-seven. In this same year, 1907, [Dr.] J. T. Searcy reported nine cases from the Bryce Memorial Hospital in [Tuscaloosa,] Alabama. . . . The importance of Searcy's work can hardly be overestimated. Through the help of his report in the *Journal of the American Medical Association* within a few weeks the disease was recognized in a half dozen states and its identity with the Italian pellagra irrefutably established. Our increasing knowledge of the disease . . . has added little to the description of Searcy. This observation was accurate and complete.[45]

These Alabama physicians were the first to diagnose pellagra in the United States, and Dr. George Searcy's studies showed that diet was a principal factor in its occurrence and prevention. Economic conditions in the state hindered the implementation of this finding. A posthumous citation was presented to Dr. George Searcy by the Medical Association of the State of Alabama on February 21, 1940, recognizing his important work on pellagra.

Complaint of Patient Mistreatment

In 1907, a complaint of mistreatment of patients at Bryce Hospital resulted in a legislative investigation. Governor B. B. Comer appointed a committee of three members of the State Legislature, and the trustees asked Judge J. M. Chilton to represent them at the hearing. No basis for the complaint was found. Judge Chilton expressed the consensus of the investigative committee to the Board of Trustees:

> It is a matter of extreme regret to the friends of your institution that this investigation was ever ordered. Its only result has been to injure the most

beneficent institution in the State—one that has stood for years in the front rank of hospitals of this character, especially in the advances made in the matter of scientific treatment of the insane.

Your honored Superintendent has devoted practically his whole life to the welfare of the Hospital, and it is a poor reward, after these years of devoted service, that an investigation so grossly impugning his conduct of the institution should have been summarily ordered without even a preliminary hearing before a committee of the Legislature.[46]

Dr. Searcy Resigns

Ill health forced Dr. Searcy to resign in June, 1919. He was eighty years of age at the time of his death on April 6, 1920. The black population of the city of Tuscaloosa paid tribute to Dr. Searcy in appreciation for the work he had done for their race by establishing the hospital at Mount Vernon. In 1919, this hospital was renamed by legislative act, The Searcy Hospital.[47]

Dr. William Dempsey Partlow (1877–1953) succeeded Dr. Searcy as superintendent. Dr. Partlow, a native of Alabama, received his M.D. degree in 1901 from the medical department of the University of Alabama. In addition to his considerable capabilities as a physician, Dr. Partlow was a man of action and a social planner with a political astuteness rarely found in medically trained individuals. His comprehension of the scope of the mental hygiene movement motivated him to involve others in this field. He encouraged prominent individuals in the national mental health field to visit Alabama and continued to cultivate the interest of civic groups and individuals in the state.

The Russell Sage Foundation Evaluates the Hospitals

At the request of Governor Charles Henderson, the Russell Sage Foundation of New York City conducted an evaluation of the Alabama Hospitals for the Insane as well as other social agencies in Alabama. The foundation's goal is "the improvement of social and living conditions in the United States."[48] Mr. Hastings H. Hart of this foundation visited Alabama in 1918 and published a study entitled "Social Problems of Alabama," which gave a detailed observation on the two hospitals. It said in part:

The two hospitals for insane are doing social work of the highest quality. I have visited many insane hospitals, but I have never seen a more careful diagnosis or a better co-ordination of the medical work and the social work than is found in these two hospitals; but their equipment is painfully inadequate. . . .

The Alabama Bryce Hospital for the Insane was established in 1860. Its superintendent, the late Dr. Bryce, was one of the leading alienists of the United States and under his leadership, the hospital became recognized as one of the best institutions in the United States. Upon the death of Dr. Bryce, his assistant, Dr. James T. Searcy, became superintendent, and, under his leadership, the high standards of the hospital have been fully maintained.[49]

Mr. Hart went on to state that he had been familiar with hospitals for the insane for the past 35 years, but he had never observed an institution in which more regard was paid both to the medical and the human side of the problem of the mentally ill than that found in the Alabama facilities.

The Russell Sage Foundation conducted a follow-up survey of these facilities in 1922.[50] The second study was entitled "Social Progress of Alabama" and was again carried out by Mr. Hart. He reported that he found "an amazing forward movement" in both care and facilities for treatment of the mentally ill.

The Establishment of the Alabama Home for Mental Deficients

Unquestionably, Dr. W. D. Partlow was the moving force behind the establishment of the Alabama Home for Mental Deficients. At the annual meeting of the State Medical Association in 1914, he appealed for aid in the establishment of such a facility. The Association responded by appointing a committee to study the feasibility of such a home.

The Committee for the Protection of Feebleminded Children, as it was called, became a reality with Dr. C. M. Rudolph of Birmingham serving as chairman and Drs. J. S. McLester and A. F. Toole as members. It was estimated that at the time there were some 7,000 mental defectives in the state. A pamphlet was compiled detailing the need for such an institution. Copies of the pamphlet entitled "A Plea for Better Care of Alabama's Feebleminded" were mailed to each senator and representative, to newspapers, and to the president of every civic and women's club in the state. The committee gave a report at the annual meeting of the Medical Association of the State of Alabama on April 20, 1915. The report was accompanied by a proposed bill entitled "An Act—To Establish and Maintain a School for the Education and Care of Feebleminded Children, to be Known as 'The Alabama School for the Feebleminded.' "[51] The bill provided for the location and organization of the school and designated the type of patients to be admitted. The bill was introduced in the State Legislature on January 28, 1915, but failed to pass because of insufficient funds. However, the members of the Alabama Society for Mental Hygiene and the State Medical Association and other interested individuals continued to stress the need for such an institution.

In 1915, after all efforts to obtain funds to establish a school for the feebleminded had failed, Dr. W. D. Partlow convened a group of prominent citizens representing the State Medical Association, the Alabama Society for Mental Hygiene, women's clubs, and other interested organizations. He urged them to join in a petition to the 1919 Legislature to establish such an institution. The retiring governor, the Honorable Charles Henderson, in his address to the State Legislature on January 14, 1919, spoke of the problem of the feebleminded in the state and his interest in the effort to establish a home for their care and treatment.

On January 23, 1919, Representative George Ross of Jefferson County introduced a bill in the State Legislature, "To provide for the establishment and maintenance of a home for mental inferiors in Alabama."[52] The bill defined mental inferiors, provided for their care, treatment, and training and appropriated the necessary funds.[53] The bill was passed and was approved by the new governor, Thomas E. Kilby (governor of Alabama, 1919–1923).

The bill became law, but again due to a chronic shortage of funds in the state treasury, construction of the Alabama Home was delayed until 1921.[54] In 1920, the Board of Trustees of the Alabama Hospitals for the Insane, who had jurisdiction over the proposed school, appointed a Board of Managers for the Alabama Home for Mental Defectives. The Board of Managers sent C. B. Verner, chairman of the Board, Mrs. R. Dupont Thompson (Birmingham), and Sam'l Will John (Birmingham) accompanied by Dr. Partlow to inspect the outstanding schools for the feebleminded in the northeastern states.

A site for the facility was purchased. It consisted of 108 acres adjoining the eastern boundary of the Bryce Hospital property. The new buildings were ready for occupancy July 1, 1922, but the State Legislature had not provided funds for water supply, equipment, and maintenance.[55] The home was finally opened on September 1, 1923, and 118 children were admitted during the first month. Due to the lack of proper facilities, applications from children who required special care were declined. There were no facilities for black children. In 1927, the institution was renamed by the State Legislature the Partlow School for Mental Defectives, thus honoring Dr. W. D. Partlow for his work.

Dr. Partlow repeatedly cited the need to establish an institution for feebleminded black children. In 1946, a new dormitory for 200 mentally deficient black children was constructed using the labor of the resident white boys. This facility was opened in 1948.

By 1948, the population at the Partlow State School had exceeded 1,000 patients, and Dr. Partlow expressed concern that the public was making more and more demands to place children in the school. In 1950, there were 1,219 patients at Partlow, but the families of only fifteen patients were financially able to pay for such care.

The Young Men's Business Club of Birmingham decided that their civic project for the club's 1952 program would be to educate the public as to the needs of Bryce Hospital and Partlow State School. Mr. Harry V. Harding organized a parents' auxiliary for the Partlow School.[56] This auxiliary met on April 6, 1952, and elected to call themselves "Patrons of Partlow State School." The aims of the group were stated in the constitution and were as follows:

1. To aid and comfort relatives of children domiciled at the school.
2. Work for the best interests of patients and operate fully all programs to promote understanding of all mentally defective children.
3. Promote understanding between relatives and staff.
4. Promote public interest in the school.
5. Co-operate in every possible way in raising the standard of care, treatment and training of the children.[57]

In 1959–1960, the patrons established a Discretionary Fund, which enabled the school to secure dentures, eye glasses, hospitalization, surgical and medical consultations, and laboratory tests when these were necessary. This aided in providing proper medical care of these patients.

The Sterilization Controversy

Dr. Partlow exerted much of his considerable talent in an effort to establish a facility for the care of the mentally deficient.[58] It was his belief that almost all feeblemindedness was hereditary. Dr. Partlow felt that such individuals should be confined in an institution and if discharged should be sterilized.

There were several efforts made in Alabama to include persons other than the feebleminded in mandatory sterilization. In 1935, Dr. Partlow outlined the contents of a proposed sterilization bill that he recommended to the State Legislature. The bill would permit legalized sterilization for the following:

1. mental deficients,
2. any [individual] constantly or habitually dependent on public relief . . . in which such dependency may be due to mental deficiency which may be transmitted to offspring,
3. criminals who, in the opinion of the chief medical officer of the Convict Department demonstrated behavior that was sadistic, homosexual, masochistic, sodomistic or in any way an act of sexual perversion, . . .

4. persons who had been committed to a state penitentiary three times or more, or any charge of a reform school, industrial school, training school, or reformatory whom the person in charge had reason to suspect "is delinquent or dependent because of constitutional mental or moral deficiency or degeneracy which may be transmitted to offspring,"

5. . . . persons who were "constitutional psychopathic personalities."[59]

The proposed law would empower the chairman of the County Board of Censors of the local county medical society to authorize sterilization of anyone thought to be mentally deficient. The bill for sterilization passed both the House and Senate in the 1935 session of the State Legislature. However, Governor Bibb Graves (governor of Alabama, 1927–1931; 1935–1939) vetoed it due to his concern over the surgical risks that would be involved.

In 1935, Dr. Partlow reported 124 boys and 86 girls had been sterilized at Partlow State School.[60] At the March, 1939, annual session of the Alabama Society of Mental Health (founded 1915), Dr. Partlow again sought aid to have a bill passed to provide for sterilization of mental deficients. Apparently nothing further was accomplished in this regard.

The Hospitals during the Great Depression

Dr. Partlow's financial acumen resulted in saving considerable money in the management of the Alabama Hospitals for the Insane. Amazingly enough, he was able to keep them operating during the financial strain of the depression in the 1930s. In addition, he was able to cope with all the adversities that occurred with the advent of World War II and the inflation that followed.

As the depression intensified, the number of applications for admission increased. The hospitals were unable to expand, and waiting lists increased. In 1930, a survey of the patient population at Bryce Hospital revealed that there were 582 more patients confined than could be properly handled at Bryce. Searcy Hospital was also overcrowded.

Colonel Murfee's Citizens' Committee

Colonel Hopson Owen Murfee, a civic leader who had been interested in the subject of mental hygiene, was a strong ally of Dr. Partlow.[61] The Alabama Citizens' Committee for the State Hospitals and Public Health was formed in 1936 by Colonel Murfee, who served as secretary and prime mover. His committee was composed of prominent men of the state and included Harry M. Ayers, William O. Baldwin, Albert P. Bush,

Donald Comer, E. D. Dunlap, Victor H. Hanson, Robert Jemison, Jr., Hugh Mallory, Hugh Mallory, Jr., H. A. Pharr, and Marion Rushton. These men were willing to give freely of their time and money to improve the hospitals for mental disease.

This committee was instrumental in obtaining a construction grant from the Federal Emergency Administration of Public Works for additional hospital facilities to alleviate some of the overcrowding. This was accomplished at a cost of more than $1,599,975, of which only $250,000 came from a special appropriation by the State Legislature. The remainder was from federal funds. The cost of labor during construction was kept at a minimum by employing the physically able patients.

The program for the prevention of mental diseases in Alabama was a principal goal of the Murfee Committee. One of its recommendations was that the public school systems of Alabama should have Child Guidance Clinics. Colonel Murfee appeared before the Medical Association of the State of Alabama and other professional, educational, and civic groups seeking their support for such a program.

Facility for Treatment of Alcoholics Proposed

Just as Dr. Partlow had been interested in heredity and its effect on mental disease, he was also concerned about alcoholism in the populace. He attributed the excessive use of alcohol to the "many degenerating effects of standards of behavior." Like Dr. Bryce, Dr. Partlow repeatedly requested the State Legislature to provide a special building on the campus of Bryce Hospital for the treatment of inebriates. Dr. Partlow's statistics on patients admitted to the hospital included the degree of alcohol use. He classified them as abstainers, temperate, and intemperate. In 1939, in a paper before the State Medical Association on "The Habitual Use of Alcohol in Alabama," he stated that whereas alcohol was formerly regarded as "a danger and a menace," today it has free entrée into all circles.

Alcoholism was recognized more and more as a national problem. The 1936 United States census report showed that 14,936 alcoholics had been admitted as patients to the various state mental hospitals. These patients comprised 12.4 percent of the total admissions for the year. In Alabama, despite the hospital's policy of declining most alcoholics, the number of applications as well as the number of admissions were increasing. The number of white male patients admitted with alcoholism between 1924 and 1934 ranged from five to forty. No women were included in this figure. By 1935, 73 had been admitted; in 1936, 93; in 1937, 144; and by April, 1938, 175 alcoholic patients had been admitted to the hospitals, and many of these were women. Crimes associated with alcoholism were on the increase in Alabama. In Dr. Partlow's opinion, alcoholism was both a social and a psychiatric problem. As a partial solution he suggested education of the people as to the dangers and deleterious effects of alcohol. He further stated that "the state will be compelled to deal specifically with the problem of treatment, cure, and discipline of the habitual drunkard."[62] The exigencies of the state's finances, however, did not allow such an expansion of the mental health facilities.

Facilities for the Criminally Insane

As early as October 12, 1851, a report from the physicians employed at the Alabama State Prison at Wetumpka stated:

> Before concluding, I would suggest that an apartment be prepared for the reception of those cases of partial insanity, which we often meet among the convicts. Without such an apartment those cases, of which there are several now, cannot be properly treated.[63]

At that time, Alabama made no legal provision for the criminally insane but sent them to prison along with those held mentally responsible for their crimes. Unfortunately, the repeated recommendations of the physicians of the state for a hospital for the criminally insane were to no avail. It would be more than a century before such a facility was built.

Dr. Peter Bryce, Dr. James Searcy, and later Dr. William Partlow repeatedly complained that the criminally insane patients were being referred for admission to the hospital. These physicians were emphatic that the hospital should not be used as a prison and recommended that a separate facility be built for the treatment of the criminally insane. The nonrestraint method of treatment in use for the mentally ill could not always be used with criminals.

By 1942, the problem of housing the criminally insane with other patients in the hospitals had become so critical that the Board of Trustees of the hospital recommended the following:

> [Establishment of] a Department of the Alabama State Hospitals for the distinct purpose of receiving, treating, detaining, caring for and employing criminals who might be committed as insane either by parole from the State Convict Department or by courts of jurisdiction in the various ways provided by law in Alabama for the commitment of those who might be adjudged or suspected of being insane who are charged with crime or indicted for crime, and those who are charged with the offense of chronic alcoholism or drug addiction.[64]

Such a department was not immediately forthcoming. It was only in 1978 that the construction contract was awarded for this desperately needed facility.

Hospitals for the Insane after 1950

After the retirement of Dr. W. D. Partlow, Dr. James Sidney Tarwater (1897–1974) was appointed superintendent of the hospitals on January 1, 1950, and served until 1970. The 1950s were great years for the hospital, years in which improvement continued to be made in the care of the patients. Dr. Tarwater instituted an outpatient clinic for diagnosis and treatment of mental diseases, staffed by physicians at Bryce Hospital. However, the clinic soon closed due to a shortage of personnel.

In 1952, a clinical psychologist and a chaplain were added to the staff at Bryce Hospital. An inpatient program for treatment of alcoholics was

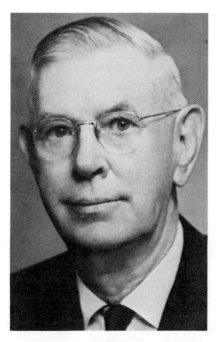

James Sidney Tarwater, M.D., 1897–1974
(Courtesy of Mrs. James Sidney
Tarwater, Tuscaloosa, Alabama)

begun. The School of Dentistry at the Medical Center at The University of Alabama in Birmingham made dental care available to the patients at both mental hospitals and at Partlow School. Recreational activities were increased, and a full-time recreational director for the hospitals was employed.

A school for training attendants to care for the insane and a training program in psychiatric nursing were established at Bryce Hospital. Students from other nursing schools in Alabama could now receive their psychiatric training in Alabama. Heretofore, they had gone out of state for this part of their training.

At Bryce Hospital, there were only seven members of the medical staff in addition to the superintendent and his assistant. A large turnover of the medical staff in the hospitals added to the difficulties. A severe overload of patients was a chronic problem in both Bryce and Searcy hospitals. The hospitals had a census of 6,501 in 1950; 7,569 in 1961; and by the end of 1962, 7,568.[65]

Soon after his appointment, Dr. Tarwater requested an appropriation from the state of $300,000 for much needed repairs and renovations at Bryce Hospital and $800,000 for the construction of a 150-bed ward for patients with tuberculosis. Infectious diseases, especially tuberculosis, had long been a problem in the hospitals. As early as 1914, the hospitals had established separate wards and buildings for the care of the tubercular and other patients who suffered from infectious diseases. Searcy Hospital was also badly in need of repairs and renovations, and $220,000 was requested for these. A like sum was requested to establish an 80-bed ward for tubercular patients at Searcy. Due to lack of funds, the State Building Commission was unable to support these projects. In 1956, a $4 million building program was approved, and the Alabama voters voted a bond issue for this purpose. Work on the hospitals began in 1957.

The greatest problem of the hospitals continued to be financial. New drugs effective in the treatment of patients with mental illness cost an average of $10 per patient per month. Many of the patients were elderly and destitute while some apparently had no family or were abandoned by their families; hence, private funds needed for drugs were not forthcoming.

When available, the new drugs often proved beneficial in the treatment of chronically disturbed patients, and with their use these individuals frequently could be discharged. Electric shock treatment proved effective in treating severe depression. During the 1930s, shock treatment and so-called psychosurgery were introduced in schizophrenia and depressions, that is, psychoses of unknown origin. Reports of successes were undoubtedly often exaggerated. Fortunately, the "psychopharmacy" (Serpasil, chlorpromazine, and other like drugs) appearing during the 1950s made it possible to forego these rather brutal methods. The tranquilizers have, by controlling the excited patient, completely changed the physiognomy of mental institutions.[66]

The tubercular patients responded well to the new antituberculosis agents. Syphilis of the nervous system and pellagra, both causes of insanity, had declined. Progress had also been made in the control of epilepsy. Probably one of the most significant advances had been the education of the public regarding the understanding of mental disease.

In 1958, an aftercare program was established for patients who were returning home with drug treatment, and plans were made for their reintroduction into society. The local mental health association purchased the drugs for outpatient treatment of the discharged patient; and the State Vocational Rehabilitation Service attempted to obtain employment for these individuals. Recreation and counseling were furnished by local social agencies.

The Organization of the Alabama Society for Mental Health

At the April, 1915, meeting of the State Medical Association, Dr. W. D. Partlow recommended the formation of a state mental hygiene society. Mr. Clifford Beers, executive secretary and founder of the National Committee of Mental Hygiene, was a guest speaker at this meeting. Mr. Beer's book, *A Mind That Found Itself*, had resulted in an increased nationwide interest in mental health.*

Dr. Thomas W. Salmon, who was then medical director of the National Committee for Mental Health, also spoke at this meeting. He stressed the importance of the prevention of mental illness through public education, public school clinics, social hygiene, and temperance organizations. Both men addressed the Association urging the physicians of the state to lend their support in organizing a state society for mental hygiene.

Mrs. Dupont Thompson of Birmingham, a well-known civic leader, also addressed the State Medical Association urging the physicians of Alabama to give their support to this movement. She pointed out that state laws could help by prohibiting the marriage of feebleminded individuals and requiring all persons planning marriage to obtain a health certificate.

---

*Clifford Beers, *A Mind That Found Itself* (Garden City, New York: Doubleday, Doran & Company, Inc., 1908).

The Alabama Society for Mental Hygiene came into being on June 16, 1915. Interested professional and lay individuals met at Bryce Hospital and adopted a constitution.[67] The constitution outlined the purpose of the organization:

> To work for the conservation of Mental Health; for the prevention of brain diseases and deficiencies and for the improvement in facilities for the care and treatment of those suffering from nervous and mental diseases or deficiency.[68]

The Alabama Society for Mental Hygiene acquired the services of Dr. Thomas H. Haines of the Medical College of Ohio State University to make a study of the incidence of mental deficiencies in Alabama. Dr. Haines made a survey of mentally defective children who were in Alabama state institutions. In July, 1920, the results of the survey were published in the *Ohio State Medical Journal.*[69] Feeblemindedness was defined as:

> an incapacity for self-direction of such a degree that it endangers the safety and happiness, either of the individual himself, or of others. Such cases as these demand state custody, because they are children in mind.[70]

The percentages of feebleminded at institutions covered by the study were: the Boy's Industrial School, 14 percent; 23 percent at the State Training School for Girls; 13 percent at the Mercy Home Industrial School for Black Girls; and 20 percent at the Mt. Meigs School for Black Boys. The committee concluded:

> Considering half the borderline cases as likely to prove feebleminded, and adding these and the constitutional inferiors and psychopaths, to the feebleminded, we find 167, or about 25 per cent of these 672 boys and girls who cannot be trained so as to become suitable cases for parole. These boys and girls should not, therefore, be in any industrial school.[71]

In March, 1921, the Alabama Society for Mental Hygiene met jointly with the Alabama Education Association in Montgomery. This began a long and profitable association of these two groups. During the next several decades, professional and civic-minded individuals spearheaded the effort for prevention, identification, and treatment of the mentally ill in Alabama. Among those active in the Alabama Society for Mental Hygiene were Drs. I. R. Obenchain, W. S. Littlejohn, E. L. Morphet, and Mr. B. R. Showalter. Dr. Obenchain was the psychologist for the Birmingham City Schools and served as president of the society in 1928. In 1931, plans were outlined for a general survey of available resources for diagnosis and treatment of patients with mental illness. Dr. W. S.

Littlejohn of Birmingham, chairman of the Committee for Mental Hygiene for the State Medical Association, cited an urgent need for mental hygiene clinics where patients could be referred for observation, classification, and management. In 1932, Dr. E. L. Morphet, who was on the faculty at the University of Alabama in Tuscaloosa, became President of the Alabama Society. In the same year, the society recommended that special classes be instituted in the public schools of Alabama and that statewide mental hygiene clinics be established for the diagnosis and treatment of serious behavioral problems. Also, Dr. Morphet felt that there should be institutional training for all idiots and imbecile children and adults, and that institutional care should be mandatory for the insane who would be a menace to society. It was suggested that all persons who might have abnormal children be sterilized before being released from an institution. It was also recommended that a juvenile court be established to handle youthful offenders and a domestic relations court be established that would handle problems of marital adjustments.

The early years of World War II were times of intense civic concern for better mental health. An institute for training teachers and social workers in psychiatric methods of child care was organized and held in the fall and winter of 1941. The Jefferson County Coordinating Council of Social Forces sponsored this institute.

The National Committee for Mental Hygiene was involved in coordinating national health and welfare activities with national defense. The Family Welfare Association of America and the National Selective Service Administration established a cooperative program to aid Selective Service draftees found to have mental health problems. The county Red Cross units, the State Department of Public Welfare and its local units were instrumental in implementing this program in Alabama as there were no mental health clinics to which persons might be referred.

During the war years, the nation began to realize the great need for research in the field of mental health. The organization of two new groups, the People's Committee for Mental Health in 1945 and the National Mental Health Foundation in 1946, reflected an increased national interest in mental health.[72]

The National Mental Health Act of 1946 provided funds for research, training of personnel, and aid to the states in establishing mental health programs that could deal with the preventive phases of this problem. The provisions of the act were written so that the first concern of such a program would be the care and treatment of serious mental illnesses. Before 1946, Alabama had no publicly supported preventive program, and passage of the act now meant such programs could be subsidized by the federal government.

In 1948, the constitution of the Alabama Society for Mental Hygiene was revised and the name changed to the Alabama Society for Mental Health.

The State Department of Mental Health

The Alabama Society for Mental Health had repeatedly recommended establishing an independent Department of Mental Health in Alabama. Prior to this time, the Division of Mental Health in the State Department of Health directed all mental health activities, with the exception of the Alabama Hospitals for the Insane and Partlow School. These were operated as a separate unit directly responsible to a board of trustees. The 1965 session of the State Legislature passed a law "providing for the establishment of a single state agency to coordinate operations and activities of the state government related to mental health," that is, a separate Department of Mental Health to have headquarters in Montgomery.[73]

On September 3, 1965, Act 881 was approved, creating the State Department of Mental Health. The new department took over the functions of the Board of Trustees of the Alabama Hospitals for the Insane, the Board of Managers of Partlow State School, the Commission on Alcoholism, the Division of Mental Health Planning, and the Mental Health Hygiene of the State Board of Health.[74]

The State Mental Health Board, which had overall supervisory control of the mental health activities, was to have a membership evenly divided between physicians and laymen. All the state hospitals for the mentally ill and the mentally retarded, the Commission on Alcoholism, and the Division of Mental Hygiene in the State Department of Health would be under its supervision. The Board of Trustees of the Partlow School, Bryce and Searcy hospitals would be abolished. Additional appropriations for the hospitals as well as the Department of Mental Health were to be funded by a tax on cigarettes.

Mental health activities in the state increased substantially. In 1965, there were mental health clinics in Anniston, Birmingham, Decatur, Dothan, Florence, Gadsden, Huntsville, Shamut, Mobile, Montgomery, Opelika, Auburn, Selma, Sylacauga, Talladega, Troy, Tuscaloosa, Tuscumbia, and Tuskegee; most of them were operating part-time. Under a new plan of statewide coordination, these became full-time operations.

The Alabama Commission on Alcoholism had established treatment clinics in Decatur, Birmingham, Florence, Montgomery, Mobile, Opelika, and Tuscaloosa. Most of these operated on a full-time basis.

This new unified system for diagnosis and treatment of mental illness provided screening for detection of the mentally disturbed as well as for their treatment. At long last, the state of Alabama had a viable functioning Mental Health Program. Peter Bryce's dream was finally becoming a reality.

Mental Health in Alabama After 1970

Bryce Hospital

Dr. James Sidney Tarwater retired in 1970 as superintendent of the Alabama Hospitals for the Insane. There have been six superintendents since that time.

Dr. J. Donald Smith, who followed Dr. Tarwater as superintendent, served from 1970 to 1971. Dr. Smith had been at Bryce for more than 21 years and had served as a physician, assistant superintendent, and chief of staff. Although he resigned as superintendent in 1971, he remained as chief of staff until 1975.

Dr. James Cannon Folsom was appointed superintendent and served from 1971 to 1972. He had served as director of the Veterans Administration Hospital in Tuscaloosa for six years. He is known for his methods of treatment, principally "reality orientation" and "attitude therapy." He resigned in 1972.

Dr. James E. Morris, a psychiatrist at Bryce, served as interim superintendent from 1972 until 1973. Mr. Rod Clelland was engaged in July of 1973 and served until 1975. Mr. Clelland was the first superintendent at Bryce who was not a physician. He had a degree in business administration and had served as superintendent for Administration at the State Hospital in Milledgeville, Georgia.

Dr. Harold W. Heller was appointed superintendent in February, 1975, after Mr. Clelland resigned for health reasons. Dr. Heller had been head of the Department of Special Education at the University of Alabama. He was superintendent from 1975 until 1977.

Mr. T. J. Callander, who replaced Dr. Heller as superintendent in July, 1978, also had a background in special education. Mr. Callander had been director of the mental illness section of the Department of Mental Health prior to becoming superintendent.

In 1972, Bryce Hospital was placed under the *Wyatt* v. *Stickney* federal court order, which established standards of treatment and set staffing ratios.

In 1975, the commitment laws of Alabama were changed by the *Lynch* v. *Baxley* federal court order. It stated that in order to be committed involuntarily to a hospital for the insane, it must be proven in a court of law with evidence that is "clear, convincing and unequivocal" that the person:

1. is mentally ill,
2. threatens harm to himself or others,
3. has committed some recent overt act demonstrating danger,
4. that treatment is available for the person, and
5. that Bryce Hospital is the least restrictive alternative to help the person recover from mental illness.

Bryce Hospital had 5,200 patients in 1970; but by 1975, the patient population had decreased to 1,900. A treatment program was begun at Bryce in which patients were placed according to their levels of functioning.

On December 7, 1977, Bryce was reorganized into geographic treatment areas, which aided in further reduction of the patient population. This plan also helped to assure that all patients receive adequate treatment. The hospital is organized by levels of functioning and by a geographic system. Patients who stay longer than ninety days are placed in an extended care region. These regions are determined geographically, according to the forty-seven counties in the Bryce Hospital catchment area. Each county, in turn, is divided into four regions. Specialty areas in the hospital include behavioral therapy, geriatrics, adolescents, forensic, alcohol, and drug programs.

Bryce Hospital's extensive Patient Education Program includes the Psychological Learning Center (PLC). Patients who are admitted to the hospital and whose illnesses are considered to have a biochemical basis— such as schizophrenia or manic-depressive illness—are assigned to a "responsible patient" class. These patients are taught the rights and obligations or responsibilities that they should know about their illness and are urged to participate in treatment planning and in following treatment routines.[75]

Searcy Hospital

Searcy Hospital was reorganized as an independent unit in 1970.[76] Prior to that time, it had been under the supervision of Bryce Hospital, and its chief officer had had the title of assistant superintendent at Bryce.

In July, 1969, Searcy desegregated its patient population and ceased to be a custodial institution, becoming a full-service treatment hospital for the mentally ill. At the present time, the treatment program at Searcy has as its primary objective helping patients return to and function adequately in their communities. Special programs have been developed in vocational rehabilitation, alcoholism, drug abuse, and adolescent and adult behavior problems.

Searcy Hospital also serves as the admissions center for two satellite adjustment facilities. The Eufaula Adolescents Adjustment Center and the Thomasville Adult Adjustment Center facilities serve individuals from the entire state, particularly those who do not require long-term care. An aftercare center was organized in 1975 in Andalusia, called the Ellie P. Dixon Aftercare Center. Here the program takes a humanistic approach; it focuses on enhancing the patient's ability to meet the fundamental needs in life. This center makes an effort to introduce the patients into community life with the help of professional and social organizations.

Partlow State School and Hospital

In 1968, the black and white resident patient population in the Partlow School was fully integrated.[77] The training program had been integrated previously. A major administrative change was made during the fiscal year 1975 when a Division of Mental Retardation was created in the Department of Mental Health. The Partlow State School and Hospital was removed from the Division of Hospitals and placed in this new division.

Significant improvements were made in 1972. The state of Alabama and the Department of Mental Health made drastic changes in staffing, physical plant, and methods of service delivery at Partlow State School and Hospital due to a federal district court order. The court appointed a Human Rights Committee to monitor the institution's progress toward compliance with the court ordered standards. The radical changes caused tension and unstable conditions, so that almost all the physicians resigned. But after much effort the medical department again gradually increased to seven physicians.

The severe overcrowding that prevailed in Partlow prior to 1972 was gradually eliminated. The population was reduced from 2,300 to 1,110 patients.

The medical services also improved. Among these new medical services were a pharmacy with a registered pharmacist and two assistant pharmacists, consultants in the various disciplines, a better system of monitoring medications, and increased funding. Much-needed remedial surgery is now possible due to the increased funding.

From 1972 until 1975, significant improvements were made at Partlow. The annual budget increased from $8,500,390 to $16,500,000. On August 1, 1975, there was a total of 1,845 staff members employed as compared with the March 1, 1972, total employment of 882. The resident patient population declined from 2,246 to 1,309. All training and living areas have been air-conditioned and renovated to meet recognized fire and safety standards.

Notes

1. Katherine Vickery, *A History of Mental Health in Alabama* (Montgomery: Ala. Dept. of Mental Health, 1972[?]), p. 8.

2. Ibid., p. 9.

3. Ibid.

4. Ibid., pp. 9–10.

5. Ibid., p. 10.

6. Whether Miss Dix met with Drs. Mabry and Fair is not known.

7. Vickery, p. 17.

8. *Alabama Tribune*, 2 December 1847, p. 2, col. 1.

9. Dr. Mabry also gives Dr. Drewry Fair of Selma as a representative to the General Assembly.

10. Vickery, p. 18.

11. Seale Harris states that Dr. J. Marion Sims, living in Montgomery at that time, was a friend of Miss Dix and aided her in her efforts. Seale Harris, *Woman's Surgeon, The Life Story of J. Marion Sims* (New York: Macmillan Co., 1950), p. 111.

12. Vickery, p. 23.

13. Ibid., p. 28.

14. Acts of Alabama, 6 February 1852, pp. 10–19.

15. Ibid., Section 7, p. 12.

16. Vickery, pp. 32–33.

17. Ibid., p. 34.

18. In 1901, the Board became self-perpetuating.

19. James S. Tarwater, *The Alabama State Hospitals and the Partlow State School and Hospital, A Brief History* (New York: Newcomen Society in North America, 1964), p. 10.

20. Vickery, p. 35.

21. Patrick Kehoe and Ellen Barry were married in 1864.

22. Tarwater, p. 4.

23. Vickery, p. 36.

24. Ibid., p. 36. Probably those trustees living in Tuscaloosa.

25. Vickery, pp. 37–38.

26. Ibid., p. 38.

27. Ibid.

28. Ibid., p. 40.

29. Ibid., p. 41.

30. Ibid., pp. 46–47.

31. Ibid., p. 40.

32. Ibid., p. 51.

33. Ibid., pp. 47–48.

34. Ibid., p. 49.

35. Ibid., pp. 55–56.

36. Tarwater, p. 16.

37. Frank Kay, "Historical Background of Alabama Psychiatry, Part 2," *De Hist. Med.* 5 (Aug. 1961): 6.

38. Tarwater, pp. 16–17.

39. Vickery, pp. 66–67.

40. Ibid., p. 81.

41. Acts of Alabama, 11 December 1900, p. 363.

42. Ibid., pp. 361–62.

43. Ibid., p. 363.

44. Ibid.

45. Edward Jenner Wood, *A Treatise on Pellagra* (New York: D. Appleton and Co., 1912), pp. 29–30.

46. Vickery, pp. 76–77.

47. Ibid., p. 92.

48. Marianna O. Lewis, ed., *The Foundation Directory*, 6th ed. (New York: The Foundation Center, 1977), p. 354.

49. Vickery, p. 91.

50. Ibid., p. 159.

51. Ibid., p. 96.

52. Acts of Alabama, 29 September 1919, pp. 1023–29.

53. Idiots were defined as those with a mental age of less than two years; imbeciles with mental ages ranging from two to seven years; morons with a mental age from eight to ten years.

54. "Alabama Home and School for Mental Deficients," *Mental Hygiene* 4 (Jan. 1920): 201–02.

55. Vickery, p. 103.

56. Ibid., p. 108.

57. Ibid.

58. Ibid., pp. 153–54.

59. Ibid., p. 156.

60. Ibid., p. 155.

61. Ibid., pp. 168–69.

62. Ibid., p. 157.

63. Ibid., p. 15.

64. Ibid., p. 176.

65. Ibid., p. 291.

66. Erwin H. Ackernecht, *A Short History of Medicine* (New York: Ronald Press Co., 1968).

67. A copy of the original constitution is on file at Bryce Hospital, Tuscaloosa, Alabama, and another in the Alabama Department of Archives and History, Montgomery, Alabama.

68. Vickery, p. 114.

69. A reprint is on file at the Reynolds Historical Library at The University of Alabama in Birmingham.

70. Vickery, p. 122.

71. Ibid., pp. 122–23.

72. Ibid., p. 139.

73. Ibid., p. 307.

74. Milo B. Howard, Jr., Director of State of Alabama Department of Archives and History, Montgomery, Ala., letter, 28 February 1980.

75. Steve Davis, director of Public Affairs, Bryce Hospital, letter, 18 August 1978.

76. Belinda Jones, Public Information, Mount Vernon, Ala., letter, 29 March 1979. Included is a typescript, "Searcy—Past, Present and Future (A Brief Progressive Chronological Account)."

77. "History of Partlow State School and Hospital, 1923–1975," TS, pp. 3–4. Copy in the author's possession.

Chapter 14

The History of Dentistry in Alabama

In pioneer Alabama, dentists found the same problems physicians found: a public that was unable or unwilling to distinguish a professional from a charlatan. The early measures taken by dentists to improve the quality of their profession in Alabama were similar to those taken by the medical profession. There were never many dentists in the state. The towns were small and usually unable to attract a well-trained dentist. Unlike an appendix, a troublesome tooth could be easily removed by a professional toothpuller, a neighbor, or the local physician. It was not until after the Civil War that the dental profession began to organize.

The Alabama Dental Association

The Alabama Dental Association was organized on October 6, 1869, through the efforts of Alabama dentists.[1] These individuals were interested in forming an organization that would protect the general public against quackery, charlatans, and mountebanks, as well as benefit dentists themselves. An organizational meeting was held in the office of Dr. R. M. Hereford of Montgomery. Those attending were Drs. J. S. McAuley of Selma, P. L. Ulmer of Pleasant Hill, E. H. Locke and H. D. Boyd of Troy, W. W. Evans of Union Springs, and Samuel Rambo, A. H. C. Walker, W. J. Reese, and R. M. Hereford of Montgomery. The meeting was the result of an earlier call issued by these dentists. Drs. L. M. Rush of Tuskegee and W. N. Bush of Prattville joined the organizational group the following day.

A constitution was drafted, and Dr. McAuley of Selma was elected president. Membership dues were three dollars, and all Alabama dentists in good standing were invited to become members of the fledgling organization. Students of dentistry were also invited to join, and special regulations were drafted for them. A certificate of membership bearing a seal of the association was adopted. This seal consisted of an antique

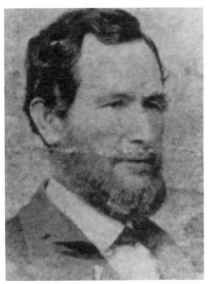 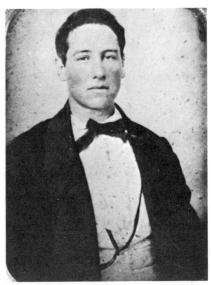

Samuel Rambo, M.D., D.D.S. (Cour-   J. S. McAuley, M.D., D.D.S. (Courtesy
tesy of the Alabama Dental Associa-   of the Alabama State Department of
tion, Montgomery, Alabama)   Archives and History)

lamp resting on a book with the motto *Nihil Sine Labore*, "never without work." The organization was small, but even at this early date, provisions were made in the constitution for impeachment of members.

Organizational matters did not occupy all the time at the first meeting. A paper was presented entitled "Filling Teeth Requiring the Destruction of the Nerve and the Treatment of Alveolar Abscess."

On August 17, 1870, the second annual meeting was held in Selma. Interest still lagged, but a few new members were added to the rolls. No formal papers were presented, and discussions were unsatisfactory. The meeting for the most part was desultory, but a format for future programs, to include formal papers, was agreed on. Dr. Samuel Rambo was elected president for the next year, and the association selected Mobile for the next meeting.

Interest in the association continued to lag; the president was unable to attend the meeting in 1871. By 1873, so little interest was shown in the annual meeting that Dr. McAuley sent a circular letter addressed to all the dentists in Alabama to see if there was any real interest in continuing the organization. A combined meeting with the Mississippi and New

Orleans dental societies was suggested, but this came to naught. The Alabama Dental Association appeared moribund. The 1874 meeting, which was to be held in Mobile, was cancelled due to a yellow fever epidemic in that city. No meetings were held for the next five years, but the records were carefully preserved during the interregnum, which indicated the continued existence of the Alabama Dental Association.

In 1879, during a meeting of the Southern Dental Association in Augusta, Georgia, Dr. T. M. Allen of Eufaula and Dr. E. S. Chisholm of Tuscaloosa decided either to revive the old society or to organize a new one. At the time, the last elected president of the Alabama Dental Association had moved out of the state, and all the other officers, except the first vice-president, Dr. W. Dunlap of Selma, had also moved away. Dr. Dunlap assumed the presidency, appointed Dr. Allen secretary pro tempore, then issued a call for a meeting to be held in Montgomery on July 20, 1880.

A small but devoted group of dentists, including some of the charter members of the original Alabama Dental Association, met in the Medical Hall at Montgomery on that date. The Association adopted a new constitution and bylaws. Dues were reduced to a dollar, and the dues for the years when there had been no meetings were remitted. Ten new dentists were approved for membership. The Association was off to a new beginning.

One of the continuing problems of the Association was the small membership, due to the fact that not all eligible dentists were interested. In 1901, there were only 95 members out of 300 licensed dentists in Alabama. Dentists who passed the examination of the State Board of Dental Examiners were eligible for membership in the Association and were encouraged to join. The Association, despite its need for members, did not hesitate to expel members who violated the association's code of ethics. The most frequent reason for expulsion was improper advertising and association with the New York and Boston Painless Dentist Parlors.

The first lady dentist was admitted to membership in 1900; the following year she was joined by a second. Both were chivalrously admitted to membership without dues.

In 1883, the association began to publish the *Transactions of the Alabama Dental Association,* which contained the papers presented and were made available to all dentists in Alabama and elsewhere. Three hundred and twenty-five copies of the first issue were printed. The size of the *Transactions* increased during a fifteen-year period as did the cost of printing. Deficits were made up personally by the Association's officers or by special collection at the annual meetings. It soon became necessary, however, to raise the members' dues to three dollars. This sum was enough to allow for the printing of the *Transactions* but not too much to discourage new members. The annual volume of the *Transactions* was replaced by a quarterly bulletin in 1917; and it continues today as the *Journal of the Alabama Dental Association*.

In addition to the Alabama Dental Association, dentists have organized eight district societies over the state. These societies meet frequently and are very active. A number of the state's dentists have been elected to office in the national organization, and some have been awarded Fellowships in the American College of Dentists.[2]

Regulation of the Practice of Dentistry

The Alabama Dental Association has had several goals, but one of the principal ones has been the regulation of dental practice in the state. There was little hope of any real control until unethical practice could be punished in the state's courts. The display of dental diplomas, licenses, or certificates of membership in the State Dental Association was considered advertising. Also, very little prestige was gained by membership in the association; and expulsion, insofar as the general public was concerned, carried little or no stigma. Therefore, the Association's ability to police practitioners of the dental profession was limited.[3]

Alabama was the first state to pass an act regulating the practice of dentistry. The General Assembly approved Act No. 26, which regulated the practice of dental surgery, on December 31, 1841.[4] This law provided that any applicant who wanted to practice dental surgery had to be examined by the local medical boards. These dentists were subject to the same restrictions and regulations as those who applied for a license to practice medicine.

The famous "1823 Law" for regulation of the practice of medicine had been passed by the General Assembly meeting in Cahaba. This statute provided for a local board composed of physicians who were authorized to examine applicants and issue licenses to practice medicine. Apparently this board also granted dentists license to practice. It soon became evident that applicants for a dental license should be examined by someone with a knowledge of dentistry. The original medical licensure law, which was revised in 1841, stated that it should be the duty of these medical licensure boards to elect a "professional dentist" as a member. The dentist was to assist them in the examination, but this was not always possible.[5]

There was a penalty for those who practiced dentistry without a license. A fine could be assessed but could not be in excess of fifty dollars for each offense. This sum was divided equally between the county in which the arrest was made and the informer. Another provision of the law was that any bonds, notes, or promissory obligations for services rendered by a person practicing dentistry without a license were void.

There was not a retroactive feature or "grandfather clause" in this first law; therefore all individuals who were already practicing dentistry in Alabama were required to take the examination. But medical practitioners who were either licensed by one of the state medical boards or who held a diploma from a "constituted Medical Institution in the United States" were free to practice medicine without an examination. It is possible, then, that many individuals continued to practice dentistry in Alabama without obtaining a license.

In 1877, the law was amended again, placing the licensing of dentists under the State Medical Association, which had been responsible for the legislation. The dental association, which had temporarily lapsed as a functioning organization, could take little or no credit for this legislation.[6]

Sentiment grew demanding separate licensing boards. One of the purposes for organizing the Alabama Dental Association in 1869 was to seek the passage of a new law creating a separate Board of Dental Examiners.[7] Such a law was prepared during the winter of 1880. This law removed dental licensure from the hands of the medical profession and established a Board of Dental Examiners.[8] On February 11, 1881, the statute was passed, Act No. 90, and the authority to regulate the practice of dentistry in Alabama was placed in the hands of the dental profession.[9]

The law provided for a separate Board of Dental Examiners consisting of five dental practitioners. These dentists had been licensed by a state medical board, but, in the future, those who served on the board would be licensed by the dental board organized under this act. To receive a license, the applicant had to have been practicing dentistry in Alabama for a minimum of three years and had to be a member in good standing of the Alabama Dental Association.[10] The members of the executive committee of the Alabama Dental Association comprised the first board. They were to serve until the next meeting of this association, at which time a dental board would be elected for a two-year term. Drs. W. D. Dunlap, E. S. Chisholm, W. R. McWilliams, T. M. Allen, and G. M. Rousseau composed a temporary board, but this board never served. This was due to the fact that on the first day of the meeting of the Alabama Dental Association held in Selma on July 19–21, 1881, the members requested that a regular board be elected immediately. The first regular board members were Drs. Dunlap, Chisholm, McWilliams, and Allen. Dr. J. S. McAuley replaced Dr. Rousseau.[11]

In implementing the licensing law, the board stipulated that (1) all dentists who could provide proof that they had been engaged in the practice of dentistry for at least five years prior to the passage of this act were automatically mailed a license without any fee; (2) any dentist who had been granted a license by a state medical board could obtain a license without examination or fee; and (3) any applicant who could provide evidence of having received a diploma from any incorporated dental college was to be given a license without a fee or examination.[12]

The law had some unique features such as (1) the Licensure Board was to prescribe a course of reading for dental students who were receiving private instruction, (2) a board member could issue to any individual a temporary license that was valid until the next board meeting, and (3) violators of the law were subject to fines of not less than $50 nor more than $300.[13] The law also specified that nothing in the act should be construed to prevent any individual who wished to extract teeth from doing so. Indeed, oral surgery must have been a very difficult field to establish in those days, with everyone free to extract teeth. Until 1888, the board members served a two-year term. From that year on, the present system of electing one new member for a five-year term was instituted.[14]

Alabama was one of the first states to pass a law regulating the practice of dental hygiene by auxiliary personnel. This was approved September 29, 1919. The Act, No. 526, stated that "Any person who shall hereafter desire to practice dental hygiene in this state shall pass an examination given by the Board of Dental Examiners of this state under such rules and regulations as said board deems fit and proper to promulgate." Nine women were licensed on July 25, 1920, although only fifteen additional hygienists were licensed under this law during the next seven years.[15]

In September of 1927, the State Legislature passed Act No. 637, which provided that any dentist legally qualified to practice in Alabama could apply for a yearly permit to employ a dental hygienist. The hygienist could be required by the board to take an examination. Also, the board could require the dentist to take an examination to determine his capability of teaching the dental hygienist. No licenses were issued, however, to dental hygienists for the next eleven years. In 1935, the portion of the law that permitted the board to examine the practicing dentist for competence in teaching the hygienist was repealed. In 1939, a written and practical examination for dental hygienists was instituted.[16]

In 1940, section 117 was added to Chapter 5, Title 46, of the *Code of Alabama*. This statute outlined the requirements of a dental hygienist: (1) a person of good moral character, (2) at least 21 years of age; (3) the person must have had at least one year's experience as a dental assistant in the office of a licensed dentist; (4) the person must be a high school graduate; and (5) the person must pass a written and practical examination. Alabama is among the few states that require no formal training by the dental hygienist before qualifying for the board examination.[17]

Alabama holds the distinction of being the only state in the Union whose law provides that the state association elect the members of the Board of Dental Examiners. The members of the board must also be members of the State Dental Association. "This wise provision frees [the board] from appointment by governors, a hazard other states are subjected to, and places the problem of selection in the hands of the one body capable of making a wise choice."[18]

Dental Education

Alabama's education of dentists left a great deal to be desired in that if any individual wished to study dentistry in the state, he had to study with a preceptor, a practicing dentist, and apply himself to studying such books as those the Board of Dental Examiners recommended.[19] If he rejected this course of study, his only other alternative was to go to Atlanta, Nashville, Knoxville, Memphis, or even farther away to study. The Alabama Dental Association requested that Vanderbilt University, the University of Tennessee, and later, the University of Illinois provide scholarships to Alabamians. A student who received a scholarship had certain fees remitted or reduced each year, and the student was assured that his acceptance of a scholarship would be kept confidential.

Alabama may not have been in the forefront in dental education, but it did take the lead in trying to instill in the general public a need for better dental health. In 1892, the *Transactions* had printed a paper by Dr. S. W. Foster of Tuscaloosa that was a culmination of a discussion concerning the need for teaching children and adults the proper care for teeth. In an effort to implement this recommendation, speeches were made in schools throughout the state on proper dental care, and the program was recommended to all other dental associations in the country.

Alabama College of Dental Surgery

This school was organized at Bridgeport in 1893.[20] Very little is known concerning its organization, faculty, or curriculum. There were three graduate students in 1893. The school closed that same year.

Birmingham Dental College

A charter to establish the Birmingham Dental College was issued on July 19, 1893.[21] William Berney, S. E. Green, Joseph F. Johnston, Frank P. O'Brien, Rufus N. Rhodes, Joseph R. Smith, and William A. Walker; and Drs. H. M. Caldwell and B. F. Riley were the organizing group and became the trustees of the school. The first class matriculated in the fall of 1895. The Board of Trustees established bylaws stating that the faculty should have no less than nine professors. These professors were to teach the following subjects: operative dentistry, dental surgery, dental pathology and therapeutics, mechanical and clinical dentistry, materia medica and therapeutics, orthodontia, crown and bridgework, chemistry and metallurgy, physiology and history, anatomy, and dental jurisprudence. The board was allowed to create other chairs if they were deemed necessary to maintain the school's standard. Within the next twelve years, the school, originally located at 209 North 21st Street, moved five times.

The faculty varied from year to year. The 1898 Birmingham Dental College directory listed the following as faculty:

Dean T. M. Allen, D.D.S.—operative dentistry and materia medica
Charles A. Merrill, D.D.S.—pathology and therapeutics
R. Augustus Jones, D.D.S.—mechanical dentistry, and in charge of infirmary
G. M. Lathem, D.D.S.—[materia] medica and therapeutics, operative dentistry, and dental technic
W. B. Fulton, D.D.S.—chemistry and metallurgy
A. Eubanks, D.D.S.—orthodontia, crown and bridgework
J. H. McCarty, M.D.—physiology and histology
D. G. Copeland, M.D.—anatomy and general surgery
L. G. Woodson, M.D.—eye, ear, nose and throat
R. G. Berry, M.D.—histology and microscopy

The outlined curriculum was for three academic years of seven months each. The classes were freshman, junior, and senior. The 1895 catalog specified the admission requirements, which were to include one of the following: a college degree, a high school diploma, a teacher's certificate, passing a preliminary examination, or having a certificate from another dental college recognized by the faculty. If medical students wished to be admitted to the junior dental class, they had to attend 75 percent of a five-month term in medical school and satisfactorily pass an examination on the studies of the freshman dental year.[22] It is interesting to note that women were to be admitted on the same basis as men; however, no evidence can be found showing that a woman student was ever accepted. In order to graduate, a candidate had to be twenty-one years of age, of good moral character, and have completed successfully the outlined course of study.

According to the catalog, the instruments that were recommended for the three-year course would also be sufficient for practice after graduation. Among the textbooks used were *Gray's Anatomy*, *Dorland's Medical Dictionary*, *Black's Anatomy of the Teeth*, and *MacFarland's Bacteriology*.

The requirements for freshmen were restoration of carious lesions on extracted teeth with tin, silver amalgam, gold foil, gutta-percha, and oxyphosphate of zinc cement. The freshman, upon completion of five restorations approved by the staff, was admitted to the infirmary to practice dentistry.

Junior class requirements were the completion of fifteen restorations on clinic patients, performance of any surgical operation in the mouth that was necessary, construction of three rubber and two metal dentures, one of which had to be a practical case, and finally, the successful waxing and casting of four crowns and two pieces of bridgework. The restorations were done with contemporary restorative materials. The juniors had to receive a satisfactory grade on all procedures from the departmental professor before they were promoted. The requirements for seniors were similar to those for the juniors. A strict rule was that all student work had to be accomplished within the college building. The patients admitted to the clinic were treated free of charge other than that of the cost of the materials used. Extractions were performed free of charge, but without the use of anesthesia. If a patient wanted anesthesia, he was charged twenty-five cents.

The student failure and dropout rate was extraordinarily high: only three out of twenty-seven students in the class of 1893 graduated; the next year only one graduated out of a class of twenty-four. When all of the students in the classes from 1893 to 1910 are taken into consideration, one finds that only one out of five entering students completed the course.

From 1895 until 1911, the Birmingham Dental College operated as an independent proprietary institution. In 1911, the school was purchased by the Birmingham Medical College for the sum of $1,041 and functioned as a part of this college until 1915.

Proprietary schools had been criticized for years for not being adequately staffed or equipped to train physicians and dentists. Therefore, the profitable operation of proprietary schools was made more difficult due to this disfavor and also to the rising costs of providing professional training. In 1915, the Birmingham Medical, Dental, and Pharmaceutical College, due to its financial instability and difficulty in maintaining compulsory professonal standards, was forced to close its doors. For the next thirty-three years, Alabama had no school of dentistry.

State Dental School Urged

In 1945, Governor Chauncey Sparks was urged to support the establishment of a dental school in Alabama by Dr. Moren Fuller.[23] Dr. Fuller was an advisor to the governor, and upon Dr. Fuller's advice the governor requested the necessary legislation. Other dentists who were instrumental in founding the dental school were Drs. Charles Bray, Olin Kirkland, and John Sullivan. The State Legislature, however, authorized

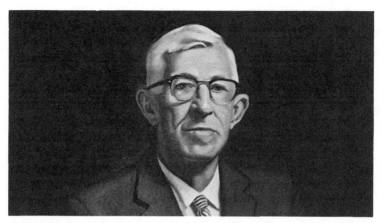

H. Moren Fuller, D.D.S., D.Sc. (Courtesy of the University of Alabama School of Dentistry, The University of Alabama in Birmingham)

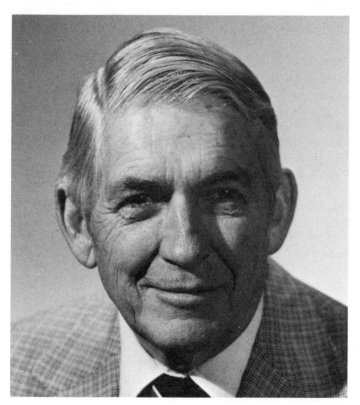

Joseph Francis Volker, D.D.S., Ph.D. (The University of Alabama in Birmingham, Department of Photography)

only $300,000, and no further steps were taken at that time to establish a dental school. In 1946, several World War II veterans who were enrolled in a predental course at the University of Alabama were discouraged by the admission rejections they had received from the dental schools to which they had applied. They were aware of the 1945 legislative action and, therefore, decided that if they wanted to become dentists, a dental school should be established in Alabama. Dr. Ralph Adams, acting president of the University of Alabama, Mr. Fred Taylor of the *Birmingham News*, Dr. Fuller, and a number of other prominent Alabamians encouraged them in their endeavors. In 1947, Governor James Folsom (governor of Alabama, 1947–1951; 1955–1959) and a number of legislators gave their support to establishing a school of dentistry. Due to their support, the 1947 Legislature appropriated the necessary funds for establishing the school, which was to be managed by the Board of Trustees of the University of Alabama.

The dental school was authorized by the State Legislature and was granted $300,000; it also received $325,000 in construction funds that were contributed by the State Building Commission. Also, an annual appropriation of $150,000 for the school's operation was granted. This assured the school's establishment.

In the spring of 1948, the Alabama Dental Association's annual meeting was in Birmingham. The Dean of Tufts University Dental School in Boston, Dr. Joseph F. Volker, participated in the Association's program. While here, he was offered the deanship of the new dental school. He accepted, provided that he be allowed to finish the academic year 1948–1949 at Tufts. Dr. Volker served both schools during the 1948–1949 academic year by commuting between Boston and Birmingham.

The State Building Commission made arrangements for the school to be temporarily housed in the old Hillman Hospital, which the Jefferson County Health Department had previously used. A staff was selected, equipment purchased, and the first class accepted in an unbelievably short time.

Dental School Established

The University of Alabama School of Dentistry opened in early October, 1948, with a class of fifty-two students.[24] The basic science faculty, most of whom were affiliated with the medical school, began an aggressive program in spite of the fact that the facilities were barely adequate. Drs. Joseph F. Volker, Perry Hitchcock, and Dominick Andronaco constituted the first full-time clinical faculty. Later, the faculty was joined by part-time members Drs. Boyd W. Tarpley, Polly Ayers,

Edward Brannon, V. D. Cooper, Robert Evans, Leon Farnum, and Charles Lokey, Jr. Drs. Joseph P. Lazansky, H. J. Tebo, and Leonard Robinson joined the full-time faculty during the school's second year of operation. Shortly after the school was opened, an oral surgery program was begun.

One of the attractions that brought Dr. Joseph Volker to Birmingham was that the University of Alabama had no experience in dental education and no preconceived ideas regarding the establishment and operation of a dental school. This appealed to him, in that he believed that until dental education was totally integrated into a medical center it could not be effective. The fact that the four-year University of Alabama Medical School was new facilitated the sharing of basic science faculty and facilities. In striving for excellence in teaching dental students, the school decided early that first, the dental school's admission requirements would be that the applicant's background should approximate those for medical students; and second, that a basic science curriculum comparable to that for medicine should be developed. The philosophy of the new dental school was that it would be balanced in education, service, and research. This philosophy has proved to be very effective. The school initiated intern and residency programs in the dental specialties and assumed the responsibility for continuing education of the dental profession in Alabama and the Southeast.

In 1949, construction was begun on the present dental school building. The dental clinic building was the first and perhaps the only dental clinic building to be funded by the Hill-Burton Hospital Construction Act. When the building—designed for about 200 students—was completed in 1951, it was one of the most modern dental schools in the country. Until 1967, fifty-two freshmen were accepted annually, but in that year the number was increased to fifty-seven. Today, preference is given to qualified residents of Alabama, but a few exceptionally well-qualified students from neighboring states are accepted each year. The School of Dentistry requires all students to take the National Board Examination, Parts 1 and 2. The students' scores have been well above average because of the broadly based and intensively taught basic science and clinical programs. At present, the dental student's knowledge of diagnosis and treatment planning is evaluated as closely as his technical ability.

The school has endeavored to encourage its graduates to further their training, and it has done so successfully in that the number of Alabama graduates studying for Masters, Ph.D., or M.D. degrees have been exceptionally high. The same is true of those entering specialty training. A program that allows selected students to receive both D.M.D. and Ph.D. degrees after seven years of training was inaugurated to develop teachers and research scientists for the dental profession. Repeatedly, the school has received international acclaim for its programs.

Dr. McCallum Appointed Dean

In 1961, Dr. Volker was promoted to vice-president for Health Affairs of the University of Alabama. This appointment gave him administrative responsibility over the entire Medical Center in Birmingham. Dr. Charles A. McCallum was appointed dean of the School of Dentistry.[25] Dr. McCallum, who had served as chairman of the Department of Oral Surgery, had received his dental degree from Tufts and a medical degree from the University of Alabama.

Dr. Volker had become chancellor of the University of Alabama System on June 15, 1976. On September 1, 1977, Dr. McCallum was appointed vice-president for Health Affairs of the University of Alabama. Dr. S. Richardson Hill, Jr., had become president of The University of Alabama in Birmingham in February, 1977.

On January 1, 1978, Dr. Leonard Robinson was appointed dean of the School of Dentistry. Dr. Robinson received his D.M.D. degree in 1943 from Tufts College Dental School and his M.D. from the University of Alabama School of Medicine in 1954.

Notes

1. Milo B. Howard, Jr., "The History of the Alabama Dental Association, Part One, 1869–1917," *The First Hundred Years, 1869–1969: A Story of the Dental Profession in Alabama* (Birmingham: n.p., 1969), pp. 6–10.

2. Marie Bankhead Owen, *The Story of Alabama: A History of the State* (New York: Lewis Historical Pub. Co., Inc., 1949), 2: 573.

3. Howard, p. 10.

4. "Early History of Alabama Dental Laws," *Bull. Ala. Dent. Assoc.* 40 (July 1956): 20–24 (hereafter cited as "Early History").

5. Ibid., p. 20.

6. Howard, pp. 10–11.

7. "Early History," p. 20.

8. Ibid., p. 21.

9. Acts of Alabama, 11 February 1881, p. 82.

10. Ibid., pp. 82–83.

11. "Early History," p. 21.

12. Ibid., p. 21.

13. In order to be in violation of the law, they had to be practicing dentistry for a fee or a reward.

14. "Early History," pp. 21–22.

15. Ibid., p. 22.

16. Ibid.

17. Ibid., pp. 22–23.

18. Owen, p. 573.

19. Howard, pp. 13, 16.

20. Owen, p. 573.

21. E. M. Speed, "A Resume of the History of Dental Education in Alabama," *The First Hundred Years, 1869–1969: A Story of the Dental Profession in Alabama* (Birmingham: n.p., 1969), pp. 101–04.

22. This began a policy of accepting students who had failed in medicine as dental students, and this policy was continued by most dental schools after World War II. This policy was never practiced by The University of Alabama in Birmingham.

23. Speed, pp. 104–05.

24. Ibid., pp. 105–06.

25. Ibid., p. 107.

Chapter 15

The Development of Pharmacy as a Profession in Alabama

Practice of Pharmacy in Early Alabama

During the French and Spanish colonial period, drugs were available to the colonists in Mobile and along the Gulf Coast. They were mostly imported from Europe, and no doubt pharmacies existed. Although drugs had been peddled to Indians along the Gulf Coast for years, until St. Stephens and Huntsville were founded there were no English-speaking settlements of any consequence where a drug-dispensing establishment could be found. Some of the other products found in these settlements were French perfume, olive oil, British ale, and something called Turlington's Balsam of Life. Newspapers advertised drugs as early as 1818 and offered for sale remedies compounded by physicians: Taylor's Balsam of Liverwort, Dr. Hewe's Bone and Nerve Remedy, Mother's Comfort, and Doctor Barclay's Syrup of Cubebs and Sarsaparilla were among such creations.[1]

Even without pharmacies, drugs were usually available in the early towns of Alabama. Frequently, they were a part of the stock in a general store, which included everything from farming implements to food, clothing, and drugs. This practice continued well into the twentieth century. Around 1825, general merchandise stores in the larger towns handled the retail distribution of drugs and supplied drugs to the smaller merchants and physicians.[2]

Pharmacists were among the earliest settlers of Alabama. The facilities they established, in pioneer Montgomery for instance, had a unique place in the life of the town, for each store was a center where people came daily. Here they discussed the news of the day, exchanged gossip, formulated policies and politics, and exchanged medical and scientific information. In 1818, Dr. James Morrow, a physician, established a drugstore on Dexter Avenue in Montgomery. This was probably one of the first apothecaries established in the Alabama territory. The first advertisement of a drugstore as such in Montgomery was in 1830. This advertisement listed a complete inventory of merchandise to be sold for cash or barter.[3]

The records of pharmacies in Montgomery illustrated the most commonly used medicines of the 1820s. The items that appeared most frequently in their stock lists were quinine, castor oil, tincture of opium, blue mass pills, salts of tartar, camphor, Epsom salts, paregoric, alum, alcohol, and mercurial ointment. The sale of medical instruments also reflected the current medical practices. Spring and thumb lancets for bleeding were in constant demand, along with syringes for the universal practice of "flushing out the patient's bowels."[4]

During this period, bloodletting was one of the great medical standbys. There were few who questioned its basic value even though the quantity of blood taken from the patient varied not only from time to time, but from physician to physician. The more drastic bloodletters favored venesection, but the moderate physicians usually resorted to scarification, cupping, and leeching. For this reason, one of the pharmacist's chief stocks in trade was always leeches. The figures on the importation of leeches into Alabama are not available. However, Duffy cites "a survey of the [New Orleans] Customs House Archives from May 2 to December 10, 1828, reveals that 7,500 leeches by count plus another three boxes, seven tubs, fifteen barrels, and four cases of leeches arrived in New Orleans, and were distributed to twelve druggists."[5] Mobile, as a busy port, no doubt received a similar supply of leeches. They were in turn shipped to physicians and pharmacists in the river towns.

There existed from the earliest time a close relationship between the physician and the pharmacist. Both were often trained by the preceptor system. The physician's nameplate was frequently hung in the drugstore nearest his office. Because there were no telephones, messages were sent in writing to the druggist, and often were written on slates which could be erased and reused. Some physicians had a part of their office set aside for the preparation and dispensation of remedies for their own patients and every physician carried in his saddlebag vials and bottles of items necessary to practice. Early drugs most frequently prescribed were castor oil, calomel, quinine, sulphur, camphor, turpentine, and C.C. (compound carthartic) pills. These were supplemented frequently by powders and teas prepared by the local inhabitants from herbs, roots, and leaves. Antiseptics were unknown.[6]

Alabama's first-known pharmaceutical chemist was Robert Armistead. In 1826, he used a machine to express castor oil from the castor bean. He lived in Madison County and probably sold his wares in Huntsville, as drugstores had existed there since 1818. In the 1820s, visionaries, living 100 miles to the south, founded an apothecary in the woods where Ashville would be located in 1832.[7]

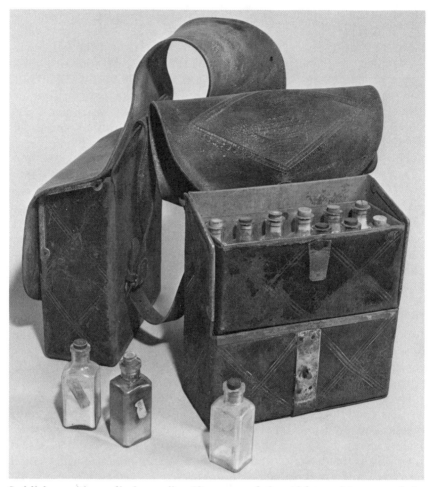

Saddlebag with medical supplies (Courtesy of the Alabama Museum of the
Health Sciences, Lister Hill Library, Medical Center, The University of Alabama
in Birmingham)

The firm of I. C. DuBose and H. C. Roff, located in Mobile, was the
first wholesale pharmacy in Alabama. The company was organized in
1834. The first Mobile city directory published after the Civil War
indicated that the business had been reorganized and named I. C.
DuBose and Company. In 1889, DuBose and Company, together with
Samuel Eichold and George Quarles, formed the Mobile Drug Com-

pany. The corporate successor to the DuBose and Mobile Drug companies is The Durr Drug Company of Mobile, which was organized in 1959 as a subsidiary of Durr Drug Company of Montgomery.[8]

In 1849, Dr. Benjamin Rush Jones announced the opening of his new pharmacy in a Montgomery newspaper. It read,

> we have a full stock of commodities, also morphine, quinine, chinoidine, codliver oil, surgeons instruments, cupping and injecting instruments, among them Pratt's celebrated nursing bottles and nipple shield, and this is an entirely new article. Dentist's forceps, excavating and plugging instruments, gold and tin foil, cosmetics, dentifrices, brushes, etc. To invalides we offer choice brands of Port, Madeira, Porter, Claret, Copenhagen, Cherry Cordial, French Brandy, all selected with care for the sick.[9]

A newspaper notice from this pharmacy appeared the next year, stating that "they had just received for sale theorem and striping brushes, amadine [sic] for chapped hands, shaving creams, fancy soaps, bear's oil, cologne and other articles."[10] It called attention to

> [their] large assortment of fancy articles fresh from Northern and Foreign markets, among which could be found rich plated and gilt shell, pearl and velvet Port Monnaes, ivory, shell, buffalo and inlaid hair brushes; assorted French Perfumery in boxes for the toilet; Ashard's Perfumed Oriental Spirit of Flowers, a new fashionable article for the handkerchief; and Lubin Extracts, Pomatums, French Colognes.[11]

These items presaged the advent of the sundries available in pharmacies today.

The most famous of all folk remedies, whiskey, was sold in large quantities and was used both as a preventive and a remedy. With opium selling for fifty cents an ounce and whiskey going for one dollar a gallon, it is easy to understand which painkiller was most frequently used. Brandy was another favorite staple. The manufacture of brandy long antedated that of whiskey; and brandy continued to retain its reputation as a medicinal stimulant on the American frontier.[12]

Accounts with pharmacies in this era were usually settled in the fall when the crops were gathered. A system of reduced rates for cash was instituted in early Montgomery. This could be viewed as an early version of the modern discount drugstore.

The early pharmacies offered homeopathic medicine chests, which were German preparations made in Leipzig. A "Family Guide" in each chest described the most common diseases and the recommended treatment.[13]

Families often had to rely on their own ingenuity, for physicians lived miles away and the roads were frequently impassable. Patent medicines were widely used, and every family had its own favorite. The frequent

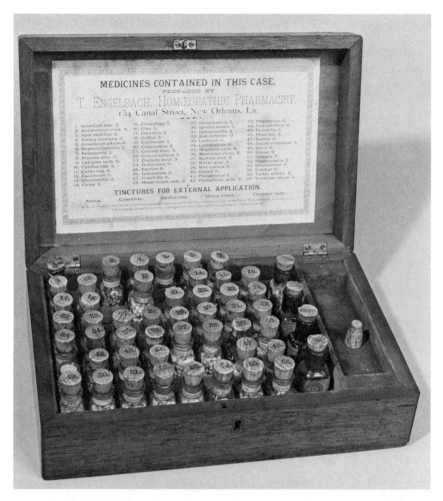

Homeopathic Medicine Chest (Courtesy of the Alabama Museum of the Health Sciences, Lister Hill Library, Medical Center, The University of Alabama in Birmingham)

appearance of large and sensational advertisements in newspapers would seem to indicate both that these concoctions were much in demand and that they provided the newspapers with additional income.

Examples of these sensational claims made in patent medicine advertisements are shown in the following promotions:

> Dr. Lins Celestial China Balm for piles, sore throat, and chest. [Another], Dr. R. Hooper's Hygean Tonic Mixture for Female Complaints, [extolled]

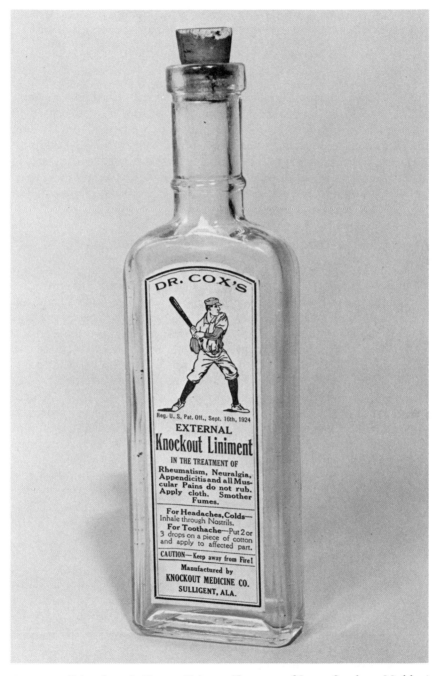

Patent medicine from Sulligent, Alabama (Courtesy of James Stephens Maddox)

'Thy wife shall be as a fruitful vine upon the walls on thine house.' This mixture, when regularly taken and directions strictly attended; if *THERE BE NO MALFORMATION* of the anatomical structure, or the person *BE NOT BEYOND THAT CERTAIN AGE* will be found a never-failing antidote for sterility or barrenness.[14]

The virtues of patent medicines such as Cardui, 666, Lydia E. Pinkham's Compound, and Sloan's Liniment were not only advertised in newspapers and magazines of the day but were trumpeted from signs on the roadside, the sides and roofs of barns and other available buildings.

Between 1820 and the outbreak of the Civil War, pharmacies sprang up all over the state of Alabama. Some of the earliest locations were in Mobile, Montgomery, Demopolis, Huntsville, Tuscaloosa, Selma, and in Sumter and Barbour counties.

Alabama Pharmaceutical Association

The Alabama Pharmaceutical Association was organized in 1881 as a voluntary professional organization whose objects were "to unite the reputable druggists and pharmacists of the state; to establish fraternal feeling and cooperation among its members; to improve the science and art of pharmacy; [and apothecaries]." The association was organized at a conference held in Birmingham, August 11, 1881, largely through the efforts of Dr. P. C. Candidus. The first officers were P. C. Candidus, Mobile, president; J. L. Davis, Birmingham, first vice-president; G. C. Stollenwerck, Greensboro, second vice-president; E. P. Galt, Selma, treasurer; and S. W. Gillespie, Birmingham, secretary.[15] In 1884, the association was chartered by the General Assembly. The constant aim of the organization has been and continues to be for better legal safeguards for the practicing pharmacist.

There are three classes of membership: *active members*—pharmacists, druggists, and teachers of pharmacy, chemistry, and botany; *associate members*—the pharmaceutical representatives; and *honorary members*—the wives and daughters of members and other persons approved by the executive committee.

One of the primary purposes in organizing the Alabama Pharmaceutical Association was to remove the practice of pharmacy from the control of the State Medical Association and place it under a pharmacy board. The association believed that the lives and health of the people of Alabama depended not only upon the physician, but also upon the competence and integrity of the pharmacist. Furthermore, the association felt that pharmacy should be raised to the dignity of a professsion.[16] "The Association's Code of Ethics includes the obligation of the pharmacist to the public, the obligation of the pharmacist to the physician, the

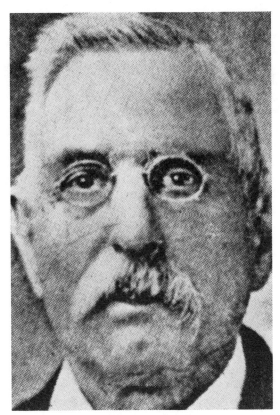

P. C. Candidus (Courtesy of the Alabama
Pharmaceutical Association, Birmingham, Alabama)

obligation of the pharmacist to each other and to [the profession of]
pharmacy."

The Birmingham Retail Druggists Association, which is now known as
the Jefferson County Chapter of the Alabama Pharmaceutical Association, was organized fifty years after the Alabama Association.[17]

In the free enterprise milieu of nineteenth-century America, a trained
or untrained person could simply declare himself a pharmacist and set
himself up in practice. To protect the public welfare, regulation became
essential.[18] Organized originally to correct some of pharmacy's problems, the Alabama Pharmaceutical Association soon found that an
organization alone was not sufficient; that there was a need to monitor
legislation, as well as a need to formulate and sponsor needed legislation.
In 1884, a permanent legislative committee was established for this

purpose. The association has sponsored laws pertaining to the practice of pharmacy, has worked for the enforcement of laws regulating the sale of narcotics, and has promoted more stringent control of amphetamines and barbiturates.[19] Many reforms in health and drug legislation have been proposed by the Alabama Pharmaceutical Association throughout its history. The association has successfully opposed many bills that would have adversely affected the profession.

In 1937, the association revised its organization to make itself more democratic, and to stimulate interest among the pharmacists of the state. The organization was divided according to congressional districts, and representatives to the executive board were elected from each district. This revision of the governing body of the association has been changed several times in subsequent years. In 1971, the association established a house of delegates made up of county association representatives, members of the board of trustees, and subdivision delegates. The association's policy, set by the House of Delegates, was then implemented by the Board of Trustees. This board was composed of state association officers, eight trustees elected at the district level, two trustees selected by the board itself, the speaker of the house of delegates, and representatives of the association's Academy of Institutional Practice (organized in 1973) and Academy of Chain Store Practice (organized in 1974). The latter two were created to give representation to special areas within the profession of pharmacy.[20]

In 1938, Thelma Morris Coburn was employed as executive secretary. She had served the Birmingham Retail Druggists Association as secretary since 1931. Mrs. Coburn was eminently qualified to guide the association through its period of greatest growth.[21]

Although the pharmacy profession still faces old challenges, many new ones have arisen. The association's role in the area of continuing education and public relations has been implemented. It has become involved in the new areas of third-party payment programs, that is, government involvement in pharmacy with its increased regulations. In 1943, a scholarship foundation was established to provide interest-free loans to needy pharmacy students. In 1971, the association became an affiliate of the American Pharmaceutical Association. This reciprocal membership increases the stature and influence of pharmacy on society.[22]

Alabama State Board of Pharmacy

One of the first acts of the state association was to draw up a pharmacy regulatory law and submit it to the General Assembly of 1882–1883. Colonel Sam Will John of Selma was the bill's sponsor and staunch

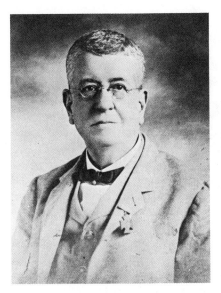

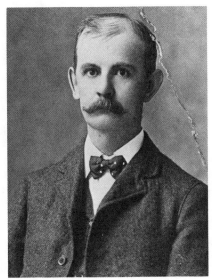

E. P. Galt (Courtesy of Mrs. Lela Legare, Montgomery, Alabama)

W. F. Dent, Montgomery, president of
the Alabama Pharmaceutical Association, 1895–1897 (Courtesy of Mrs.
Lela Legare, Montgomery, Alabama)

supporter. It was through his efforts that a law was passed. However, it
did take several years of consistent and constructive work by the Alabama Pharmaceutical Association before the law passed on February 28,
1887.

The law made it mandatory for the governor of Alabama to appoint a
Board of Pharmacy to regulate the practice of pharmacy in the state.
The Alabama State Board of Pharmacy then became the enforcement
body of the Alabama Pharmaceutical Association. This board was composed of three pharmacists who had had at least five years of practical
experience and who were to serve one, two, and three years respectively.
The Board of Pharmacy appointed by Governor Thomas Seay (governor of Alabama, 1886–1890) on March 21, 1887, consisted of P. C.
Candidus, E. P. Galt, and James Milner. The original law applied only to
towns with populations of more than 1,000. In 1907, a general law made
the provisions of the act applicable only to towns with a population of
more than 900. This left the small villages with no regulation.[23]

An act of the General Assembly in 1895 permitted graduate physicians to "fill prescriptions . . ., compound medicines and poisons, . . . and to carry on the business of a druggist, or drug store, or apothecary shop."[24]

By 1909, the pharmacy laws needed to be updated. Pharmaceutical work was becoming more complicated as new drugs were developed; and, more importantly, there were fewer physicians who were preparing their own prescriptions. An enlarged and revised pharmacy act, which contained several important changes, was passed by the State Legislature on August 26, 1909. These changes were: (1) only registered pharmacists could operate businesses in towns of more than 800 people, (2) licensed assistant pharmacists could operate in smaller towns, and (3) all pharmacists then working in Alabama had to renew their licenses annually.[25]

The Board of Pharmacy now had some influence over academic programs. It had authority to accept only graduates from schools that were recognized by the board. Practicing pharmacists rather than academic instructors comprised the Board of Pharmacy. These provisions insured that the state's pharmacists would receive the education required to meet changing needs.[26]

The 1909 Act enlarged the board to five members. These were all members of the Alabama Pharmaceutical Association, were not connected with any school of pharmacy, were licensed as pharmacists with at least ten years of practical experience, and were actively engaged in the practice of pharmacy in the state.[27]

On several occasions since 1909 the act has been expanded; but, the basic organization of the board has not been changed. The board is still made up of five members who are charged with the responsibility of examining the state's pharmacists and seeing to the proper handling of drugs and poisons.[28]

In 1937, the method of selecting nominees for the Alabama State Board of Pharmacy was revised by the association so that no member would be permitted to serve more than one full regular term on the board. Prior to that time, an individual could remain on the Board of Pharmacy from fifteen to twenty-five years.[29]

Alabama Pharmacy Schools

Medical College of Alabama

The history of the schools of pharmacy in Alabama parallels advances in medicine and science within the state.[30] The first school of pharmacy was founded in Mobile in conjunction with the medical college there.

The annual announcement of the Medical College of Alabama in Mobile for the session 1882–1883 carried the following:

> To meet a want which is making itself more and more felt, the Faculty have established a Chair of Pharmacy in connection with the College, and to that end have secured the services of a practical pharmaceutist, who is a regular graduate in that branch. Students taking this Course will be required to attend the regular lectures on Chemistry and Materia Medica.[31]

Two students received the degree of Graduate in Pharmacy on March 20, 1884; the commencement was held in Temperance Hall in Mobile. Very little is known concerning the operation of this department of the Medical School.[32]

A Department of Pharmacy was continued after the Medical College of Alabama came under the auspices of the University of Alabama in 1897.[33] The course of study was two years; usually there were about fifteen students in the first-year class and about ten students in the second-year class. Until the Medical College of Alabama in Mobile closed in 1920, the Department of Pharmacy remained an integral part of the University.[34]

The Birmingham Medical College

In 1894, when the Birmingham Medical College was organized, the college provided instruction in dentistry and pharmacy. Many of the pharmacy faculty taught in both the Medical College and the Dental College. Dr. E. P. Hogan, Associate Professor of Gynecology and Abdominal Surgery in Birmingham, served as secretary of both the Dental College and the Medical College. He served also in the Department of Pharmacy and Pharmaceutical Chemistry. Dr. J. D. Heacock was Professor of Dental Jurisprudence and Hygiene in the Dental College and Professor of Hygiene and Pharmaceutical Jurisprudence in the Department of Pharmacy. In 1910, Dr. A. Richard Bliss was appointed chairman of the Department of Pharmacy. The catalog for 1913–1914 listed three courses of instruction leading to the following degrees: Graduate in Pharmacy, Ph.G.; Pharmaceutical Chemist, Ph.C.; and Doctor of Pharmacy, Phm.D. The Birmingham Medical, Dental, and Pharmaceutical College closed in 1915.[35] The College was transformed into the Graduate School of Medicine of the University of Alabama that same year.

Montezuma University

The following announcement appeared in the 1896–1897 bulletin of the Montezuma University of Bessemer:

SCHOOL OF PHARMACY

The position of Pharmacist is always lucrative, and the well equipped 'Drug Clerk' need not be out of employment. Recent legal restrictions, in almost every State of the Union, make a thorough Pharmaceutical training an absolute necessity. The advantages afforded in this school are superior in every respect. The Professor of Pharmacy and Materia Medica is maturely up in both the theory and practice of the business, and his co-laborers are specially fitted for the positions they occupy.

Young men of limited education can enter our school of Pharmacy and at the same time pursue any needed branches of study in the University Literary courses.

Students of Pharmacy will have special training in the Medical College free Dispensary.

The degree of Graduate of Pharmacy will be conferred upon all worthy students who complete the studies in this department. The candidate for graduation must have a good moral character, and have attained the age of twenty-one years.

He must have attended two full courses of instruction in some reputable college of Pharmacy, the last of which must have been in this college, and he must have had a practical experience in Pharmacy, including the period of attendance at college.[36]

J. A. B. Lovett, A.M., Ph.D., served as president of Montezuma University, as well as Professor of Botany in the School of Pharmacy. W. H. Johnson, M.D., was dean of the School of Pharmacy and Professor of Materia Medica and Pharmacy. Frank A. Adams, Ph.Gr., was Professor of Medical Chemistry.[37]

Nothing more is known concerning the number of students and graduates. The pharmacy school was not mentioned again in the 1898–1899 catalog. The school was destroyed by fire on May 23, 1898.[38]

Auburn University

Instruction in pharmacy at the Alabama Polytechnic Institute (Auburn University) was authorized by the Board of Trustees in 1885.[39] The authorizing statement read in part: "A special course of instruction in pharmacy . . . to qualify young men, by systematic work in chemistry and other sciences, to become practical pharmacists and chemical manufacturers."

In 1895, President W. LeRoy Broun, to strengthen the pharmacy course, employed Dr. Emerson R. Miller, who had been educated at the University of Michigan and was highly qualified in pharmacy. After his appointment, a junior class in pharmacy was organized. A student could receive the Bachelor of Science degree in pharmacy following a four-year course of study.

In 1899, Auburn introduced a two-year curriculum in pharmacy for those students who were unable to pursue the four-year degree course. The student who completed this two-year course received a certificate as a graduate pharmacist. The two-year course was discontinued in 1924, and in that same year, a three-year course was offered, which led to the degree of pharmaceutical chemist. In 1932, this three-year course was discontinued in order to comply with the requirements of the American Association of Colleges of Pharmacy. Since then, a four-year course leading to the degree of Bachelor of Science in Pharmacy has been offered by Auburn.

Dr. Emerson R. Miller resigned in 1913, and another graduate of the University of Michigan, Lynn Stanford Blake was employed to replace him. In 1941, Professor Blake was appointed dean of the School of Pharmacy and served in this capacity until his death in 1959. B. O. Shiflett, who had operated his own school of pharmacy in Birmingham from 1919 to 1927, joined the faculty of the School of Pharmacy at Auburn in January, 1947, as an assistant professor.

Enrollment in the School of Pharmacy reached twenty-seven students in the second year of operation and gradually increased to fifty-five students by 1910. An all-time record was reached in 1949, following World War II, when 329 students matriculated. The enrollment has since been approximately 250 students per year. The School of Pharmacy at Auburn has conferred degrees on more than 1,100 individuals.

Auburn has now established five divisions: Pharmacy, Pharmaceutical Chemistry, Pharmacology, Pharmacognosy, and Pharmaceutical Economics. The first four divisions offer postgraduate work leading to the Master of Science degree.[40]

B. O. Shiflett's School

One of the early alumni of Auburn's School of Pharmacy, Mr. Barry O'Neal Shiflett, organized a private school of pharmacy in Birmingham in 1919: the B. O. Shiflett School of Pharmacy. The school's first class graduated early in 1921.[41] The school offered two four-month courses per year and catered to individuals working in local drugstores who had either not enrolled in a regular college course in pharmacy or had not become registered pharmacists. The catalog of the school stated that the course was not to be compared with schools whose courses were "merely quiz courses," but that daily laboratory work was a most important part of the curriculum in the new school. The school filled more than a local need, and students came from many states. The school provided night classes, which had been requested by many area drug clerks. A correspondence course was offered, but Mr. Shiflett advised everyone to attend the school and take the regular course with all its available laboratory facilities, even if it meant a business sacrifice. As early as 1923, records of the graduates' success were such that the school made an absolute money-back guarantee that those graduating would pass the State Board Examination if they met requirements of the Alabama State Pharmacy Law: that is, if they were twenty-one years of age and had completed at least two years of high school. A new law became effective January 1, 1927, requiring pharmacy students to complete a three-year course in pharmacy plus one year of practical experience in drugstore work. These new requirements forced the closure of Mr. Shiflett's school in December, 1926.[42]

In 1931, an act of the Alabama State Legislature allowed persons holding licenses as assistant pharmacists and those who had been in the drug business for the past ten years to take the examination given by the Alabama State Board of Pharmacy. If they passed, they were to be issued a license to practice pharmacy.[43]

This licensure law created a demand for a refresher course or a "cram" course in pharmacy. Mr. Shiflett reopened his school and taught not only daytime classes but also night classes for those who were employed during the daytime.

Birmingham-Southern College

Prior to closing his school, Mr. Shiflett consulted with Dr. Guy E. Snavely, president of Birmingham-Southern College. Dr. Snavely was making plans to establish a department of pharmacy at Birmingham-Southern College. On January 31, 1927, a department of pharmacy was opened, and Dr. W. C. Jones was appointed head of the department and Professor of Pharmacology. Mr. Shiflett was appointed Instructor of Pharmacy and was to have charge of all practical pharmaceutical courses.[44]

Mr. Shiflett also established a journal, *The Birmingham Bulletin of Pharmacy*, which he edited and published under the sponsorship of Birmingham-Southern College. Due to rising costs and the failure of the college to support the project financially, the publication was discontinued after several issues.

The Department of Pharmacy at Birmingham-Southern operated for two years and then it, too, was discontinued due to a lack of funds. On September 7, 1928, President Snavely wrote Mr. Shiflett a letter stating that Birmingham-Southern College was discontinuing the department of pharmacy. Mr. Shiflett later became associated with Howard College (Samford University) of Birmingham.[45]

Samford University

The administration of Howard College in Birmingham had been petitioned to establish a department of pharmacy. On November 16, 1926, the trustees' report to the Alabama Baptist State Convention stated that the Department of Pharmacy would be established as of January 31, 1927.[46] The new state licensure law, which had become operative in September, 1927, was attractive to the Howard College Administration in that it required pharmacy students to complete a three-year pharmacy course plus one year of practical experience in drugstore work. In Birmingham at that time, there were 200 drugstores that could be made available for students' practical experience. Also, Alabama Polytechnic Institute's Department of Pharmacy, then the only School of Pharmacy in Alabama, did not have accommodations for the practical training required by the law.

The Howard College Bulletin, April, 1927, stated that Dr. James L. Brakefield was head of the Department of Biology and Pharmacy and Mr. W. R. Little, Ph.C., was Professor of Pharmacy.[47] The bulletin of April, 1929, mentioned B. O. Shiflett as Instructor in Pharmacy. After four years, pharmacy ceased to be offered at Howard. Neither the Department of Pharmacy nor any pharmacy courses were mentioned in the 1931 bulletin of the College.

The Department of Pharmacy at Howard College was reinstituted in 1932, and two new instructors were appointed. First-year classes began in September, 1932. The pharmacy faculty was strengthened when Dr. A. Richard Bliss, Jr., joined the staff on September 1, 1934, and a third- and fourth-year specialized course was offered.

According to a more recent college bulletin, the department is now listed as a Division of Pharmacy. In September, 1957, the Division of Pharmacy moved into the new Robert I. Ingalls Hall on the new campus.[48] Two courses of study were offered: the four-year course for students training as retail, hospital, wholesale, and manufacturing pharmacists; and the five-year course for those who desired training as pharmaceutical analysts, inspectors in government bureaus, pharmaceutical journalists; and for those who sought a background for graduate study in pharmacy.

Summary

Of the six departments or schools of pharmacy in the state of Alabama, two are still functioning. One is at Auburn University and the other at Samford University. The American Council on Pharmaceutical

Education has accredited both schools and has given each a grade A rating. Auburn and Samford are members of the American Association of Colleges of Pharmacy.

Notes

1. Alabama Pharmaceutical Association, *Profiles of Alabama Pharmacy* (Collegedale, Tenn.: College Press, 1974), p. 5 (hereafter cited as *Profiles*).
2. Ibid., p. 61.
3. Lela Legare, "History of Pharmacy in Alabama," MS., pp. 15–16.
4. John Duffy, ed., *The Rudolph Matas History of Medicine in Louisiana* (Baton Rouge: Louisiana State University Press, 1962), 2: 28.
5. Ibid., pp. 30–31.
6. *Profiles*, pp. 61, 63.
7. Ibid., p. 5.
8. Ibid., p. 149.
9. Legare, p. 35.
10. Ibid.
11. Ibid., p. 36.
12. Duffy, p. 30.
13. Legare, p. 45.
14. Ibid., p. 67.
15. *Profiles*, pp. 60–61; and Legare, p. 373.
16. *Profiles*, p. 61.
17. Legare, p. 373.
18. *Profiles*, p. 63.
19. Ibid.
20. Ibid.
21. Ibid., pp. 63–64.
22. Ibid., pp. 68–69.
23. Legare, pp. 372–74.
24. Acts of Alabama, 14 February 1895, p. 569.
25. Acts of Alabama, 26 August 1909, pp. 215–16.
26. *Profiles*, pp. 87–88.
27. Ibid., p. 88.
28. Ibid.
29. Ibid., p. 63.
30. Emmett B. Carmichael, "Pharmacy Schools in Alabama," *J. Ala. Acad. Sci.* 32 (1961): 531–38.
31. Medical College of Alabama, Catalogue, 1882–1883, p. 13.
32. Ibid., 1883–1884, p. 16.
33. University of Alabama, Catalogues, 1907–1918.
34. Carmichael, p. 531.
35. Birmingham Medical College, Catalogue, 1913–1914.
36. Montezuma University, Catalogue, 1896–1897, p. 18.
37. Ibid.

38. James A. Thompson and Michael R. Kronenfeld, "The Montezuma University Medical College," *Ala. J. Med. Sci.* 16 (1979): 68.

39. L. S. Blake, "Pharmacy at Alabama Polytechnic Institute," MS., cited in Carmichael, pp. 532–33.

40. Graduate Program, "Auburn Alumnus," p. 4, May 1954, cited in Carmichael, p. 533.

41. B. O. Shiflett's School of Pharmacy, General Catalogue, 1921–1922.

42. Alabama Pharmacy Law, Regular Session, No. 423, 1923, cited in Carmichael, p. 534.

43. "Requirements for Registration as Pharmacist," enacted by the Legislature of Alabama, 1931, cited in Carmichael, pp. 535–36.

44. Birmingham-Southern College, Bulletin, 1927–1928.

45. Ibid., 1928–1929.

46. *Annual of the Alabama Baptist State Convention* (Atlanta: Foote & Davies Co., 1926), pp. 65–66.

47. Howard College, Bulletins, 1927–1931.

48. Howard College became Samford University in 1965.

Epilogue

The Use of the Past in the Study of Medicine

"The past isn't dead. It's not even past."—William Faulkner

The story of medicine is . . . closely interwoven with the story of peoples, of civilizations, and of the human mind. It deals with great men and small . . . philosophers and scientists, with monarchs and ecclesiastics, with scoundrels and humbugs. On the one hand, it springs from folk-ways, legends, credulity, and superstition; on the other from intelligence, culture, labor, valor, and truth. And always it seems to reflect the character and progress of the people with whom for the time it is lodged—be they reactionary or . . . progressive. Whatever else it is, the history of medicine is never dull.[1]

For medical students and physicians, and for those in related fields, the study of the history of a profession, dealing as it does with all aspects of human culture, affords one of the soundest bases for forming and relating ideas. It is also an excellent counteraction to the daily grind and to the mental staleness that can result from narrow specialization.

The spectacle of the contemporary scene and the temper of the times are apt to distract the attention of those in the medical professions. The result is a tendency to observe conditions solely as they are at the moment. Perspective is lost, and man seems to exist only in the immediate present. A knowledge of medical history is essential to provide this perspective and serves as a corrective for the systematic amassing of facts that passes for education today. Developments in science-based medicine should continue redirecting our attention to the often forgotten work of the past or to a reevaluation of observations with which we have long been familiar. It is a truism that any profession worthy of the name must be forever strengthening and recreating its traditions.

The early days in Alabama medicine are gone, but they are not really dead. Pioneer physicians have vanished, but they enriched our continuing tradition with enduring values. They were courageous men of dedication and compassion facing disease, pestilence, and death. Riding horseback in all types of weather, risking their lives and their fortunes, they ministered to the sick and dying. They fought disease with all they had at their command, which indeed was very little. Nevertheless, their appearance on the scene when illness occurred brought hope and encouragement. These men were aware of their deficiencies. They sought knowledge wherever they could find it; indeed, many studied at more than one medical school. Some pursued knowledge in the great medical centers of Europe. It was their fervent desire that medicine would evolve out of its darkness. That wish, combined with that of fellow physicians around the world, has resulted in a scientific revolution that has ushered in a veritable golden age of medicine.

For the physician then, "the realization that only in a humble awareness of the past, with its errors and triumphs, a sensitiveness to high values, a sense of compassion, and a rendering to material power of not a whit more than belongs to it, is our hope for the future."[2]

Notes

1. F. H. Garrison, *Introduction to the History of Medicine,* 4th ed. (Philadelphia: W. B. Saunders Co., 1929), p. 10.

2. Earle C. Scarlett, *In Sickness and In Health,* Charles G. Roland, ed., (Toronto, Canada: McClelland and Stewart Limited, 1972), p. 252.

Table of Abbreviations

Alabama Historical Quarterly—Ala. Hist. Quart.
Alabama Journal of Medical Sciences—Ala. J. Med. Sci.
Alabama Lawyer—Ala. Lawyer
Alabama Medical Journal—Ala. Med. J.
Alabama Review—Ala. Rev.
American Heritage—Amer. Heritage
American Journal of Medical Sciences—Amer. J. Med. Sci.
American Journal of Roentgenology, Radium Therapy and Nuclear Medicine—Amer. J.
   Roentgen., Radium Therapy & Nuclear Med.
Annals of Medical History—Ann. Med. Hist.
Annals of Surgery—Ann. Surg.
Bulletin of the Alabama Dental Association—Bull. Ala. Dent. Assoc.
Bulletin of the History of Medicine—Bull. Hist. Med.
De Historia Medicinae—De Hist. Med.
Florida Historical Quarterly—Fla. Hist. Quart.
Journal of the Alabama Academy of Science—J. Ala. Acad. Sci.
Journal of the American Medical Association—JAMA
Journal of the Birmingham Historical Society—J. B'ham Hist. Soc.
Journal of the History of Medicine and Allied Sciences—J. Hist. Med. & Allied Sci.
Journal of the Medical Association of the State of Alabama—J. M. A. Ala.
Journal of the National Medical Association—J. Nat. Med. Assoc.
Journal of Southern History—J. South. Hist.
Medical Record—Med. Record
Mobile Medical and Surgical Journal—Mobile Med. & Surg. J.
New England Journal of Medicine—NEJM
New Orleans Medical and Surgical Journal—New Orleans Med. & Surg. J.
Quarterly of Phi Beta Pi Medical Fraternity—Quart. Phi Beta Pi Med. Frat.
Southeast Alabama Medical Center Newsletter—SAMC Newsletter
Southern Journal of Medicine and Pharmacy—South. J. Med. & Pharm.
Southern Medical Journal—South. Med. J.
Southern Medical Reports—South. Med. Reports
Southern Surgeon—South. Surg.
Transactions of the American Medical Association—Trans. Amer. Med. Assoc.
Transactions of the Association of the American Physicians—Trans. Assoc. Amer. Phys.
Transactions of the Medical Association of the State of Alabama—Trans.
Transactions of the Southern Surgical and Gynecological Association—Trans. South.
   Surg. & Gyn. Assoc.
Transactions of the Southern Surgical Association—Trans. South. Surg. Assoc.
University of Alabama Medical Center Bulletin—U. Ala. Med. Center Bull.
Virginia Magazine of History and Biography—Va. Mag. Hist. Biog.
Alabama Collection, Lister Hill Library, The University of Alabama in Birmingham, Birmingham, Alabama—Alabama Collection.

Alabama Museum of the Health Sciences, Lister Hill Library, The University of Alabama in Birmingham, Birmingham, Alabama — Alabama Museum of the Health Sciences.

Medical Association of the State of Alabama—MASA.

Reynolds Historical Library, Lister Hill Library, The University of Alabama in Birmingham, Birmingham, Alabama—Reynolds Historical Library.

Bibliography

Note: Interviews, letters, pamphlets and leaflets have not been included.

Principal Sources

PUBLIC DOCUMENTS

Acts of Alabama. 22 December 1823, pp. 45–47.
_____. 28 April 1841, p. 14.
_____. 21 December 1841, pp. 74–75.
_____. 4 March 1848, p. 394.
_____. 1 February 1850, p. 314.
_____. 6 February 1852, pp. 10–19.
_____. 7 February 1852, p. 260.
_____. 10 February 1852, p. 259.
_____. 15 February 1854, pp. 58–59.
_____. 11 February 1856, pp. 72–73.
_____. 21 February 1860, pp. 450–51.
_____. 8 February 1866, pp. 263–64.
_____. 28 January 1867, p. 247.
_____. 9 February 1877, pp. 80–82.
_____. 11 February 1881, pp. 82–84.
_____. 14 February 1895, p. 569.
_____. 16 February 1897, pp. 1186–89.
_____. 11 December 1900, pp. 358–73.
_____. 26 August 1909, pp. 215–28.
_____. 29 September 1919, pp. 909–45; pp. 1023–29.
Annual Report, Alabama Department of Health. 1963, p. 5.
_____. 1965, p. 35.
Brodie, Surgeon R. L. Medical Director, Division of the West, Inspection Report, 26 December 1864. State of Alabama Department of Archives and History, Montgomery, Alabama.
Code of Alabama 1852. title 13, chap. 2, "Physicians, Surgeons and Dentists," sect. 971. Montgomery: Brittan and DeWolf, State Printer, 1852.
Code of Alabama 1907. Chapter 32, "Municipal Corporations," article 19, "Powers, Authorities and Duties of Municipalities," section 1289, "Diseases, contagious, vaccination, etc." Nashville, Tennessee: Marshall and Bruce Co. Printers and Binders, 1907.
Code of Alabama 1923. Chapter 52, "Physicians," article 1. Atlanta, Georgia: Foote and Davies Co., 1923.
Code of Alabama 1975. vol. 18, title 34 (Professions and Businesses), chapter 24, "Physicians and Other Practitioners of Healing Arts." Charlottesville, Virginia: Michie Company, Bobbs-Merrill Law Publishing, Law Publishers, 1977.
Code of Ordinances of the City of Birmingham. 1905, section 914, p. 354.
Directory for the City of Mobile, For 1861, Mobile: Farrow and Dennett, 1861.
Rowland, D. and A. G. Sanders, eds. *Mississippi Provincial Archives, 1704–1743, French Dominion.* vol. 3. Jackson, Mississippi: Press of the Mississippi Department of Archives and History, 1932.

Toulmin, H., ed. *Digest of the Laws of the State of Alabama: Containing the Statutes and Resolution in Force at the End of the General Assembly in January, 1823.* Cahawba, Alabama: Ginn & Curtis, 1823.

NEWSPAPERS

Alabama Tribune, Mobile, Ala., 2 December 1847, p. 2, col. 1; 3 December 1847, p. 2, col. 1.

"Two Doctors Organized City's First Hospital." *Anniston Star*, 27 February 1977, sect. 2B.

Birmingham Age-Herald, 19 September 1912.

Birmingham News, 5 November 1973; 6 November 1973.

Boone Aiken. "Meet Man Who Put UAB on the Map of Medicine." *Birmingham News*, Tuesday, 30 October 1979, p. 31.

Birmingham Post-Herald, 13 February 1953.

Dallas Gazette, 9 August 1859, p. 1.

"A Medical Examination." *Dallas Gazette*, 30 September 1859, p. 1, col. 5.

"To the Medical Men in Huntsville." *Huntsville Republican*, 15 June 1821.

"Old Marine Hospital Now Historic Place." *Mobile Press*, 9 July 1974.

Crozier, Natalie. "New Life Planned For Keeler Memorial Hospital." *Mobile Register*, 12 June 1974, sect. A.

Mobile Weekly Register, 10 March 1860.

Montgomery Advertiser and State Gazette, 21 June 1851; 21 June 1859.

"Medical." *Southern Advocate of Huntsville*, 7 December 1827.

MANUSCRIPTS AND TYPESCRIPTS

Brown, Virginia P. and Jane P. Nabers. "The History of the Anti-Tuberculosis Movement in Alabama." TS, 24 pages. Copy in the author's possession.

Conley, Catherine. "The History and Trends of Public Health Nursing in Alabama." TS. Lecture to the Jefferson-Hillman Nurses, 20 February 1952. Copy in the author's possession.

Doron, T. Director of Public Relations, Carraway Methodist Medical Center, Birmingham, Alabama. "Carraway Methodist Medical Center." TS. 15 September 1972. Copy in the author's possession.

Emerson, Geraldine. "A Spanish Lady in Alabama, 1918–1919." MS. 1980.

Falkenberry, Eleanor R. Selma, Alabama. TS. 30 April 1980.

_____. Selma, Alabama. TS. December 1980.

Gibson, J.M. "Dr. Cochran's Dream & Your Health." Transcript of radio talk, 6 December 1951, in Library of the State of Alabama Department of Public Health, Montgomery, Alabama.

Graves, Stuart. "Medical College of Alabama 1920–1945." Nott Memorial Program Exercises. Alabama Museum of the Health Sciences.

_____. "Medical College of Alabama: Notes from Old Catalogs." MS. Alabama Museum of the Health Sciences.

"History of Partlow State School and Hospital, 1923–1975." TS. Copy in the author's possession.

Jones, Belinda. Public Information, Searcy Hospital, Mount Vernon, Alabama. "Searcy—Past, Present and Future (A Brief Progressive Chronological Account)." TS. Copy in the author's possession.

Legare, Lela. TS on Dr. R. S. Hill, which includes a personal interview with Mrs. Carney Laslie, Senator Hill's sister, n.d. Copy in the author's possession.

――――. "History of Pharmacy in Alabama." MS. Copy in the author's possession.

―――― and T. Brannon Hubbard. TS on Watkins Infirmary.

Lott, Janie. Publications Director for Baptist Medical Centers, Birmingham, Alabama. "Baptist Medical Centers: Short Historical Sketch." TS, 21 September 1972. Copy in the author's possession.

Ludden, Forest E. *The History of Public Health in Alabama (1941–1968).* Ph.D. dissertation, The University of Alabama, 1970. Alabama Collection, Lister Hill Library, The University of Alabama in Birmingham, Birmingham, Alabama. Published by The Alabama Department of Public Health, 1970.

Marriner, Jessie L. "History of Public Health Nursing in Alabama." MS. Library of the State of Alabama Department of Public Health, Montgomery, Alabama. Copy in the author's possession.

Minutes of the Board of Managers of Hillman Hospital, 1 September 1893. Jefferson-Hillman Hospital Papers, Alabama Museum of the Health Sciences.

Minutes of a Called Meeting of the Board of Directors of the Birmingham Medical College, 20 October 1909. Alabama Museum of the Health Sciences.

Minutes of the Jefferson County Anti-Tuberculosis Association, 24 June 1910, 19 October 1910, 17 January 1911, in office of Jefferson County Tuberculosis Association.

Minutes of the Mobile Medical Society, 8 April 1847, Mobile Medical Society, Mobile, Alabama. Copy in the author's possession.

Morin, Father Paul A. "Good Samaritan Hospital." TS.

Pritchett, Mary. Administrative Assistant II to Robert A. Kreisberg, M.D., Dean, University of South Alabama College of Medicine, Mobile, Alabama. Letter includes typescript, 8 August 1979. Copy in the author's possession.

"Resolution of the Board of Trustees of the University of Alabama, 1912." Alabama Museum of the Health Sciences.

"A Short History of Eliza Coffee Memorial Hospital." Florence, Alabama. TS, n.d. Copy in the author's possession.

Stabler, Carey V. "The History of the Alabama Public Health System." Ph.D. dissertation, Duke University, 1944.

――――. "Medicine—Forward March: Physicians and Preventive Medicine." TS, 1945. Alabama Collection.

ARTICLES

"Address of Dr. Weatherly on Medical Education." *Trans.* (1871), pp. 32–45.

"Alabama Home and School for Mental Deficients." *Mental Hygiene* 4 (January 1920): 201–02.

"The American Tuberculosis Exhibition." Editorial. *Ala. Med. J.* 20 (April 1908): 301–02.

Ames, Silas. "Report on the Diseases of Montgomery County in 1849." *Trans.* (1851), pp. 39–41.

Anderson, L. H. "On the Summer and Autumnal Fevers of South Alabama: To which are appended some remarks on the Diagnosis and Treatment of Typhoid Fever." *Trans.* (1852), pp. 97–157.

———. "Report on Surgery." *Trans.* (1852), pp. 38–49.

Anderson, Wm. H. "The Annual Message of the President." *Trans.* (1881), pp. 10-36.

———. "Report on the Diseases of Mobile." *Trans.* (1850), pp. 68–76.

———. "Report on the Diseases of Mobile." *Trans.* (1854), pp. 39–50.

"Annual Session of 1868." *Trans.* (1869), pp. 5–7.

Ariel, Irving M. "George T. Pack, M.D., 1898–1969, A Tribute." *Amer. J. Roentgen., Radium Therapy & Nuclear Med.* 107 (1969): 443–46.

Baker, J. N. "Sulfanilamide." *J.M.A. Ala.* 7 (1937): 192–93.

Barnes, J. P. "Report on the Number, Character, etc. of Practitioners of Medicine." *Trans.* (1852), pp. 163–64.

Bell, W. H. "Announcement." Editorial. *Ala. Med. J.* 19 (December 1906), 51–52.

Berman, Alex. "Neo-Thomsonianism in the United States." *J. Hist. Med. & Allied Sci.* 11 (1956), 133–55.

———. "The Thomsonian Movement and Its Relation to American Pharmacy and Medicine, Part I." *Bull. Hist. Med.* 25 (1951), 405–28.

Birmingham Medical College. Catalogues, 1894–1895, 1899–1900, 1910–1911, 1913–1914. Alabama Museum of the Health Sciences.

———. "Statistical Report," 1912. Alabama Museum of the Health Sciences.

Birmingham-Southern College. Bulletins, 1927–1928, 1928–1929. Birmingham-Southern College, Birmingham, Alabama.

Blow, John W. "Micro-Organisms and Their Relation to Disease." *Trans.* (1882), pp. 429–47.

Board of Censors of the Medical Association of the State of Alabama. "Our New Venture." Editorial. *J.M.A. Ala.* 1 (1931): 20.

Boling, W. "Review of P. H. Lewis, 'Medical History of Alabama.' "*New Orleans Med. & Surg. J.* (1847), pp. 459–91.

Bondurant, E. D. "The Message of the President." *Trans.* (1906), pp. 12–24.

———. "Some of the Therapeutic Uses of the X-Ray." *Trans.* (1902), pp. 283–87.

Brantley, William H., Jr. "Alabama Doctor." *Ala. Lawyer* 6 (1945): 247–85.

———. "An Alabama Medical Review." *Ala. J. Med. Sci.* 4 (1967), 185–207.

Breeden, James O. "Thomsonianism in Virginia." *Va. Mag. Hist. Biog.* 82 (April 1974): 150–80.

Brown, George Summers. "Appendicitis." *Trans.* (1899), pp. 415–33.

———. "Appendicitis." *Trans.* (1900), pp. 449–59.

Cannon, D. L. "Alabama's Eighty-Nine Years of Medical Organization, A Brief History of the Association." *J.M.A. Ala.* 5 (1936): 313–22, Part 1; 348–56, Part 2; 385–93, Part 3.

Carmichael, Emmett B. "Nathan Bozeman." *Ala. J. Med. Sci.* 6 (1969): 233–36.

———. "Luther Leonidas Hill." *South. Surg.* 14 (1948): 659–69.

———. "William Joseph Holt." *Ala. J. Med. Sci.* 1 (1964): 451–54.

————. "George Augustus Ketchum—Teacher—Administrator—Physician." *Ala. J. Med. Sci.* 5 (1968): 511–14.

————. "Roy Rachford Kracke." *Quart. Phi Beta Pi Med. Frat.* 45 (1948): 157–60, 167–68.

————. "Robert Archibald Lambert: Pathologist—Teacher—Physician." *J.M.A. Ala.* 32 (1963): 232–34.

————. "Albert Gallatin Mabry." *J.M.A. Ala.* 38 (1969): 1015–21.

————. "James Sommerville McLester: Nutritionist—Physician." *Bull. Hist. Med.* 36 (1962): 141–47.

————. "The Medical Association of the State of Alabama." *J.M.A. Ala.* 30 (1961): 587–88.

————. "Lloyd Noland—Sanitarian, Surgeon and Hospital Administrator." *Ala. J. Med. Sci.* 7 (1970): 114–17.

————. "Pharmacy Schools in Alabama." *J. Ala. Acad. Sci.* 32 (1961): 531–38.

————. "Charles Alexander Pope." *Ann. Med. Hist.* 3rd series 2 (1940): 422–31.

"Dr. Cochran's Address on Medical Education." *Trans.* (1870), pp. 171–78.

"Dr. Cochran's Paper on Public Hygiene." *Trans.* (1872), pp. 18–27.

Cochran, Jerome. "Yellow Fever in Relation to Its Cause." *Trans.* (1877), pp. 129–57.

Comer, B. B. "Address of Welcome." *Trans.* (1908), pp. 12–13.

Confederate States Medical and Surgical Journal. Vols. 1, 2. 1864 and 1865. Reynolds Historical Library.

Crawford, J. W. "Report on the Diseases of Centreville and Vicinity." *Trans.* (1855), pp. 53–55.

————. "A Report on the Number and Character of Physicians of Bibb County." *Trans.* (1854), p. 148.

Dark, Virgil and Fred Boswell. "Results Observed in 125 Cases of Deep Seated Malignancies Treated with High Voltage X-Rays." *Trans.* (1923), pp. 330–36.

Davis, John D. S. "Blood Transfusion." *Trans.* (1909), pp. 499–510.

————. "An Experimental Study of Intestinal Anastomosis." *Trans. South. Surg. & Gyn. Assoc.* 2 (1889): 142–73.

————. "The President's Message." *Trans.* (1928), pp. 7–22.

Davis, W. E. B. "Annual Address of the President." *Trans. South. Surg. & Gyn. Assoc.* 15 (1902): 1–20.

"Deaths." *JAMA* 101 (July 1933): 154.

Diard, Francois Ludger, ed. *The Tablet.* Vol. 2, no. 12 (Mobile, Alabama: n.p., 1961), pp. 1–8.

Dibble, Eugene H., Jr.; Louis A. Rabb; and Ruth B. Ballard. "John A. Andrew Memorial Hospital." *J. Nat. Med. Assoc.* 53 (March 1961): 103–18.

"Discussion." *Trans.* (1905), pp. 375–80.

Donald, J.M. "James Monroe Mason, 1871–1952." *Trans. South. Surg. Assoc.* 64 (1952): 406–09.

Donald, W. J. "Alabama Confederate Hospitals." *Ala. Rev.* 15 (1962): 271–81; Part 2, 16 (1963): 64–78.

Drennen, Earle. "Blood Transfusion." *Trans.* (1920), pp. 143–49.

Dubose, F. G. "Local Anaesthesia in Major Surgery with Report of Cases." *Trans.* (1914), pp. 445–57.

Duffy, John. "Sectional Conflict and Medical Education in Louisiana." *J. South. Hist.* 23 (1957): 289–306.

Dunn, W. L. "Some Lessons to be Learned from Results of Treatment of Pulmonary Tuberculosis." *Trans.* (1912), pp. 483–504.

Earle, E. P. "Typhlitis, Peri-Typhlitis, and Appendicitis." *Trans.* (1887), pp. 351–58.

"Early History of Alabama Dental Laws." *Bull. Ala. Dent. Assoc.* 40 (July 1956): 20–24.

Edmondson, John H. "The Present Status of the X-Ray in Diagnosis." *Trans.* (1922), pp. 214–17.

———. "X-Ray Diagnosis in Colon." *Trans.* (1912), pp. 514–19.

Ellman, Michael H. "William Crawford Gorgas and the American Medical Association." *JAMA* 243 (15 February 1980), 659–60.

Fisher, W. "Physicians and Slavery in the Antebellum Southern Medical Journal." *J. Hist. Med. & Allied Sci.* 23 (1968): 36–49.

Gaines, T. "The President's Message." *J.M.A. Ala.* 1 (1932), 445–54.

"Golden Anniversary, Southern Medical Association." *J.M.A. Ala.* 26 (1956): 76–77.

Griffith, Lucille. "Mrs. Juliet Opie Hopkins and Alabama Military Hospitals." *Ala. Rev.* 6 (1953): 99–120.

Grote, C. A. "A Two Year Public Health Campaign in a Rural County." *South. Med. J.* 9 (1916): 320–24.

Halstead, F. G. "A First-Hand Account of a Treatment by Thomsonian Medicine in the 1830's." *Bull. Hist. Med.* 10 (1941): 680–87.

Harrell, L. D. S. "Colonial Medical Practice in British West Florida, 1763–1781." *Bull. Hist. Med.* 41 (1967): 539–58.

———. "Preventive Medicine in the Mississippi Territory, 1799–1802." *Bull. Hist. Med.* 40 (1966): 364–75.

Harris, J. C. "Influence of Temperature in the Production of Various Forms of Fever." *Trans.* (1851), pp. 28–32.

Harris, Robert P. "The Operation of Gastro-Hysterotomy (True Cesarean Section), Viewed in the Light of American Experience and Success; With the History and Results of Sewing Up the Uterine Wound; and a Full Tabular Record of the Cesarean Operations Performed in the United States, Many of Them not Hitherto Reported." *Amer. J. Med. Sci.* 75 (April 1878): 313–42.

Harris, Seale. "Clyde Porter Loranz and The Southern Medical Association." *South. Med. J.* 42 (1949): 1–4.

Heustis, James Fountain. "Recent Progress in Surgery." *Trans.* (1882), pp. 329–70.

———. "Surgical Cases." *Trans.* (1881), pp. 498–508.

Hill, Luther Leonidas. "Beacon Lights in Alabama." *J.M.A. Ala.* 46 (1976): 17, 20.

———. "Progress in Surgery." *Trans.* (1893), pp. 327–41.

———. "A Report of a Case of Successful Suturing of the Heart, and Table of Thirty-seven Other Cases of Suturing by Different Operators with Various Terminations, and the Conclusions Drawn." *Med. Record* 62 (29 November 1902), 846–48.

————. "Wounds of the Heart with a Report of Seventeen Cases of Heart Suture." *Med. Record* 58 (15 December 1900): 921–24.

Hogan, E. P. "The Appendix Problem." *Trans.* (1928), pp. 491–99.

Hogan, Robert S. "Edgar Poe Hogan—Physician, Surgeon and Public Servant." *Ala. J. Med. Sci.* 2 (1965): 99–100.

Holley, Howard L. "A Century and a Half of the History of the Life Sciences in Alabama; Cholera in Birmingham." *Ala. J. Med. Sci.* 15 (1978): 288–89.

————. "A Century and a Half of the History of the Life Sciences in Alabama; Smallpox Epidemic in Jefferson County." *Ala. J. Med. Sci.* 16 (1979): 140–42.

————. "Medical Education in Alabama." *Ala. Rev.* 7 (1954): 245–64.

————. "Narration: The Civil War: The AMA and Embargo on Medicine for the Confederacy." *JAMA* 182 (December 1962): 204, 208.

————. "A Study in Courage." *New Physician* 14 (1965): 161.

————. "Lawrence Reynolds, M.D., 1889–1961: An Appreciation." *J.M.A. Ala.* 31 (1961): 210.

———— and Eugenia Blount Dabney. "The History of the Hillman Hospital, The Hospital of the United Charities, Part 1." *De Hist. Med.* 5 (1961): 9–16.

———— and Velimir Luketic. "The History of the Hillman Hospital, Part 2." *Ala. J. Med. Sci.* 6 (1969): 228–32.

Holmes, J. D. L., ed. "Fort Stoddard in 1799: Seven Letters of Captain Bartholomew Schaumburgh." *Ala. Hist. Quart.* 26 (1964): 231–52.

————. "Medical Practice in the Lower Mississippi Valley During the Spanish Period, 1769–1803." *Ala. J. Med. Sci.* 1 (1964): 332–40.

Howard College. Bulletins, 1927–1931. Samford University, Birmingham, Alabama.

Howard, Milo B., Jr. "Health Problems in Colonial Alabama." *J.M.A. Ala.* 39 (1970): 1051–52, 1055–57.

"The International Congress on Tuberculosis." Editorial. *Ala. Med. J.* 20 (1908): 546–47.

Irons, G. V. "Howard College as a Confederate Military Hospital." *Ala. Rev.* 9 (1956): 22–32.

Jackson, W. R. "Complications of Acute Appendicitis Due to Delayed Operation." *Trans.* (1922), pp. 236–43.

James, Thomas N. "Walter B. Frommeyer, Jr., 1916–1979." *Forum on Medicine* 2 (1979): 230.

Johns, L. J. "Appendicitis in Children." *Trans.* (1929), pp. 222–30.

Jones, C. C. "The Message of the President." *Trans.* (1905), pp. 13–23.

Jones, J. Paul. "Report on Surgery in Wilcox County." *Trans.* (1869), pp. 111–18.

Kay, Frank A. "Historical Background of Alabama Psychiatry, Part 2." *De Hist. Med.* 5 (August 1961): 3–10.

Ketchum, G. A. "Memorial Meeting." *Trans.* (1897), pp. 91–101.

————. "Report on the Diseases of Mobile for 1854." *Trans.* (1855), pp. 99–117.

Klaw, Spencer. "Belly-My-Grizzle." *American Heritage* 28 (June 1977): 97–105.

Kracke, R. R. and Wm. G. Kracke. "The University of Alabama Medical Center, The Past, The Present and The Future." *Ala. J. Med. Sci.* 4 (1967): 315–30.

"Karl Landsteiner." *Dictionary of Scientific Biography.* Vol. 7. New York: Charles Scribner's Sons, 1973.

Lamonte, Edward S. "The Mercy Home and Private Charities in Early Birmingham," *J. B'ham Hist. Soc.* 5 (July 1978): 5–15.

"The Legal Requirements Exacted of Medical Practitioners in the Several States of the Union (and in other Countries)." *Trans. Amer. Med. Assoc.* 2 (1849): 326–36.

Levi, Irwin P. "The Roentgen Ray as an Aid to Diagnosis in Cardiac Lesions." *Trans.* (1923), pp. 341–53.

Lewis, P. H. "Medical History of Alabama." *New Orleans Med. & Surg. J.* Part 1 (May 1847), pp. 691–706; Part 2 (July 1847), pp. 1–34; Part 3 (Sept. 1847), pp. 151–77.

———. "Sketch of Yellow Fever of Mobile with a Brief Analysis of the Epidemic of 1843." *New Orleans Med. & Surg. J.* (1845), pp. 281–301, 413–34.

Luketic, Velimir. "Abraham Flexner and Medical Education in Alabama." *J.M.A. Ala.* 38 (1969): 699–707.

———. "The Birmingham Medical College." *Ala. J. Med. Sci.* 6 (1969): 447–54.

———. "Early Medical Journals in Alabama." *Ala. J. Med. Sci.* 6 (1969), 422–24.

Maples, W. C. "Prevention of Tuberculosis." *Trans.* (1900), pp. 369–87.

Maréchal, E. L. Editorial. *Mobile Med. & Surg. J.* 1 (January 1902): 32–33.

Marks, J. C. "Report on the Number, Character, etc., of Practitioners of Medicine in Dallas County." *Trans.* (1854), pp. 147–48.

McDaniel, E. D. "Report on the Topography, Climatology and Diseases, of Wilcox County." *Trans.* (1869), pp. 97–110.

"Medical Center Observes 23rd Anniversary." *SAMC Newsletter*, (September-October, 1980), pp. 2, 5.

Medical College of Alabama. Catalogues, 1882–1883, 1883–1884. Alabama Museum of the Health Sciences.

Mitchell, M. C. "Health and the Medical Profession in the Lower South, 1845–1860." *J. South. Hist.* 10 (1944): 424–46.

Montezuma University Medical College. Catalogues, 1896–1897, 1897–1898, 1898–1899. Alabama Museum of the Health Sciences.

Moore, Robert M. "The Davis Brothers of Birmingham and the Southern Surgical and Gynecological Association." *Trans. South. Surg. Assoc.* 74 (1962): 1–13; reprint *Ann. Surg.* 157 (1963): 657–69.

Moss, P. B. "Some Practical Points on Blood Transfusion." *Trans.* (1917), pp. 480–83.

Murfee, Hopson Owen. "An Alabama State Medical Center." *Ala. J. Med. Sci.* 13 (1976): 215–39.

Neva, Franklin A. "Malaria—Recent Progress and Problems." *NEJM* 277 (7 December 1967): 1241–52.

Nevins, Allan. "The Glorious and the Terrible." *Saturday Review* 44 (2 September 1961): 9–11, 46–48.

Niedermeier, William. "Tom D. Spies: Physician, Scientist, Humanitarian, A Biographical Note." *Ala. J. Med. Sci.* 1 (1964) 329–31.

Nott, J. C. "Thoughts on Acclimation and Adaptation of Races of Climates." *Amer. J. Med. Sci.* 32 (October 1856): 320–34.

———. "Yellow Fever Contrasted with Bilious Fever—Reasons for Believing it a Disease *Sui Generis*—Its Mode of Propagation—Remote Cause—Probable Insect or Animalcular Origin, etc." *New Orleans Med. & Surg. J.* (March 1848), pp. 563–601.

Oates, William H. "The Value of the X-Rays in Diagnosis." *Trans.* (1910) pp. 455–66.

"The Omnibus Discussion, Antiseptic Surgery." *Trans.* (1886), pp. 96–100.

Partin, R. "Alabama's Yellow Fever Epidemic of 1878." *Ala. Rev.* 10 (1957): 31–51.

Physicians' Charges as described in a fee schedule in the Art Lewis' Modest Museum, Selma, Alabama.

Pittman, James A., Jr. "Tinsley Randolph Harrison, 1900–1979 [1978]." *Trans. Assoc. Amer. Phys.* 92 (1979): 30–32.

Pritchett, J. A. "Tuberculosis in the Negro." *Trans.* (1893), pp. 352–70.

Program of the Annual Session—Symposium on Tuberculosis. *Trans.* (1905), pp. 5–6.

Pullen, John J. "Gentlemen, *This* Is Not Humbug." *American Heritage* 30 (August/September 1979): 81–96.

Pusey, Wm. Allen. "The Present Status of Roentgentherapy." *Trans.* (1906), pp. 418–31.

Rea, Robert R. " 'Graveyard for Britons,' West Florida, 1763–1781." *Fla. Hist. Quart.* 47 (1969): 345–64.

Reese, W. P. "Notes on Maramus, Pertussis and Typhoid Fever." *Trans.* (1850), pp. 112–17.

————. "Report of the Diseases of Selma for 1854." *Trans.* (1855), pp. 91–93.

"Report on the Council." *Trans. South. Surg. Assoc.* 29 (1916): 1ii-1viii.

"Report on the Number, Character, etc., of Practitioners of Medicine." *Trans.* (1852), pp. 163–66.

Reynolds, Lawrence. "The Evolution of the Lawrence Reynolds Library." *De Hist. Med.* 5 (October 1958): 12–15.

Riggs, B. H. "The History of the Yellow Fever Epidemic in Selma in 1853." *Trans.* (1882), pp. 400–25.

Robinson, E. Bryce, Jr. "Lloyd Noland and T.C.I." *De Hist. Med.* 4 (August 1959): 3–24.

Rogan, B. B. "The Responsibility of the General Practitioner in Reference to Syphilis." *Trans.* (1924), pp. 210–13.

Schoonover, S. G. "Alabama Public Health Campaign, 1900–1919." *Ala. Rev.* 28 (1975): 218–33.

Sears, John William. "The Birmingham Epidemic of Jaundice." *Trans.* (1882), pp. 472–80.

Sheridan, Richard C. "Alabama Chemists in the Civil War." *Ala. Hist. Quart.* 37 (1975): 265–74.

B. O. Shiflett's School of Pharmacy. General Catalogue, 1921–1922. Alabama Museum of the Health Sciences.

Shryock, Richard H. "Quackery and Sectarianism in American Medicine." *Scalpel* 19 (May 1949): 91–96.

Simms, B. B. "Annual Message of the President." *Trans.* (1915), pp. 8–19.

Sisk, G. N. "Diseases in the Alabama Black Belt, 1875–1917." *Ala. Hist. Quart.* 24 (Spring 1962): 52–61.

Smith, Eli P. "The Prevention of Tuberculosis." *Ala. Med. J.* 19 (December 1906): 35–41.

Smith, J. R. "Remarks on Typhoid Fever, as it Appeared in Jefferson County, Ala." *West Lancet* 4 (1845–1846): 433–38.

Southern University. Catalogues, 1874, 1879. Alabama Museum of the Health Sciences.

Stiles, C. W. "The Significance of the Recently Recognized American Hookworm Disease for the Alabama Practitioner." *Trans.* (1903), pp. 300–63.

"Symposium to Honor Dr. Tom Spies." *U. Ala. Med. Center Bull.* 10 (March 1966): 5.

Taylor, W. "Report on Surgery—Talladega County." *Trans.* (1855), pp. 88–90.

_____. "Valedictory Address." *Trans.* (1854), pp. 149–55.

Thomas, D. H. "Fort Toulouse." *Ala. Hist. Quart.* 22 (1960): 141–230.

Thompson, James A. and Michael R. Kronenfeld. "The Montezuma University Medical College." *Ala. J. Med. Sci.* 16 (1979): 67–68.

Toole, B. W. "The Annual Message of the President (Historical Sketch of the Medical Association of the State of Alabama)." *Trans.* (1897), pp. 15–41.

Torchia, Marion M. "Tuberculosis Among American Negroes: Medical Research on a Racial Disease, 1830–1950." *J. Hist. Med. & Allied Sci.* 32 (1977): 252–79.

Turner, Roy H. "Graefenberg, The Shepard Family's Medical School." *Ann. Med. Hist.* N.S. 5 (1933): 548–60.

University of Alabama. Catalogues, 1907–1918.

_____. Graduate School of Medicine. "First Announcement." 1 September 1913.

Waite, F. C. "American Sectarian Medical Colleges Before the Civil War." *Bull. Hist. Med.* 19 (1946): 148–66.

Weed, Walter A. "The Present Status of the Local Application of Radium and X-Rays." *Trans.* (1917), pp. 434–41.

_____. "The Value of the X-Ray in the Diagnosis of Incipient Tuberculosis." *Trans.* (1916), pp. 420–27.

Welch, S. W. "Annual Message of the President." *Trans.* (1908), pp. 14–27.

_____. "Public Health Administration in Alabama." *Trans.* (1918), pp. 195–204.

Wilder, William H. "Report of the Epidemic of Smallpox in Jefferson County in 1897 and 1898." *Trans.* (1898), pp. 288–99.

Wilkinson, James Anthony. "Some Thoughts on Our Modern Therapeutics." *Trans.* (1890), pp. 311–18.

Wooten, H. V. "Diseases etc. of Lowndesboro,' (Ala.) and Its Vicinity—Reported 1850." *Trans.* (1850), pp. 77–94.

Wyman, B. L. "Annual Message of the President." *Trans.* (1909), pp. 13–30.

BOOKS

Ackernecht, Erwin H. *A Short History of Medicine*. New York: Ronald Press Co., 1968.

Alabama Pharmaceutical Association. *Profiles of Alabama Pharmacy*. Collegedale, Tennessee: College Press, 1974.

Alexander, Dan Dale. *Arthritis and Common Sense*. 3rd ed. Hartford: Witkower Press Inc., 1954.

"William H. Anderson." *Representative Men of the South*. Philadelphia: Charles Robson Co., 1880, pp. 136–43.

Annual of the Alabama Baptist State Convention. Atlanta: Foote & Davies Co., 1926, pp. 65–66.

Augustin, G. *History of Yellow Fever*. New Orleans: Searcy and Pfaff Ltd., 1909.

Baldwin, Joseph G. *The Flush Times of Alabama and Mississippi*. New York: D. Appleton and Co., 1853.

Bartram, William. *Travels Through North and South Carolina, Georgia, East and West Florida*. Philadephia: James & Johnson, 1791.

Bassett, John Y. "Report on the Topography, Climate and Diseases of Madison County, Ala." *South. Med. Reports* (1850), pp. 256–81. Reprinted in *The Medical Reports of John Y. Bassett, M.D.*, D. C. Elkin, ed., Memaska, Wisconsin: Charles C. Thomas, 1941, pp. 3–42.

Beers, Clifford. *A Mind That Found Itself*. Garden City, New York: Doubleday, Doran & Company, Inc., 1908.

Bethea, Helen. *The Hillman Hospital—A Story of the Growth and Development of the First Hospital in Birmingham: 1888–1907*. [Birmingham]: n.p., 1928.

Breeden, James O. *Joseph Jones, M.D.: Scientist of the Old South*. Lexington: University Press of Kentucky, 1975.

Clark, Willis G. *History of Education in Alabama 1702–1889*. Bureau of Education Circular Information, no. 3. Washington, D.C.: GPO, 1889.

Cochran, Jerome. "The Medical Profession." *Memorial Record of Alabama*: *Historical and Biographical*. Vol. 2. Madison, Wisconsin: Brant and Fuller, 1893.

A Compend for the Members of the Organized Medical Profession of Alabama. Montgomery, Alabama: Brown Printing Co., 1928.

Craighead, Erwin. *Mobile: Fact and Tradition*. Mobile, Alabama: Powers Printing Co., 1930.

Cumming, Kate. *Kate: The Journal of a Confederate Nurse*. Baton Rouge: Louisiana State University Press, 1959.

Cunningham, H. H. *Doctors in Gray: The Confederate Medical Service*. Baton Rouge: Louisiana State University Press, 1958.

Davis, John D. S. "The Medical Profession." *Jefferson County and Birmingham*. n.p.: Southern Historical Press, 1887, pp. 97–119.

Delaney, Caldwell. *Craighead's Mobile*. Mobile: The Haunted Bookshop, 1968.

Duffy, John. *The Healers, A History of American Medicine*. Chicago: University of Illinois Press, (Illini Books edition, 1979).

_____, ed. *The Rudolph Matas History of Medicine in Louisiana*. Vols. 1, 2. Baton Rouge: Louisiana State University Press, 1958, 1962.

England, Ann D. *A Compilation of Documented Information About the Confederate Hospital in Marion, Alabama, May 20, 1863–May 20, 1865*. [Marion]: n.p., circa 1950.

Etheridge, E. W. *The Butterfly Caste; Social History of Pellagra in the South*. Westport: Greenwood Publishers, 1972.

Flexner, Abraham. *Medical Education in United States and Canada*. New York: D. B. Updike; Boston: Merrymount Press, 1910.

Garrison, F. H. *Introduction to the History of Medicine.* 4th ed. Philadelphia: W. B. Saunders Co., 1929.

The Graduates and Friends of the Graefenberg Medical Institute. *The Celebration of the Birthday and Life of Professor P. M. Shephard.* Dadeville, Alabama: n.p., 1859.

Griffith, Lucille. *Alabama: A Documentary History to 1900.* University, Alabama: University of Alabama Press, 1972.

Hamilton, Peter J. *Colonial Mobile, A Historical Study.* New York: Houghton, Mifflin & Co.; Cambridge: Riverside Press, 1897.

Hanlon, John J. *Principles of Public Health Administration.* St. Louis: C. V. Mosby Co., 1960.

Harris, Seale. *Woman's Surgeon, The Life Story of J. Marion Sims.* New York: The Macmillan Company, 1950.

Heustis, Jabez W. *Physical Observations and Medical Tracts and Researches, on the Topography and Diseases of Louisiana.* New York: T. & J. Swords, 1817. Reynolds Historical Library.

Higginbotham, Jay. *Old Mobile, Fort Louis de la Louisiane, 1702–1711.* [Mobile]: Museum of the City of Mobile, 1977.

Holmes, J. D. L. *A History of the University of Alabama Hospitals.* Birmingham: University of Alabama in Birmingham Print Shop, 1974.

Howard, Milo B., Jr. "The History of the Alabama Dental Association, Part One, 1869–1917." *The First Hundred Years, 1869-1969: A Story of the Dental Profession in Alabama.* Birmingham: n.p., 1969.

Jackson, W. M. *The Story of Selma.* Birmingham: Birmingham Printing Co., 1954.

Jemison, E. Grace. *Historic Tales of Talladega.* Montgomery, Alabama: Paragon Press, 1959.

Jones, Joseph. "Outline of Observations on Hospital Gangrene as It Manifested Itself in the Confederate Armies, During the American Civil War, 1861–1865." New Orleans, Louisiana: n.p., 1869. Cited in Breeden, James O., *Joseph Jones, M.D.* . . .

Jordan, W. T. *Ante-Bellum Alabama Town and Country.* Tallahassee: Florida State University, 1957.

Kane, J. N. *Famous First Facts—A Record of First Happenings, Discoveries and Inventions in the United States.* 3rd ed. n.p.: H. W. Wilson Co., 1964.

Kett, J. F. *The Formation of the American Medical Profession: The Role of Institutions, 1780–1860.* New Haven: Yale University Press, 1968.

Kloss, Jethro. *Back to Eden.* 5th ed. Santa Barbara, California: Woodbridge Press Publishing Co., 1975.

Lewis, Marianna O., ed. *The Foundation Directory.* 6th ed. New York: The Foundation Center, 1977.

Loranz, C. P. *Golden Anniversary—Fifty Years of Service to Physicians of the South— Southern Medical Association, October 2–3, 1906–1956.*" Birmingham: Birmingham Printing Co., September, 1960.

———. *Golden Anniversary of the Southern Medical Association, 1906–1956.* Birmingham: Southern Medical Association, 1960.

Lovelace, J. M. *A History of Siloam Baptist Church of Marion, Alabama.* Birmingham: Burroughs Pub. Co., 1943.

McMillan, M. C. *Constitutional Development in Alabama, 1798–1901: A Study in Politics, the Negro, and Sectionalism.* Chapel Hill: University of North Carolina Press, 1955.

Miller, F. T., ed. *The Photographic History of the Civil War.* Vol. 7. New York: Review of Reviews Co., 1912.

Mohr, Charles T. *Plant Life of Alabama.* Montgomery: Brown Printing Co., 1901. Reynolds Historical Library.

Moore, Albert Burton. *History of Alabama.* Tuscaloosa: Alabama Book Store, 1951.

_____. *History of Alabama and Her People.* Vol. 1. Chicago: American Historical Society, Inc., 1927.

Osler, William. *An Alabama Student.* London: Oxford University Press, 1908.

Owen, Marie Bankhead. *The Story of Alabama: A History of the State.* Vols. 1, 2. New York: Lewis Historical Pub. Co., Inc., 1949.

Owen, Thomas McAdory. *History of Alabama and Dictionary of Alabama Biography.* Vols. 1–4. Chicago: S. J. Clarke Pub. Co., 1921.

Parks, J. H. and O.C. Weaver, Jr. *Birmingham-Southern College, 1856–1956.* Nashville, Tennessee: Parthenon Press, 1957.

Report on the Quarantine on the Southern and Gulf Coasts of the United States. New York: n.p., 1873.

Roberts, B. M. *A Determination of Medical Nursing and Health Profession.* Birmingham, Alabama: n.p., 1971.

Romans, Bernard. *A Concise Natural History of East and West Florida.* New York: n.p., 1775; Reprint. New Orleans: Pelican Pub. Co., 1961.

Savitt, Todd L. *Medicine and Slavery, The Diseases and Health Care of Blacks in Antebellum Virginia.* Chicago: University of Illinois Press, 1978.

Scarlett, Earle C. *In Sickness and In Health.* Charles G. Roland, ed., Toronto, Canada: McClelland and Stewart Ltd., 1972.

Shafer, H. B. *The American Medical Profession, 1783 to 1850.* New York: Columbia University Press; London: P. S. King & Sons, Ltd., 1936.

Shryock, Richard H. *Medicine in America: Historical Essays.* Baltimore: Johns Hopkins Press, 1966.

The Southern Medical Association Yearbook, 1979–80. Birmingham: Southern Medical Association, 1979.

Speed, E. M. "A Resume of the History of Dental Education in Alabama." *The First Hundred Years, 1869–1969: A Story of the Dental Profession in Alabama.* Birmingham, Alabama: n.p., 1969.

Sullivan, M. *Our Times, The United States, 1900–1925.* Vol. 3. Chautauqua, New York: Chautauqua Press, 1931.

Sulzby, James F., Jr. *Birmingham Sketches: From 1871 Through 1921.* Birmingham, Alabama: Birmingham Printing Co., 1945.

_____. *Historic Alabama Hotels and Resorts.* University, Alabama: University of Alabama Press, 1960.

Tarwater, James S. *The Alabama State Hospitals and the Partlow State School and Hospital, A Brief History.* New York: Newcomen Society in North America, 1964.

Thompson, M.T. *History of Barbour County, Alabama.* Eufaula: n.p., 1939.

Thomson, Samuel. *A Narrative of the Life and Medical Discoveries of Samuel Thomson*. Boston: E. G. House, 1822. Reprint. New York: Arno Press & The New York Times, 1972.

Tindall, G. B. *The Emergence of the New South, 1913–1945* Vol. 10 of *A History of the South*. Wendell H. Stephenson and E. Merton Coulter, eds. Baton Rouge: Louisiana State University Press, 1967.

Vickery, Katherine. *A History of Mental Health in Alabama*. Montgomery: Alabama Department of Mental Health, 1972(?).

Waring, J. I. *A History of Medicine in South Carolina, 1825–1900*. Charleston: South Carolina Medical Association, 1967.

Wilder, Alexander. *History of Medicine*. New Sharon, Maine: New England Eclectic Pub. Co., 1901.

Wiley, Bell Irvin. *The Life of Johnny Reb, The Common Soldier of the Confederacy*. Baton Rouge: Louisiana State University Press, 1978.

Wood, Edward Jenner. *A Treatise on Pellagra*. New York: D. Appleton and Co., 1912.

Young, J. H. *The Medical Messiahs*. Princeton, New Jersey: Princeton University Press, 1967.

_____. *The Toadstool Millionaires: A Social History of Patent Medicines in America Before Federal Regulation*. Princeton, New Jersey: Princeton University Press, 1961.

Index

See also Birmingham Medical College
Birmingham Retail Druggists Association, 371, 372
Birmingham-Southern College School of Pharmacy, 378
Blacks: malaria among, 22, 180–81; typhoid among, 22; diseases among, 24, 83; tuberculosis among, 24, 178, 296, 300, 305; hospital care of, 46, 48, 50, 53, 56, 69–70, 81, 326–27; medical education of, 118, 207, 294; medical societies for, 207; mental health and, 322, 326–27, 330–33, 346. *See also* Slaves
Black faith doctors, 9
Black widow spider bites: A. W. Blair and, 121
Blair, Allan Walker, M.D., **119**, 121
Blake, Mr. Lynn S., 377
Blalock, Alfred, M.D., 113
Blankenhorn, Marion, M.D., 190
Bliss, Dr. A. Richard, 375
Bliss, Dr. A. Richard, Jr., 379
Blood banks, 165, 166, 198 (n.29)
Bloodgood, Joseph C., M.D., 153
Bloodletting. *See* Venesection, "Heroic" method of therapy
Blood transfusions, 165–66, 184
Blood types, 165
Blount County Medical Board of Botanic Physicians, 252 (n.22)
Blue, John H., M.D., 106
Board of Botanic Physicians (Alabama), 246
Bolan, Dr. A. W., 52n
Boling, William M., M.D., 13, 14, 21, 206, 214, 316
Bondurant, Eugene D., M.D., **168**, 232, 326; Medical College of Alabama (Mobile) and, 92, 108; Birmingham Medical College and, 98; neurology and, 166–67; radiology and, 173; antituberculosis movement and, 296; pellagra and, 330
Boon, John B., M.D., 77
B. O. Shiflett School of Pharmacy, 377–78
Boswell, Fred, M.D., 174–75
Botanico-Medical College of Memphis, 244
Botanic physicians, 14, 245, 252 (n.13). *See also* Thomsonianism
Botany and medicine, 5, 10, 13, 14, 80, 242. *See also* Thomsonianism
Bowel sounds: Davis brothers and, 158
Boyd, Dr. H. D., 350
Bozeman, Mathew, M.D., 206

Bozeman, Nathan, M.D., 32, **33**, 157
Brakefield, Dr. James L., 379
Brannon, Dr. Edward, 361
Bray, Dr. C. B., 107
Bray, Charles, D.D.S., 358
Brooks, Clyde, M.D., **103**, 104, 108
Broun, Dr. W. Leroy, 376
Brown, George L., M.D., 52
Brown, George S., M.D., **97**, 98, 164
Brown, N. H., 84
Bruck, Dr. Carl, 183
Bruhn, Dr. John M., 108
Bryant, H. C., M.D., 207
Bryce, Marie E. Clarkson, 318, 324
Bryce, Peter, M.D., **319**; superintendent of insane hospital, 177, 214; death of, 222–23; Bryce Hospital and, 318–26; Russell Sage Foundation and, 332; alcoholism and, 336; criminally insane and, 337
Bryce Hospital. *See* Alabama Hospitals for the Insane: Bryce Hospital
Bucher, Robert, M.D., 116
Bush, Dr. W. N., 350

Cahaba, 6; yellow fever in, 17; Medical Licensure Board of, 256, 257
Cain, J. S., M.D., 228–29
Caldwell, E. V., M.D., 106
Caldwell, H. M., 356
Callander, T. J., 344
Camp, Reverend Joseph, 323–25
Cancer, 173, 175, 196, 292; uterine/cervical, 29, 174; research in, 121, 290; breast, 154, 173; osteosarcoma, 35, 154; lung, 174; prostate, 174; "sure cures" for, 249–50; American Cancer Society and, 306
Candidus, Dr. P. C., 370, **371**, 373
Cannon, Douglas L., M.D., 288, **289**
Can't-Get-Away Club (Mobile), 19–20, 278
Carangelo, John, M.D., 108
Cardiovascular disease and surgery, 113, 159–61, 165, 174, 184, 196
Carmichael, Emmett B., Ph.D., 108, 236
Carnegie Foundation: medical education and, 91–92; Medical College of Alabama (Mobile) and, 94
Carraway, Ben, M.D., 68
Carraway, C. N., M.D., 68, 107
Carraway Methodist Medical Center (Birmingham), 68
Carroll, Dr. James, 192
Carson, J. C., M.D., 95
Carthy, Thomas L., M.D., 46
Casey, Albert, M.D., 198 (n.29)